Clinical Management of Bone and Joint Pain

The Haworth Medical Press®
Haworth Series in Clinical Pain and Symptom Palliation
Howard Smith
Senior Editor

Clinical Management of the Elderly Patient in Pain edited by Gary McCleane and Howard Smith

Cholecystokinin and Its Antagonists in Pain Management by Gary McCleane

Clinical Management of Bone and Joint Pain edited by Gary McCleane and Howard S. Smith

Clinical Management of Bone and Joint Pain

Gary McCleane, MD
Howard S. Smith, MD
Editors

HMP

The Haworth Medical Press®
An Imprint of The Haworth Press, Inc.
New York

For more information on this book or to order, visit
http://www.haworthpress.com/store/product.asp?sku=5771

or call 1-800-HAWORTH (800-429-6784) in the United States and Canada
or (607) 722-5857 outside the United States and Canada
or contact orders@HaworthPress.com

Published by

The Haworth Medical Press®, an imprint of The Haworth Press, Inc., 10 Alice Street, Binghamton, NY 13904-1580.

PUBLISHER'S NOTE
The development, preparation, and publication of this work has been undertaken with great care. However, the Publisher, employees, editors, and agents of The Haworth Press are not responsible for any errors contained herein or for consequences that may ensue from use of materials or information contained in this work. The Haworth Press is committed to the dissemination of ideas and information according to the highest standards of intellectual freedom and the free exchange of ideas. Statements made and opinions expressed in this publication do not necessarily reflect the views of the Publisher, Directors, management, or staff of The Haworth Press, Inc., or an endorsement by them.

This book has been published solely for educational purposes and is not intended to substitute for the medical advice of a treating physician. Medicine is an ever-changing science. As new research and clinical experience broaden our knowledge, changes in treatment may be required. While many potential treatment options are made herein, some or all of the options may not be applicable to a particular individual. Therefore, the author, editor and publisher do not accept responsibility in the event of negative consequences incurred as a result of the information presented in this book. We do not claim that this information is necessarily accurate by the rigid scientific and regulatory standards applied for medical treatment. **No warranty, express or implied, is furnished with respect to the material contained in this book. The reader is urged to consult with his/her personal physician with respect to the treatment of any medical condition.**

Cover design by Kerry Mack.

Library of Congress Cataloging-in-Publication Data

Clinical management of bone and joint pain / Gary McCleane, Howard S. Smith, editors.
     p. ; cm.
  Includes bibliographical references and index.
  ISBN: 978-0-7890-3145-7 (hard : alk. paper)
  ISBN: 978-0-7890-3146-4 (soft : alk. paper)
    1. Pain—Treatment. 2. Bones—Diseases. 3. Joints—Diseases. 4. Bone pain—Treatment. 5. Joint pain—Treatment. I. McCleane, Gary. II. Smith, Howard S., 1956-
    [DNLM: 1. Bone and Bones—physiology. 2. Pain—drug therapy. 3. Analgesics—therapeutic use. 4. Joints—physiology. WE 200 C641 2007]
RB127.C586 2007
616'.0472—dc22
                   2007000528

CONTENTS

PART II

PART III

ABOUT THE EDITORS

Gary McCleane, MD, is a practicing consultant in pain management in Northern Ireland. His interests include the use of cholecystokinin antagonists in pain management and the use of tricyclic antidepressants and topical analgesics. He has published a number of studies examining the analgesic effect of CCK antagonists, capsaicin, topical TCAs, and anti-epileptics, including gabapentin, lamotrigine, phenytoin, fosphenytoin, and the novel anti-epileptic SPM 927. He has published a number of review papers examining current options for the treatment of neuropathic pain and cholecystokinin antagonists in human pain management.

Howard S. Smith, MD, is Academic Director of Pain Management in the Department of Anesthesiology at Albany Medical College, Albany, New York. He has also served on the faculty at the University of Pittsburgh School of Medicine and Harvard Medical School as Director of Pain Medicine—Presbyterian University Hospital, University of Pittsburgh Medical Center, Pittsburgh, Pennsylvania, and Director of Cancer Pain—Beth Israel Deaconess Medical Center, Boston, Massachusetts, respectively. Dr. Smith also served as the Director of Pain Management and Director of Pain Fellowship at the Albany Medical College/Albany Medical Center Hospital. He is editor of the *Journal of Neuropathic Pain & Symptom Palliation* and the *Journal of Cancer Pain & Symptom Palliation* and is an editorial board member of the *American Journal of Hospice and Palliative Care.* Dr. Smith is the author of the forthcoming books *Drugs for Pain* and *A Women's Guide to Ending Pain.*

Clinical Management of Bone and Joint Pain
© 2007 by The Haworth Press, Inc. All rights reserved.
doi:10.1300/5771_a

CONTRIBUTORS

Charles Argoff, MD, Director, Cohn Pain Management Centre, North Shore University Hospital, Assistant Professor of Neurology, New York University School of Medicine, New York.

David Blake, MD, Professor of Bone and Joint Medicine, Royal National Hospital for Rheumatic Disease, Bath, UK.

Helen Cohen, MD, Royal National Hospital for Rheumatic Disease, Bath, UK.

Elizabeth Demers, MD, Department of Anesthesia, Albany Medical College, Albany, New York.

Jennifer A. Elliott, MD, Assistant Professor, Department of Anesthesiology, University of Missouri, Kansas School of Medicine, Kansas City, Missouri.

Mark Guerdan, DO, Department of Anesthesiology, Albany Medical College, Albany, New York.

Lori Lavelle, DO, Department of Rheumatology, Albany Medical College, Altoona Arthritis and Osteoporosis Centre, Albany, New York.

William Lavelle, MD, Department of Surgery—Division of Orthopedic Surgery, Albany Medical College, Albany, New York.

Denis Martin, DPil, BSc (Hons), School of Health Science and Social Care, Collegiate Crescent Campus, Sheffield, UK.

Muhammad A. Munir, MD, Assistant Professor and Program Director, Pain Medicine, Department of Anesthesiology, College of Medicine, University of Cincinnati, Ohio.

Rahul Parikh, MD, Albany Medical College, Albany, New York.

Clinical Management of Bone and Joint Pain
© 2007 by The Haworth Press, Inc. All rights reserved.
doi:10.1300/5771_b

Gira Patel, LicAc, Masters Acupuncture and Oriental Medicine, Arnold Pain Management Center, Beth Israel Deaconess Medical Center, Osher Institute Harvard Medical School.

Jana Sawynok, PhD, Professor of Pharmacology, Dalhousie University, Halifax, Nova Scotia, Canada.

Nisar Soomro, MB, Consultant Anesthetist, Lagan Valley Hospital, Lisburn, N. Ireland, UK.

Jun-Ming Zhang, MD, MSc, Associate Professor and Director of the Research, Department of Anesthesiology, College of Medicine, University of Cincinnati, Ohio.

Introduction

Gary McCleane

Remarkable advances have been made in recent years in the operative and nonoperative management of a whole range of bone and joint diseases. Similarly, dramatic improvements have been made in the understanding and treatment of pain, a symptom that almost invariably accompanies bone and joint disease. Despite these advances, we are not universally successful in our treatment of bone or joint diseases or the pain that may emanate from these structures.

Along with increased understanding of the causes and treatment of pain has come a specialization in its treatment. While few practitioners not have the alleviation of distress and discomfort as a major aim of their practice, the introduction of novel analgesics and new pain-relieving techniques, along with all the other advances occurring in their own fields, often precludes them from becoming experts in the use of these new drugs and techniques. This overload of information confronting practitioners is exacerbated by the confusion caused by the gloss and spin that accompanies the marketing of new drugs by the pharmaceutical industry. Very often, we are encouraged by the industry to use newly introduced drugs, only to later appreciate that, in fact, the compound contained by the "new" drug is already available under a different generic name, or that the drug, while genuinely new, has a mode of action and pharmacological profile identical to other currently available preparations.

So, a clear understanding of pain and the options available for its treatment is necessary for logical and effective treatment to be instituted. That said, pain management should not be the realm of the pain specialist alone. Because of their practice, pain specialists have the opportunity to become experts in the modern, evidence-based treatment

Clinical Management of Bone and Joint Pain
© 2007 by The Haworth Press, Inc. All rights reserved.
doi:10.1300/5771_01

of pain. This practice will include acquiring knowledge of, and experience in the use of, new analgesic agents. They can define when the use of these agents is indicated and when their use would be inappropriate. This knowledge and experience should then be passed on to those in the front line of clinical medicine and surgery, who are faced daily with the problems of providing effective and appropriate pain relief to their patients. This book is an attempt to gather the latest thinking about the treatment of pain associated with bone and joint disease. It is not an attempt to delve into the realms of diagnosis, which properly belongs to other specialists. Rather, it is an attempt to offer practical options for the treatment of pain associated with these conditions. These pain relief options may be used temporarily while specific medical or surgical treatment is instituted, or they may be used in the long term where pain persists despite specific disease-orientated therapy. To this end, individual treatment options are discussed separately in Part II of this book, along with specific practical information on the clinical use of these options. Because it would be a rarity for only one analgesic option to exist in any clinical scenario, the treatment of specific types of pain is explored in Part III. This section is designed to bring together the information outlined in Part II regarding individual classes of therapeutic options and to present it as a list of alternative treatments that may help in that particular situation. Part III is designed to put in context the information gathered in Part II and to emphasize that, as the "numbers needed to treat" is never one and the "numbers needed to harm" is never infinity, a range of options for any one pain problem is necessary. Because the treatment of joint pain, for example, does not depend to any great extent on the cause of that pain, it is possible to consider the treatment of joint pain as a single heading rather than present lists of alternatives for each etiological cause of joint pain.

Where possible, the pain-relieving options mentioned are included because of the evidence base that supports their use. However, other options are mentioned that lack the supportive literature needed to classify them as "evidence based" because practitioners experienced in their field find them to be efficacious and the risk associated with their use to be low. If we were to restrict the focus of this book merely to those treatments that are evidence based, it would be, of necessity, a short book that offered little additional information beyond what is already well known.

Information has been included about management of conditions not primarily arising in bone or joint but which are common accompaniments of bone or joint disease. For example, muscle spasm and pain frequently complicate diseases of bone and joint. To ignore its treatment would decrease the utility of this book. Furthermore, inclusion of these other conditions may stimulate the practitioner to attempt to define which structure is actually giving rise to the pain in question, rather than just accepting that pain felt over a bone or joint arises solely from that bone or joint. Given that the treatment of muscle pain or spasm is not always the same as that for bone or joint pain, there may be merit to this approach.

No account such as this can be entirely comprehensive or inclusive. Indeed, if an attempt were made to discuss all options for pain treatment, then the danger of excessive detail may cloud the picture. Rather, the intention is to provide the reader with practical treatment options that may enhance their ability to provide relief for those with bone and joint pain, and to offer insight into the latest thinking about the various therapeutic options that can be considered in the clinical management of bone and joint pain.

PART I

Chapter 1

Basic Pain Mechanisms

Jana Sawynok

INTRODUCTION

Pain (the human pain experience) involves multiple dimensions, which are broadly regarded as sensory (nociception), affective (emotional components), and cognitive (interpretation, context, and meaning). The neural circuitry underlying nociception (physiological pain) has been revealed by the use of a variety of nociceptive tests and further developed by the use of inflammatory and neuropathic pain models. There now is considerable information available on the neuronal circuitry of nociception; the key elements include:

1. Activation of peripheral sensory afferent nerves
2. Transmission in the spinal cord
3. Projections to supraspinal structures
4. Regulation of spinal transmission by modulatory pathways originating in the brain stem and by spinal interneurons

The affective and psychological dimensions of pain are now being elaborated by the use of brain-imaging techniques in humans, and this has revealed the involvement of a number of supraspinal regions (collectively known as the "pain matrix"). Pain generally can be regarded as acute nociceptive, inflammatory (involves peripheral inflammation), or neuropathic (involves injury to peripheral or central nerves).

Clinical Management of Bone and Joint Pain
© 2007 by The Haworth Press, Inc. All rights reserved.
doi:10.1300/5771_02

JOINT INNERVATION AND ACTIVATION

Joints are innervated by articular nerves that contain sensory afferent fibers as well as sympathetic efferent fibers. The main classes of primary afferent fibers are based on conduction velocities and fiber diameter, and have been established for some time. Detailed morphological analysis of articular nerves has shown that about 20 percent of articular afferent fibers are myelinated; most are thinly myelinated group III units (Aδ fibers; conduction velocity 2.5 to 20 msec^{-1}), some are large-diameter myelinated low-threshold group II units (Aβ fibers; conduction velocity 20 to 65 msec^{-1}). The majority of fibers consist of unmyelinated afferent fibers, with about half being group IV units (C fibers; conduction velocity <2.5 msec^{-1}) and the remainder unmyelinated sympathetic efferent units. Low-threshold non-nociceptive afferents (group II) have corpuscular endings (Ruffini, Golgi, and Pacini), which are located in fibrous joint tissues. High-threshold afferents, which transmit noxious information (groups III and IV), show little specialization, terminate as free nerve endings, and can be identified as beaded varicosities; these are located in the fibrous joint capsule, synovium, ligaments, menisci, and periosteum. Collectively, this network of primary afferent nerves detects both non-noxious and noxious stimuli.

Most joint afferents are mechanosensitive and are activated by pressure applied to the joint and by movements of the joint. Non-nociceptive fibers are activated by innocuous mechanical stimuli, such as gentle pressure applied to the joints and movement in the working range of the joint (most are group II and III fibers), while nociceptive fibers are activated only by noxious stimuli such as strong pressure applied to the joint and movement exceeding the working range of the joint (group III and IV units). Most of the latter also respond to chemical stimuli, and so are called polymodal nociceptors. Following inflammation, group II fibers exhibit acute and transient changes, while group III and IV fibers exhibit spontaneous activity and enhanced responses to mechanical stimulation. A further group of afferents do not, normally, respond to mechanical inputs, but are recruited by inflammation (silent nociceptors).

More recently, primary afferent nerve fibers have been classified according to their neuropeptide phenotype. These comprise three main groups: (a) large diameter non-nociceptive neurons that are labeled with neurofilament proteins, (b) nociceptive neurons that are isolectin B_4 (IB_4)-positive and express receptors for glial-derived neurotrophic factor (GDNF), and (c) peptidergic nociceptive neurons that contain calcitonin gene-related peptide (CGRP) and express tyrosine kinase A (TrkA) receptors for nerve growth factor (NGF); subsets of these also contain substance P (SP) (about half), and some contain other neuropeptides (e.g., somatostatin, or SOM). Whether these two classes of nociceptors have different functional properties in conveying noxious information in pathological states, as some have suggested, remains to be determined.

In the spinal cord, nociceptive afferent input is processed in the dorsal horn. Numerous afferent fibers project to single spinal cord neurons (convergence) such that the receptive field of spinal neurons is much larger than that of a single afferent unit examined in the periphery. Spinal cord neurons with joint input are either nociceptive specific (i.e., respond only to noxious compression or movement) or of wide dynamic range (i.e., respond to innocuous pressure to joints and other structures and to movements in the working range, and with more prolonged responses to noxious stimulation). Responses of spinal units are tonically regulated (inhibition or facilitation can occur) by descending modulatory systems, and such regulation can be altered by inflammation. Spinal cord neurons responding to joint input activate supraspinal pathways leading to thalamic and some brain stem structures, with further connections to a variety of structures involved in pain affect and cognition. Innocuous joint activation leads to activation of intraspinal pathways regulating reflexes and motor events, and these may contribute to events such as joint stiffness.

MODELS OF INFLAMMATION

A number of nociceptive tests have been developed to model arthritic inflammatory pain. These include: (a) complete Freund's adjuvant (CFA) model of arthritis [heat-killed *Mycobacterium butyricum* or *Mycobacterium tuberculosis* in adjuvant injected intradermally, often at the base of the tail; produces a model of mono- or polyarthritis involving inflammation of joints and soft tissue, which persists for weeks or months, and joint inflammation peaks in the first week and then resolves (monoarthritis) or enters a second phase that lasts for weeks (polyarthritis)], (b) adjuvant-induced arthritis [AIA; involves immunization with methylated bovine serum albumin (mBSA) emulsified with CFA, followed by an articular injection of mBSA; leads to knee inflammation, which can persist for months], and (c) carrageenan (CARR)/kaolin model (injected into the joint; this leads to changes in afferents in 1 to 2 hours, which continues up to 24 hours). In another model, CARR is injected locally into the hind paw to produce a subacute model of tissue inflammation (up to 1 week); this represents a more general model of inflammatory pain. In osteoarthritis, inflammation is secondary to degenerative changes, and further tests have been developed specifically to model this condition. These include chemical models (iodoacetate is injected into the joint; this leads to chondrocyte damage, cartilage loss, and perturbations of subchondral bone) and surgical models (partial meniscotomy, transection of collateral anterior cruciate ligament; also produce morphological joint changes). Each of these models produce tissue changes and behavioral effects that are consistent with various arthritic conditions and may be of value in examining the pharmacology of rheumatoid arthritis and osteoarthritis, but they are not necessarily complete models for such conditions.

PAIN IN ARTHRITIS

Pain in arthritis is characterized by spontaneous pain (pain at rest) and hyperalgesia (a response to a stimulus that would not normally produce pain, and an exaggerated response to a normally noxious stimulus). The term allodynia is reserved for the sensation of pain evoked by gentle innocuous stimuli that do not cause pain under normal conditions. The hyperalgesia of arthritis occurs when the joint is moved through its working range and when gentle pressure is applied to the joint. Inflammation of the joint leads to *peripheral sensitization* (lowered threshold to activation and increased responses of afferent neurons following activation) and *central sensitization* (hyperresponsiveness of nociceptive neurons in the CNS). Sensitization may also alter *neurogenic inflammation* (efferent neuronal processes by which the nervous system influences the inflammatory process).

Peripheral Sensitization

The molecular events involved in activation of sensory nerves by noxious modalities (heat, pressure, and chemicals) and sensitization of these processes by inflammation in general, and specific chemical inflammatory mediators in particular, are currently receiving considerable attention. While these have been identified as part of the inflammatory process in general, it is likely that many of the observations also are relevant to joint inflammation. Figure 1.1 illustrates a schematic representation of a sensory nerve ending, and depicts ion channels (top) and receptors for chemical mediators (bottom) that are important in sensory nerve activation and sensitization. While these are displayed on the nerve ending, free nerve endings *in situ* are not amenable to many forms of investigation (e.g., electrical recording), and ion channel activity and modulation of such activity have been explored in the cell body of primary afferent nerves (dorsal root ganglion, or DRG). There is direct evidence that DRG cell bodies express the same ion channels as the sensory nerve ending and that receptors produced in the cell body are transported to peripheral and central terminals. However, some have noted that isolated DRG cell bodies may be more accurate models of axotomized rather than intact sensory neurons.

Sensory Nerve Activation

Activation and depolarization of sensory afferent nerves reflects entry of Na^+ and Ca^{2+} into the nerve via a series of ion channels,

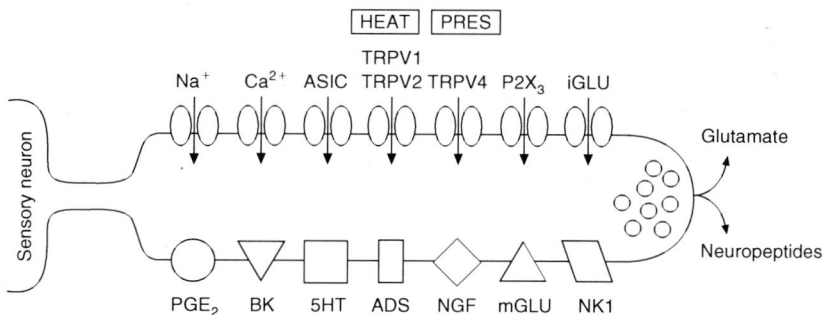

FIGURE 1.1. Schematic depiction of the nociceptive primary afferent neuron indicating ion channels (top) and receptors (bottom) involved in activation and sensitization of sensory nerves (PRES = pressure).

including voltage-dependent Na^+ and Ca^{2+} channels, acid-sensitive ion channels (ASICs) and transient receptor potential (TRP) channels. It can also result from activation of ionotropic purinergic [particularly $P2X_3$, responding to adenosine $5'$-triphosphate (ATP)] and glutamate (GLU) [NMDA, α-amino-3-hydroxy-5-methyl-4-isoxazole propionic acid (AMPA), and kainate (KA)] receptors, which respond to chemical mediators that may contribute to inflammation.

The identification and cloning of the TRPV1 (previously called vanilloid receptor-1 or VR1) receptor was a significant advance in understanding the molecular transduction of nociceptive stimuli at the level of the sensory nerve ending. There are now known to be several members of the TRP family of receptors; these respond to a wide range of different temperatures: TRPV2 > 52°C, TRPV1 > 43°C (heat receptors), TRPV3 > 32°C to 39°C, TRPV4 > 27°C to 35°C (warm receptors), TRPM8 < 25°C to 28°C, and TRPA1 (ANKTM1) < 17°C (cold receptors). All are expressed in sensory neurons of some kind, and their potential physiological roles in sensory processes have been explored by using animals in which the gene for the receptor has been deleted and observing the functional phenotype. Their presence in other cell types indicates that their physiological functions are not limited only to sensory function.

The TRPV1 receptor is the best characterized of this family of receptors; it is activated by capsaicin (vanilloid chemical structure, the pungent ingredient in hot chili peppers), resiniferotoxin (potent capsaicin analog present in cactus), lipid mediators (e.g., anandamide and *N*-arachidonyl dopamine), and protons in addition to heat. Capsaicin and other chemical mediators bind to an intracellular domain on the receptor, while protons bind to a distinct site outside the cell; heat transduction appears to involve the channel itself. TRPV1 −/− mice show normal behavioral responses to temperatures near the threshold for activation of TRPV1 receptors, although there are reduced pain behaviors at higher temperatures (>50°C to 52°C) which exceed the activation threshold. However, dissociated DRG cells from these animals show deficient moderate heat-evoked responses, and this difference between dissociated cells and intact systems invites caution in interpreting data from *in vitro* systems. In TRPV1 −/− mice, thermal hyperalgesia, in response to inflammation (carrageenan) and tissue injury (incision), is reduced, suggesting a clear role for TRPV1 receptors in inflammatory hyperalgesia. Mechanical thresholds and responses to cold are not altered in TRPV1$-/-$ mice.

Another member of the TRP family, TRPV4, is involved in sensing osmotic changes, but also appears to contribute to noxious pressure. Thus, gene deletion leads to impaired noxious pressure detection, while thermal thresholds and touch are unaltered. This channel is expressed in small (low threshold) and large (high threshold) DRG neurons, in free nerve endings, as well as at cutaneous mechanosensory terminals (including Meissner, Merkel terminals), suggesting that the sensation of pressure by mechanosensitive TRPV4 channels is transmitted by A- and C-fibers. An ion channel member of the degenerin family, mDEG (also called BNC1, or brain sodium channel-1, and ASIC-2) is involved in aspects of touch sensation, but not noxious mechanical pressure sensation. $P2X_3$ receptors are implicated in some aspects of pressure transduction, whereby ATP is released from tissue by mechanical stimulation and then activates receptors; this model represents a mechanochemical process of pressure detection. The continued exploration of gene deletion phenotypes of animals that lack specific receptors identified in sensory afferent nerves will likely lead to a further clarification of receptor entities involved in the transduction of noxious physical stimuli.

Sensory Nerve Modulation and Modification

Inflammation is a complex process involving many cell types and many chemical mediators (acute mediators, cytokines, and growth factors) whose actions are elaborated during different phases of inflammation. The functional activity of ion channels in sensory neurons can be increased (e.g., altered voltage dependence, decreased threshold to activation, and increased currents when activated) by various inflammatory mediators. This phenomenon was first recognized with prostaglandin E_2 (PGE_2), which was shown to alter activation kinetics of tetrodotoxin (TTX)-resistant Na^+ channels in DRG cells *in vitro*; subsequent studies indicated it was mediated by protein kinase A (PKA), which phosphorylated the channel protein. This form of sensitization now has been shown also to occur with TRPV1 and $P2X_3$ receptors in DRG cells and/or cell expression systems and to involve several inflammatory mediators [e.g., PGE_2, 5-hydroxytryptamine

(5-HT), bradykinin, or BK, and ATP] and PKA and protein kinase C (PKC). Pathways other than through PKA or PKC also may contribute to sensitization; thus, BK can heighten TRPV1 sensitivity via release from inhibition by an endogenous lipid (PtdIns(4,5)P2), while NGF can sensitize VR1 via a phospholipase-γ pathway. Some of the interactions demonstrated *in vitro* also have been observed *in vivo*, as pain behaviors produced by local injections (into rat hind paw) of capsaicin (activates TRPV1 receptors) and $\alpha\beta$-methylene-ATP (activates P2X$_3$ receptors) are variously enhanced by specific inflammatory mediators as well as by inflammation.

Following inflammation, significant changes in the expression of ion channels on sensory neurons occur (Table 1.1). Thus, a general upregulation (increase in receptor protein) is observed for Na$^+$ channels, ASICs and TRPV1 receptors in DRG and/or sensory nerves. Furthermore, there is an upregulation of receptors for neuropeptides released from sensory afferent nerve endings (neurokinin 1, or NK1), inflammatory mediators which regulate ion channel activity (e.g., BK and 5-HT) and neurotrophins (NGF) (Table 1.1). NGF regulates TRPV1 via p38 mitogen-activated protein kinase (MAPK) following inflammation; it can also regulate expression of Na$^+$ channels and receptors (P2X$_3$ and BK). The enhanced expression of each of these targets may play a role in the functional hypersensitivity that occurs in inflammatory states. Finally, a phenotype shift can occur following inflammation, in which A-fiber neurons begin to express SP and brain-derived neurotrophic factor (BDNF; which are normally found in C-fibers); this may account for the capacity of normally non-noxious tactile stimuli to contribute to allodynia and hyperalgesia following inflammation.

Central Sensitization

Spinal cord transmission of sensory input following tissue injury and inflammation involves a process known as central sensitization. This manifests specifically as: (a) a reduction in threshold to activation of spinal units, (b) an increased responsiveness of spinal cord units, and (c) an expansion of the receptive field and recruitment of novel inputs. Cellular elements involved in central sensitization are depicted in Figure 1.2. Spinal transmission in the normal state involves

TABLE 1.1. Ion channels and receptors on sensory neurons which are increased by inflammation.

Target	Effect (model)
Ion Channels	
Na^+	↑ α-Subunit common to all isoforms of Na^+ channels (CFA)[a]
	↑ Nav1.8 (TTX-R), ↑ Nav1.3 and Nav1.7 (TTX-S) (mRNA, immunohistochemistry, currents in DRG) (CARR)[b]
ASIC	↑ ASIC1a (but not others) in large diameter DRG neurons (CFA)[c]
TRPV1	↑ TRPV1 receptor expression, but no change in mRNA in DRGs (CARR, CFA)[d]
	↑ TRPV1 receptor immunocytochemistry in peripheral nerves (CFA)[e]
	↑ TRPV1 receptors in IB_4^+ (but not IB_4^-) neurons[f]
	↔ TRPV1 (AIA)[g]
Receptors	
P2X	↑ $P2X_2$ and ↑ $P2X_3$ receptors in DRG (CFA)[h]
GLU	↑ NMDA, AMPA, and KA receptors in cutaneous nerves (myelinated, unmyelinated) (CFA)[i]
NK1	↑ NK1 receptor and substance P immunoactivity in DRG neurons (AIA)[j]
	↑ NK1 receptors in unmyelinated nerves (CFA)[k]
Bradykinin	↑ B2 receptors (acute, chronic-phase AIA)[j]
5-HT	↑ mRNA in DRG for $5\text{-}HT_{1A}$, $5\text{-}HT_{1B}$, $5\text{-}HT_{1F}$, $5\text{-}HT_{2A}$, $5\text{-}HT_{2C}$, $5\text{-}HT_3$, $5\text{-}HT_4$, and $5\text{-}HT_7$ receptors (CFA)[l]
NGF	↑ p75 and TrkA receptors in DRG (CFA)[m]

[a]Gould et al., 1998, 69; Gould et al., 1999, 269.

[b]Black et al., 2004, 237; Tanaka et al.,1998, 967.

[c]Voilley et al., 2001, 8026.

[d]Ji et al., 2002, 57.

[e]Carlton and Coggeshall, 2001, 53.

[f]Breese et al., 2005, 37.

[g]Bär et al., 2004, 172.

[h]Xu and Huang, 2002, 93.

[i]Carlton and Coggeshall, 1999, 63.

[j]Segond von Banchet et al., 2000, 424.

[k]Carlton and Coggeshall, 2002, 29.

[l]Okamoto et al., 2002, 133; Wu et al., 2001, 183.

[m]Pezet et al., 2001, 113.

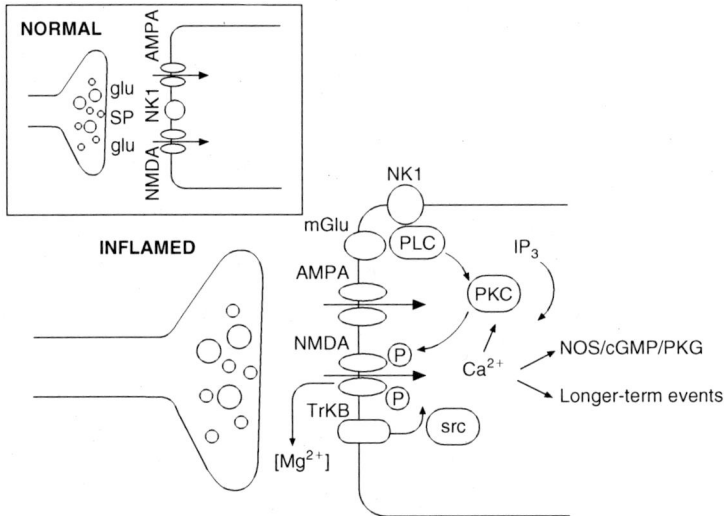

FIGURE 1.2. Schematic illustration of synaptic activity at the primary afferent synapse in the spinal cord showing activity in the normal state and following inflammation.

release of glutamate from sensory nerve terminals; glutamate then acts on postsynaptic AMPA receptors leading to cation entry and rapid depolarization. With repetitive stimulation (wind up) or more intense activity, SP is coreleased with glutamate; this leads to sustained slow depolarization and removal of the Mg^{2+} block of the NMDA receptor. The resulting NMDA receptor activation leads to increased intracellular Ca^{2+} entry and activation of a cascade of intracellular events that modulate or modify activity. Metabotropic glutamate receptors and NK receptors are coupled to inositol triphosphate (IP_3), which also leads to increased intracellular Ca^{2+} release and further contributes to activation of Ca^{2+}-dependent processes. For example, PKC (highly Ca^{2+} sensitive) is activated and phosphorylates NMDA receptor ion channels (on serine thronine residues), leading to enhanced activity. Other elements of inflammation (enhanced NGF) can also lead to phosphorylation of NMDA receptors (on tyrosine residues) and lead to the same net effect of enhanced activity of the channel (even though there may be mechanistic differences). Ca^{2+} also can activate other intracellular signaling pathways such as the nitric oxide/cyclic-GMP/protein kinase G (PKG) pathway and lead further enhancement of transmission. Activation of MAP kinases (e.g., p38 and ERK) in DRG cells and in spinal cord neurons may further regulate long-term processes that contribute to sensitization. *Induction* of central sensitization appears to result from phosphorylation of receptors (post-translational event) and prominent activation, but *maintenance* depends on transcriptional and post-translational changes that result from such activation.

Spinal release of glutamate is observed following joint inflammation, and both AMPA and NMDA receptors contribute to central sensitization in such instances. Thus, antagonists for both receptor subtypes inhibit central sensitization; these can both prevent sensitization and reverse it when it is established. Neuropeptides such as SP and CGRP are also released intraspinally when the joint is inflamed and stimulated. Antagonists for these receptors reduce responses to noxious joint stimulation following inflammation, although the antinociceptive effects of such antagonists are weaker than the effects of glutamate receptor antagonists. Neuropeptide receptors are likely to be involved in the longer-term changes in synaptic transmission that occur during inflammation.

Prostaglandins in the spinal cord also play a role in central sensitization. Thus, PGE_2 is released in the spinal cord following joint inflammation, and can facilitate responses of spinal cord neurons to mechanical stimulation of the joint. Inhibition of the production of prostaglandins leads to reduced generation of hyperexcitability, but may play a lesser role in the maintenance of hyperexcitability once established. While a potential role of glial cells in inflammatory pain has been examined following identification of a role in neuropathic pain, a prominent role for microglia in inflammatory pain states is not indicated at this time.

Neurogenic Inflammation

In addition to afferent functions, sensory fibers also subserve efferent functions, whereby they influence the inflammatory process elaborated in the periphery (neurogenic inflammation). In this regard, mediators (in particular, SP and CGRP) are released into the microenvironment from sensory nerve endings following activation of the nerve, and can influence vasodilation, vascular permeability, modify immune system activity, have trophic effects, and control vascular tone. Furthermore, sympathetic and parasympathetic efferent nerves also may contribute to inflammation, either independently or in concert with sensory nerves, by releasing specific neuropeptides. The synovial membrane is richly innervated, and peptidergic SP and CGRP fibers have been described extensively; fibers containing vasoactive intestinal polypeptide (VIP) and neuropeptide Y (NPY) also have been identified. The nerve network in the joint is complex; furthermore, neurons may undergo degeneration, regeneration, and sprouting following inflammation.

A number of experimental observations suggest a role of the peripheral nervous system in experimental arthritis; for example: (a) section of peripheral nerves decreases the severity of adjuvant arthritis, (b) destruction of unmyelinated sensory afferents with capsaicin reduces swelling, hyperalgesia and cellular inflammation in the arthritic joint, (c) antidromic stimulation of articular C-fibers contributes to inflammation in joints, (d) SP applied to the knee joint increases inflammation, and (e) at later stages in inflammation, responses to nerve stimulation and SP are lost, suggesting alterations in sympathetic and neuropeptide actions. Certain clinical observations also suggest an involvement of neurogenic mechanisms in arthritis; thus, (a) there is a bilateral involvement of joints in rheumatoid arthritis, (b) autonomic dysfunction is common in arthritis, and (c) joints in the paretic side of patients with focal neurological lesions are largely spared following the development of arthritis.

Table 1.2 summarizes various effects of neuropeptides that may contribute to pain (nociception) and inflammation. SP is synthesized in a proportion of DRG neurons (10 to 20 percent) and transported to terminals of small-diameter sensory fibers; it is generally proinflammatory and exerts effects on a number of cell types. While SP levels are increased in inflamed joints (reflecting increased synthesis in DRGs), SP does not exert strong effects on afferent transmission alone, and its actions seem dependent on the presence of other mediators. AIA leads to a bilateral upregulation of NK1 receptors in DRGs in the acute phase, while inflammation in general leads to upregulation of spinal cord NK1 receptors. CGRP is present in some primary sensory neurons that contain SP; it is a potent vasodilator and promotes

TABLE 1.2. Neuropeptide effects that may influence inflammation.

Neuropeptide	Effects
Substance P	*General:* proinflammatory, immunomodulatory, pro-nociceptive ↑ vascularization, ↑ permeability, ↑ tissue destruction
	Cellular: T-cell proliferation, B-cell stimulation; ↑ prostanoid, leukotriene, cytokine production/release from macrophages; mast cell degranulation [→ histamine, tumor necrosis factor-α (TNFα), NGF, NO release] mitogenic on fibroblasts, synoviocytes, endothelial cells
Calcitonin gene-related peptide (CGRP)	*General:* anti-inflammatory, immunomodulatory ↑ vascularization, ↑ vasodilation, ↑ edema, ↑ permeability, ↑ healing, ↑ osteogenesis, ↓ bone resorption
	Cellular: ↓ T-cell proliferation but ↑ chemotaxis; macrophage inhibition, ↓ mast cell extravasation, recruitment; ↑ osteoblasts, ↓ osteoclasts; ↓ synoviocyte proliferation; mitogenic on endothelial cells; promotes leukocyte adhesion
Somatostatin (SOM)	*General:* anti-inflammatory, analgesic immunomodulatory, neurohormone, neurotransmitter
	Cellular: antiproliferative; anti-angiogenic; autocrine or paracrine role when released from lymphocytes; neural release may modulate neurogenic inflammation
Vasoactive-intestinal polypeptide (VIP)	*General:* anti-inflammatory, immunomodulatory antagonist to SP, ↑healing, ↑ osteolysis, ↓ bone resorption
	Cellular: alters T-cell proliferation and migration, favors T-helper cells, B-cell stimulation; macrophage stimulation; osteoblast and osteoclast stimulation, ↓ proliferation of synoviocytes
Neuropeptide Y (NPY)	*General:* neuroendocrine, stress-responses ↑ vasoconstriction, ↓ extravasation hyperalgesic/NGF, neurotrophic/NGF

Source: Compiled from Nissalo et al., 2002, 384; Schaible et al., 2005, 77; D. Paran and H. Paran, 2003, 578.

edema. CGRP levels are increased in arthritis joints, and antibodies to CGRP given in the joint reduce the swelling of arthritis. While it has potent anti-inflammatory effects in some situations, it also is reported to produce some synergistic effects with SP on afferents. SOM is also found in a subset of primary afferent neurons, and can have widespread effects depending on the cellular location of receptors. Applied peripherally, it inhibits sensitized nociceptors, possibly by regulating TRPV1 activity; it exerts a tonic inhibitory effect on nociceptor activity. Intra-articular SOM has beneficial effects in experimental arthritis. In humans, somatostatin analogs have anti-inflammatory effects in rheumatoid arthritis, and there is interest in this as a potential therapy in the treatment of arthritis.

The roles of other neuropeptides present in peripheral nerves in inflammation are less elaborated. VIP is colocalized with acetylcholine in postganglionic effector fibers (parasympathetic system), and its actions are synergistic with acetylcholine in many cases. It exerts anti-inflammatory and immunomodulatory effects, with actions on a number of cell types. VIP administration in an experimental collagen-induced arthritis model leads to a notable improvement of symptoms. NPY is colocalized with noradrenaline (NA) in sympathetic postganglionic neurons, and enhances vasoconstriction produced by NA (in some cases it inhibits release by autoinhibition). It may play a role in neuroendocrine and stress responses in which the stress axis is activated. NPY is present in synovial tissue, and levels are increased in inflammatory synovial fluids.

Endogenous opioid peptides are another family of neuropeptides that may contribute to neural-immune interactions in the periphery. Multiple opioid receptors are upregulated in sensory nerves following inflammation reflecting increased synthesis in the DRG and transport to the nerve terminal; endogenous opioids (particularly β-endorphin) are released from inflammatory and immune cells, and this system may provide a substrate for immune regulation of sensory function. The intra-articular administration of morphine has been reported to have beneficial effects in both osteoarthritis and in rheumatoid arthritis, and provides a potential novel therapy for such conditions.

CONCLUSION

There is considerable progress occurring in understanding mechanisms involved in joint inflammation. This reflects several developments, including (a) development of models that specifically target rheumatoid arthritis and osteoarthritis, where inflammation may play a primary/immunological role and a secondary/degenerative role, respectively, (b) use of general models of tissue inflammation to identify fundamental molecular aspects of activation of sensory nerves and changes in peripheral nerves (modulation, modification) that occur with inflammation, (c) recognition of distinct contributions of peripheral sensitization and central sensitization, (d) recognition of the role of neuropeptides in inflammation and immunomodulatory processes, and (e) recognition of immune-nervous system communication. An appreciation of specific mechanisms involved in enhanced pain signaling that occurs following joint inflammation provides useful information in potentially identifying novel systemic or localized therapies.

BIBLIOGRAPHY

Pain Pathways and Joint Afferents

Fields HL, Basbaum AI (1999) Central nervous system mechanism of pain modulation. In: *Textbook of Pain*, 4th Edn, Ed: Wall PD, Melzack R, Churchill Livingstone, Edinburgh, pp. 309-329.

Grubb BD (2004) Activation of sensory neurons in the arthritic joint. *Novartis Foundation Symp* 260:28-48.

Millan MJ (2002) The induction of pain: An integrative review. *Prog Neurobiol* 57:1-164.

Price DD (2000) Psychological and neural mechanisms of the affective dimension of pain. *Science* 288:1769-1772.

Schaible HG (1998) The neurophysiology of pain. In: *Oxford Textbook of Rheumatology*, 2nd Edn, Vol 1, Ed: Maddison PJ, Isenberg DA, Ubo P, Glass DN, Oxford University Press, Oxford, pp. 487-499.

Schaible HG, Grubb BD (1993) Afferent and spinal mechanisms of joint pain. *Pain* 55:5-54.

Vagas H, Schaible HG (2004) Descending control of persistent pain: Inhibitory or facilitatory? *Brain Res Brain Res Rev* 46:295-309.

Models of Inflammation

Fernihough J, Gentry C, Malcangio M, Fox A, Rediske J, Pellas T, Kidd B, Bevan S, Winter J (2004) Pain related behavior in two models of osteoarthritis in the rat knee. *Pain* 112:83-93.

Griffith RJ (1992) Characterization and pharmacological sensitivity of antigen arthritis induced by methylated bovine serum albumin in the rat. *Agents Actions* 35:88-95.

Pomonis D, Boulet JM, Gottshall SL, Phillips S, Sellers R, Benton T, Walker K (2005) Development and pharmacological characterization of a rat model of osteoarthritis pain. *Pain* 114:339-346.

Segond von Banchet G, Petrow PK, Bräuer R, Schaible HG (2000) Monoarticular antigen-induced arthritis leads to pronounced bilateral upregulation of the expression of neurokinin 1 and bradykinin 2 receptors in dorsal root ganglion neurons of rats. *Arthritis Res* 2:424-427.

Walker K, Fox AJ, Urban LA (1999) Animal models for pain research. *Mol Medi Today* 5:319-321.

Pain Signaling and Sensitization

Aley KO, Messing RO, Mochly-Rosen D, Levine JD (2000) Chronic hypersensitivity for inflammatory nociceptor sensitization mediated by the ϵ isoenzyme of protein kinase C. *J Neurosci* 20:4680-4685.

Amaya F, Shimosato G, Nagano M, Ueda M, Hashimoto S, Tanaka Y, Suzuki H, Tanaka M (2004) NGF and GDNF differentially regulate TRPV1 expression that contributes to development of inflammatory thermal hyperalgesia. *Eur J Neurosci* 20:2303-2310.

Dai Y, Fukuoka T, Wang H, Yamanaka H, Obata K, Tokunaga A, Noguchi K (2004) Contribution of sensitized P2X receptors in inflamed tissue to the mechanical hypersensitivity revealed by phosphorylated ERK in DRG neurons. *Pain* 108: 258-266.

Doubell TP, Mannion RJ, Woolf CJ (1999) The dorsal horn: State-dependent sensory processing, plasticity and the generation of pain. In: *Textbook of Pain*, 4th Edn, Ed: Wall PD, Melzack R, Churchill Livingstone, Edinburgh, pp. 165-182.

Ferreira J, da Silva GL, Calixto JB (2004) Contribution of vanilloid receptors to the overt nociception induced by B2 kinin receptor activation in mice. *Brit J Pharmacol* 141:787-794.

Gold MS, Levine JD, Correa AM (1998) Modulation of TTX-R I_{Na} by PKC and PKA and their role in PGE_2-induced sensitization of rat sensory neurons in vitro. *J Neurosci* 18:10345-10355.

Gould HJ, Gould TN, England JD, Paul D, Liu ZP, Levinson SR (2000) A possible role for nerve growth factor in the augmentation of sodium channels in models of chronic pain. *Brain Res* 854:19-29.

Hamilton SG, Wade A, McMahon SB (1999) The effects of inflammation and inflammatory mediators on nociceptive behaviors induced by ATP analogues in the rat. *Brit J Pharmacol* 126:326-332.

Ji RR (2004) Peripheral and central mechanisms of inflammatory pain, with emphasis on MAP kinases. *Curr Drug Targets-Inflamm Allergy* 3:299-303.

Ji RR, Samad TA, Jin SX, Schmoll R, Woolf CJ (2002) p38 MAPK activation by NGF in primary sensory neurons after inflammation increases TRPV1 levels and maintains heat hyperalgesia. *Neuron* 36:57-68.

Jordt SE, McKemmy DD, Julius D (2003) Lessons from peppers and peppermint: the molecular logic of thermosensation. *Curr Opin Neurobiol* 13:487-492.

Julius D, Basbaum AI (2001) Molecular mechanisms of nociception. *Nature* 413: 203-210.

Levine JD, Reighling DB (1999) Peripheral mechanisms of inflammatory pain. In: *Textbook of Pain*, 4th Edn, Ed: Wall PD, Melzack R, Churchill Livingstone, Edinburgh, pp. 59-84.

Numazaki M, Tominaga M (2004) Nociception and TRP channels. *Curr Drug Targets-CNS Neurol Disord* 3:479-485.

Obata K, Noguchi K (2004) MAPK activation in nociceptive neurons and pain hypersensitivity. *Life Sci* 74:2643-2653.

Petersen M, Segond von Banchet G, Hepplemann B, Koltzenburg M (1998) Nerve growth factor regulates the expression of bradykinin binding sites on adult sensory neurons via the neurotropin receptor p75. *Neuroscience* 83:161-168.

Ramer MS, Bradbury EJ, McMahon SB (2001) Nerve growth factor induces P2X(3) expression in sensory neurons. *J Neurochem* 77:864-875.

Scholz J, Woolf CJ (2002) Can we conquer pain? *Nature Neuroscience* 5:1062-1067.

Snider WD, McMahon SB (1998) Tackling pain at the source: New ideas about nociceptors. *Neuron* 20:629-632.

Suzuki M, Mizuno A, Kodaira K, Imai M (2003) Impaired pressure sensation in mice lacking TRPV4. *J Biol Chem* 278:22664-22668.

Suzuki M, Wanatanabe Y, Oyama Y, Mizuno A, Kusano E, Hirao A, Ookawara S (2003) Localization of mechanosensitive channel TRPV4 in mouse skin. *Neurosci Lett* 353:189-192.

Woolf CJ, Costigan M (1999) Transcriptional and post-translational plasticity and the generation of inflammatory pain. *Proc Natl Acad Sci* 96:7723-7730.

Woolf CJ, Salter MW (2000) Neuronal plasticity: Increasing the gain in pain. *Science* 288:1765-1768.

Neurogenic and Neuropeptide Mechanisms

Carlton SM, Zhou S, Du J, Hargett GL, Ji G, Coggeshall RE (2004) Somatostatin modulates the transient receptor potential vanilloid 1 (TRPV1) ion channel. *Pain* 110:616-627.

Delgado M, Abad C, Martinez C, Leceta J, Gomiriz RP (2001) Vasoactive intestinal peptide prevents experimental arthritis by down regulating both autoimmune and inflammatory components of the disease. *Nat Med* 7:563-568.

Likar R, Schäfer M, Paulak F, Sittl R, Pipam W, Schalk H, Geissler D, Bernatzky G (1997) Intra-articular morphine analgesia in chronic pain patients with osteoarthritis. *Anesth Analg* 84:1313-1317.

Nissalo S, Hukkanen M, Imai S, Törnwall J, Konttinen YT (2002) Neuropeptides in experimental and degenerative arthritis. *Ann NY Acad Sci* 966:384-399.

Paran D, Paran H (2003) Somatostatin analogs in rheumatoid arthritis and other inflammatory and immune-mediated conditions. *Curr Opin Invest Drugs* 4: 578-582.

Schaible HG, Del Rosso A, Matucci-Cerinic M (2005) Neurogenic aspects of inflammation. *Rheum Dis Clin N Am* 31:77-101.

Stein A, Yassouridis A, Szopko C, Helmke K, Stein C (1999) Intraarticular morphine versus dexamethasone in chronic arthritis. *Pain* 83:525-532.

Stein C, Schäfer M, Machelska H (2003) Attacking pain at its source: New perspectives on opioids. *Nat Med* 9:1003-1008.

Chapter 2

The Physiology and Basic Science of Bone and Joints

Helen Cohen
David Blake

> ... to know them was merely to know their ailments, and the ailments were almost invariably rheumatism. Some, of course, had other bodily infirmities, but they always had rheumatism as well.

> Saki (H. H. Munro), from *The Toys of Peace*

The evolution of vertebrate organisms and the internal skeleton required the development of bone and cartilaginous tissues and of joints. When all is functioning normally, we are not even aware of our joints. However, all too commonly, degeneration or disease afflicts the joints, and then we become painfully aware of their integral nature.

This chapter will outline the developmental biology of bone, cartilage, and joints, the normal physiology of the mature human joint and its supporting structures, and relate this to dysfunction and disease.

SKELETAL DEVELOPMENTAL BIOLOGY

Embryology

The skeletal system develops from the mesoderm and the neural crest. By the fourth week, it has formed embryonic connective tissue,

Clinical Management of Bone and Joint Pain
© 2007 by The Haworth Press, Inc. All rights reserved.
doi:10.1300/5771_03

or mesenchyme. This will differentiate and migrate in many different ways, including into fibroblasts, chondroblasts, and osteoblasts. Mesenchyme has a bone-forming capacity, and may do so directly (membranous ossification, for example, skull bones) or by forming a hyaline cartilage model, which later becomes ossified (see Figures 2.1 and 2.2) (endochondral ossification, for example, long bones).

Limb buds become visible on the body wall at 4 weeks. They initially consist of a mesenchyme core covered by a layer of ectoderm, which is thickened at the limb bud tip, forming the apical ectodermal ridge (AER). The AER has an inductive influence on the adjacent underlying mesenchyme, which becomes a population of rapidly proliferating, undifferentiated cells. The more distal mesenchyme further away from the influence of the AER develops into cartilage and muscle. Thus, limbs develop in a proximodistal direction with the more proximal structures such as the glenohumeral joint developing before more distal structures such as the wrist. The upper limbs develop approximately 24 hours in advance of the lower limbs. Therefore, embryonic insults occurring at this stage affect more distal parts of the upper limbs than of the lower limbs. At 6 weeks, the distal portion of the limb bud becomes flattened, forming the hand and foot plates. Cell death in the AER separates the distal part of the plate into five parts, which will form the digits. At 7 weeks, the limbs rotate in opposite

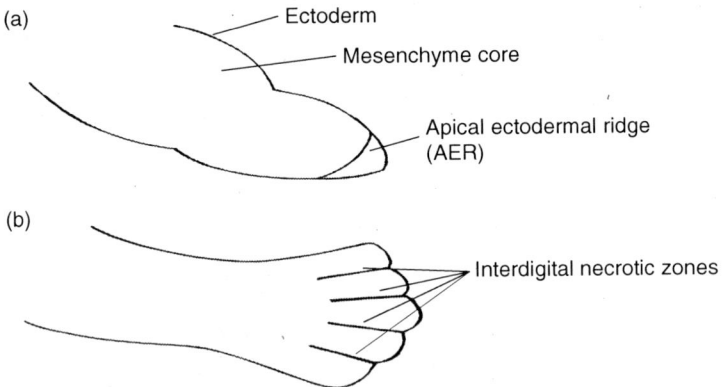

FIGURE 2.1. Embryological development of a limb. *Note:* (a) Diagrammatic representation of a human upper limb bud at the fifth week; (b) Diagrammatic representation of a human hand plate at the sixth week.

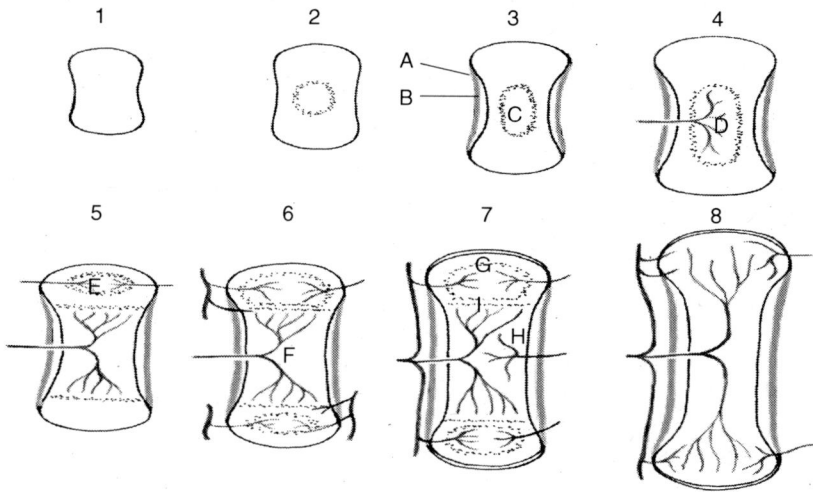

FIGURE 2.2. Endochondral ossification. *Note:* 1. Hyaline cartilage model; 2. Hypertrophy of central cells; 3. Formation of periosteum (A) periosteal collar (B) and calcification of matrix in primary center (C); 4. Invasion of primary center by periosteal buds (D); 5. Formation of secondary ossification center (E); 6. Bones at birth (F = Medullary cavity); 7. Continued growth (G = Trabecular bone, H = Compact bone, I = epiphyseal growth plate); 8. Mature long bone.

directions such that, in the upper limb, the extensor muscles lie on the posterior and lateral surfaces with a laterally positioned thumb, where, as in the lower limb, the extensor muscles lie anteriorly with a medially positioned great toe.

By 6 weeks, the mesenchyme has condensed, forming the blastema (a growing mass of mesenchyme in which definitive tissues are not distinguishable), and the hyaline cartilage model precursors of the limb bones are recognizable. Endochondral ossification begins near the end of the embryonic period at about 8 weeks, and primary ossification centers are present in the long bones at 12 weeks. At birth, the bone diaphysis is usually ossified. The epiphyses are still cartilaginous, but ossification centers soon appear in them. Between the ossification centers of the epiphysis and diaphysis lies a cartilaginous plate, the epiphyseal growth plate that allows for the continued growth of the bone. These gradually ossify and fuse throughout childhood and adolescence, the last growth plate to fuse being the proximal clavicular epiphysis at 22 years.

Synovial joints are visible by 7 to 8 weeks preceding the vascularization of epiphyseal cartilage (8 to 12 weeks), synovial villous fold formation (10 to 12 weeks), bursae (3 to 4 months), and fat pad formation (4 to 5 months). The synovial joints develop in a series of stages: condensation (blastema formation), chondrification and interzone formation, synovial mesenchyme formation, cavitation, and mature joint formation (Figure 2.3).

Synovial Mesenchyme

The joint capsule develops from a dense layer of cartilage surrounding the interzone. Some vascularized mesoderm becomes enclosed, which gives rise to the menisci, synovial lining, intracapsular ligaments, and tendons. Synovial lining cells are initially fibroblast-like type-B cells, but macrophage-like type-A cells are recruited later from the circulation. The synovium is innervated at 8 weeks, with substance P present by 11 weeks and neuropeptide Y by 13 weeks (see Figure 2.3).

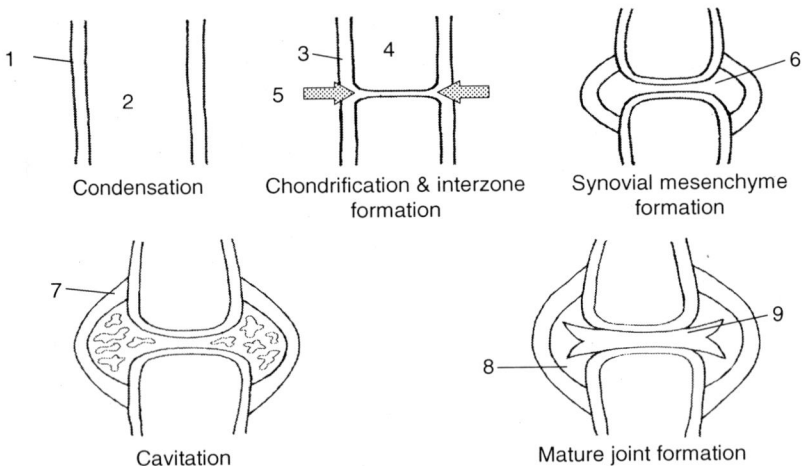

FIGURE 2.3. Synovial joint formation. *Note:* 1. Mesenchyme; 2. Blastema; 3. Perichondrium; 4. Cartilage; 5. Homogeneous interzone; 6. Synovial mesenchyme; 7. Articular capsule; 8. Synovial tissue; 9. Articular cavity.

MOLECULAR GENETICS

With the continuing advances in biosciences and molecular genetics, there have been major advances in this field. Most are beyond the scope of this chapter, so the following is a brief, simplified outline of some of the relevant research findings.

Morphogens

Cartilage and bone gradually evolve through a series of processes to their final, mature state, a transformation known as "morphogenesis." Signaling proteins are involved, and families of bone and cartilage "morphogens" and their receptors have been identified. They are believed to be involved in the signaling and induction of the various processes of morphogenesis, including initiation, maintenance, promotion, and programmed cell death by apoptosis. They are involved in functions such as mesenchymal condensation, chondrogenesis, bone morphogenesis, cartilage development, and hypertrophy and ligament and tendon development.

Bone morphogenetic proteins (BMPs) are members of the TGF-β superfamily. They first induce cartilage formation followed by bone, so it follows that all BMPs are also cartilage morphogens. As more have been identified and cloned, they have been assigned numbers, for example, BMP-1, and number up to at least 11 with undoubtedly more to follow. There are several distinct subfamilies.

Cartilage-derived morphogenetic proteins (CDMPs) were isolated after BMPs had been discovered in bone and prompted a search for similar proteins in articular cartilage. A mutation in the CDMP-1 gene locus has been found in patients with Hunter-Thompson chondrodysplasia.[1,2]

MATURE JOINT TISSUES

Classification of Joints

1. *Synarthrosis (immovable):* The bones surfaces are almost in direct contact with each other, joined by fibrous tissue or hylaline cartilage (see Table 2.1). There are four types:

- Sutura—the bone edges are joined by fibrous tissue. They are only found in the skull.
- Schindylesis—a thin plate of bone is received into a cleft or fissure in another bone. An example is the articulation of the rostrum of the sphenoid and the perpendicular plate of the ethmoid with the vomer.
- Gomphosis—this is the type of joint that seats the tooth in its socket.
- Synchondrosis—the bone edges are joined by cartilage. The epiphyseal growth plates of long bones are examples.

2. *Amphiarthrosis (slightly movable):* The bone surfaces are connected by an interposed piece of fibrocartilage. Examples include the costosternal junctions, pubic symphysis, and intervertebral discs between adjoining vertebrae.
3. *Diarthrosis (freely movable):* This is the most common form of skeletal articulation. The opposing bone surfaces are capped with articular cartilage and joined together by ligaments and a joint capsule lined by synovium. There may be an interposing articular disc or meniscus in the joint. Diartoses may be subdivided by the type of movements that they permit:
   - Uniaxial: hinge joint, e.g., elbow
   - Polyaxial: ball and socket, e.g., shoulder.

MATURE BONE

Although bone is often thought of as an inert chunk of calcium, nothing could be further from the truth. It is a metabolically active

TABLE 2.1. Classification of joints.

Class	Type	Example
Synarthrosis (immoveable)	Sutura Schindylesis Gomphosis Synchondrosis	Skull Rostrum of sphenoid Tooth socket Epiphyseal growth plate
Amphiarthrosis (slightly moveable)		Public symphysis Intervertebral discs
Diarthrosis (freely moveable)	Synovial joints –Uniaxial –Polyaxial	Elbow Shoulder

tissue, constantly turning over and responding to the physical activity and mechanical loading placed on it. Professional tennis players (larger forearm bones of the racket-hand arm) and astronauts (weightlessness and osteoporosis) illustrate these points. It responds to genetic, hormonal, nutritional, and inflammatory influences. It is intimately involved with calcium, phosphate, and vitamin D homeostasis, of which many aspects are not fully understood.

Mature bone consists of three types of cell supported by a mineralized extracellular matrix. The extracellular matrix is 35 percent organic, of which 90 percent is type-1 collagen with the remainder including osteocalcin, osteonectin, and proteoglycan. The inorganic part comprises calcium and phosphate in the form of hydroxyapatite (see Figure 2.4).

GROSS STRUCTURE

There are two types of bone present in varying amounts throughout the skeleton. Compact (dense or cortical) bone is most obvious in the shafts of long bones, and in the walls of the vertebrae and subchondral

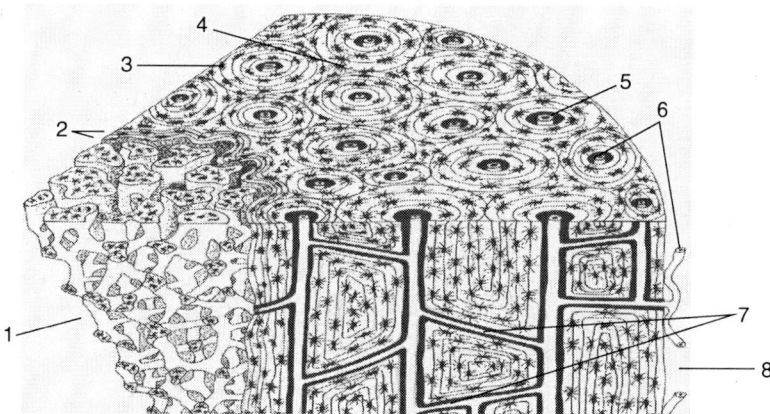

FIGURE 2.4. Compact bone. *Note:* 1. Trabecular bone; 2. Endosteal lamellae; 3. Lacuna containing an osteocyte; 4. Canaliculi; 5. Haversian canal; 6. Capillary; 7. Volkmann's canal; 8. Compact bone.

plates of the acetabulum and glenoid fossa. Trabecular (cancellous) bone is spongy in appearance when a dry bone is cut. It has a delicate, cross-linked structure that varies according to the loading of the particular bone. For example, where compressive forces are high in the patella or humeral head, it has a more chambered structure, whereas in areas of low compressive stress, it has a looser, lace-like form. The importance of the three-dimensional cross-linking of trabecular bone for maintaining bone strength has become more recognized as osteoporosis has become more widely diagnosed and treated. In osteoporosis, a major factor in bone weakness is thought to be loss of trabecular bone linkage. Most current treatment may improve bone mineral density, but the effects on linkage are usually small and poorly understood. Trabeculae are constantly undergoing remodeling though the processes of bone absorption and formation (see Figure 2.5).

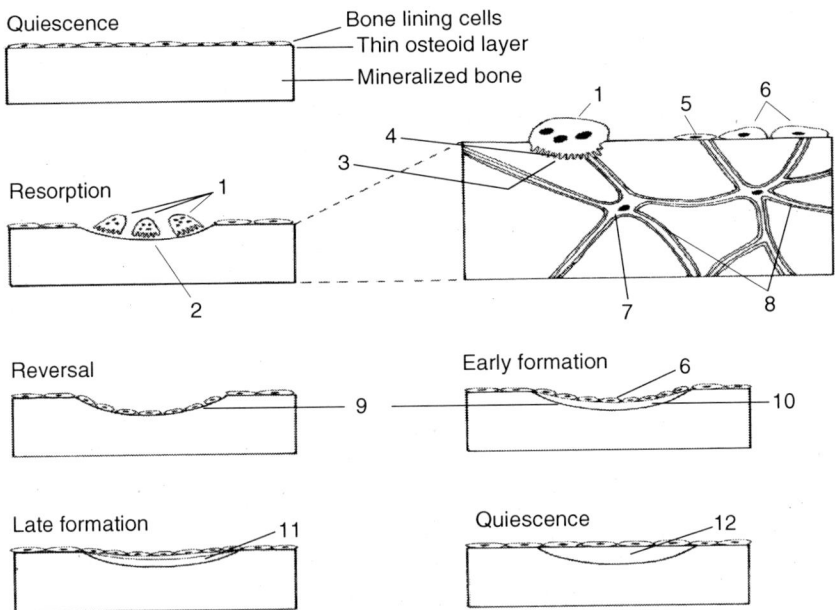

FIGURE 2.5. The bone cycle. *Source:* Based on a diagram from Ericson et al., 1989. *Note:* 1. Osteoclasts; 2. Resorption pit; 3. Howship's resorption lacuna; 4. Ruffled border; 5. Bone lining cell; 6. Osteoblasts; 7. Osteocyte; 8. Canaliculi; 9. Cement line; 10. Osteoid; 11. Mineralized osteoid; 12. Osteoid mineralization completed.

MICROSCOPIC STRUCTURE

Osteoblasts are bone-forming cells that produce organic bone matrix and control bone mineralization. They are derived from the mesenchymal stromal cell system. They influence other cell types including osteoclasts, and are sensitive to cytokines, bone morphogenetic proteins, and many other growth factors.

Osteocytes are located within a lacuna at the center of a Haversian system (Figure 2.5). They are osteoblasts that have become imprisoned within the bone matrix. Fine, cytoplasmic processes extend for some way into the canaliculi radiating out from the lacunae, and provide communication with other osteocytes via gap junctions.

Another form of osteoblast is the inactive, flattened bone-lining cell. They cover endosteal surfaces and trabeculae.

Osteoclasts are multinucleated giant cells derived from the hemopoietic cell system, responsible for bone resorption. They attach to bone and form a seal, isolating their zone of activity. Bone is resorbed by the production of a locally acidic environment through carbonic anhydrase activity and by lysosomal enzyme digestion. The bone resorption lacuna is known as Howship's lacuna.[3] A rare form of osteopetrosis is due to an absence of carbonic anhydrase II.[4] Osteoclasts are sensitive to calcitonin, oestrogen, prostaglandins, and osteoblasts. Parathyroid hormone and vitamin D effects on bone are probably mediated via osteoblasts.

The bone cycle is initiated by osteoclastic attachment and bone resorption. This is followed by a reversal phase when the cement line is deposited, and then by oteoblastic secretion of new bone matrix, which is subsequently calcified. In children, the bone formation/resorption balance is toward bone formation, it is level with constant bone mass in young adults, and tipped toward bone loss in old age.

MATURE CARTILAGE

Cartilage comprises chondrocytes and the extracellular matrix that they synthesize and maintain. Cartilage may be classified into three types according to the type and abundance of fiber within the matrix: fibrocartilage, elastic cartilage, and hyaline cartilage.

Fibrocartilage occurs where high tensile strength is required, such as the symphysis pubis, intra-articular discs, intervertebral discs, and at some entheses. It is found in close association with the dense connective tissues of tendons, ligaments, and the joint capsule at the site of insertion into the bone, and can be considered as a transitional form between cartilage and dense connective tissue merging gradually with both. Histologically it comprises bundles of dense collagenous connective tissue with areas of hyaline cartilage lying between, and lacks a perichondrium.

Elastic cartilage occurs where support with flexibility is needed such as external ear, epiglottis, and larynx. It contains collagen and elastic fibers, and is surrounded by a perichondrium.

Hyaline cartilage forms the articular surfaces of bones within joints and is also found in the costal cartilages, nose, larynx, trachea, and bronchi. The term "hyaline" originates from the Greek word "hyalos," meaning glass, as the cut surface of fresh articular cartilage is translucent and glassy in appearance. It comprises mostly water, collagen, and proteoglycans, accounting for approximately 65 to 80 percent, 10 to 30 percent, and 5 to 10 percent wet weight, respectively, with small amounts of noncollagen proteins, inorganic material, and lipids. Chondrocytes account for < 2 percent of the articular cartilage volume (see Figure 2.6).

The collagen of hyaline cartilage is largely type II (90 percent), with small amounts of types III, V, VI, IX, and XI. Type X is restricted to

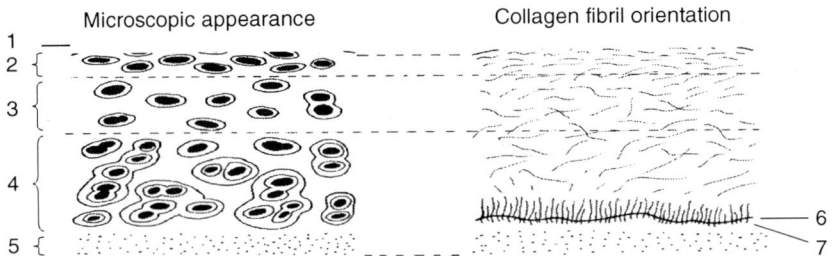

FIGURE 2.6. Diagram of the microscopic histological appearance of hyaline cartilage and collagen fibril orientation. *Note:* 1. Articular surface; 2. Superficial zone; 3. Middle zone; 4. Deep zone; 5. Subchondral bone; 6. Tidemark; 7. Calcified cartilage.

hypertrophic chondrocytes undergoing endochondral ossification such as growth plates. Mutations of type II, IX, X, and XI have been found in certain skeletal chondrodysplasias.[5-8] Poteoglycans form large polyanionic aggregates with hyaluronate that attract water but are restrained by the collagen network. The aggregates have a high density of fixed negative charge providing expansile properties like a coiled spring. Together, this helps to provide the firmness and resilience required of articular cartilage. The water content is dependent on the concentration and organization of the collagen network, and the stiffness and strength of the collagen network determined by the compaction of the proteoglycans in the matrix.

Histologically, hyaline cartilage can be divided into four zones (Figure 2.6):

1. Superficial tangential zone (or "lamina splendens; 5 to 10 percent of cartilage thickness)
2. Middle zone (40 to 60 percent)
3. Deep zone (30 percent)
4. Calcified cartilage (interface with bone)

The lamina splendens is subject to the greatest shearing forces, and its structure reflects this. The collagen fibrils are arranged at an angle to the usual direction of motion of the joint and tangentially to the articular surface. It has the highest water content (80 percent wet weight) and collagen content (85 percent dry weight), with relative amounts of collagen declining in each zone moving towards the tide mark.

William Hunter demonstrated that adult articular cartilage does not contain blood vessels in 1743.[9] Blood flow is not practical in a tissue subject to the repeated high compressive forces of weight bearing, which would cause continual occlusion to flow, and where the presence of such vessels would compromise the mechanical properties and structural integrity required. Indeed, chondrocytes may produce an inhibitor of neovascularization.[10] The exact mechanisms by which articular cartilage receives its nutrition are not clear, though two major sources seem likely. Diffusion from synovial fluid via synovial vessels, and from subchondral bone blood vessels. Articular cartilage is also lacking direct innervation.

Mechanical Properties

Articular cartilage is compliant and compressible. On loading, the cartilage indents immediately, and if the load is continued, there is a "creep" phase during which it continues to gradually indent with the load remaining constant. When the load is removed, the cartilage slowly recovers its resting volume. The initial rapid indentation is due to the efflux of water and compression of the collagen, with further water movement occurring in the creep phase. If loading is continued, eventually equilibrium will be reached, when there is no further flow of water and the entire load is taken by solid matrix. The viscoeleastic properties and compliance of cartilage help to adsorb energy during loading, thereby decreasing impact and aiding the spread of the load through the joint.

SYNOVIUM

The synovium is the soft tissue lining of synovial joints, tendon sheaths, and bursae. The normal synovium is characterized by a lack of cellularity. It consists of a continuous layer of synovial lining cells three to four cells deep, the intima, and underlying connective tissue, the subintima. Microscopically, synovium can be classified into three main types based on the subintimal structure, namely fibrous, areolar, and adipose.[11] Synovium may also be considered by functionality rather than histological appearance and divided into functional compartments comprising the intima, subintimal stroma, and vasculature (see Figure 2.7).

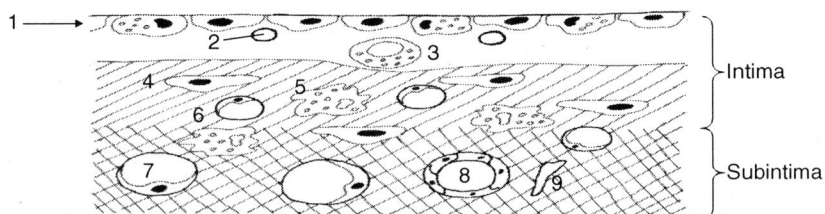

FIGURE 2.7. Schematic representation of synovium. *Source:* Based on a diagram in Rheumatology. Hochberg et al. Mosby, 3rd ed 2003. *Note:* 1. Intimal cells; 2. Capillary; 3. Mast cell; 4. Fibroblast; 5. Macrophage; 6. Small venule; 7. Venule; 8. Arteriole; 9. Lymphatic vessel.

Intima

Intimal cells loosely interdigitate, and in some areas there are gaps where intimal cells are absent. Originally, two types of intimal cell were recognized based on their electron microscopic appearances; type A macrophage-like and type B fibroblast-like.[12] In normal synovium, fibroblast-like B cells predominate with only 10 to 20 percent of macrophage-like A cells. A transitional form can be recognized and is occasionally referred to as a type C cell.[13] Type-B fibroblast-like intimal cells express the enzyme UDPGD and synthesize hyaluronan, an important constituent of synovial fluid.[14] They also express adhesion molecules[15] including VCAM-1, ICAM-1, CD44, and β1 integrins. Type-A macrophage-like intimal cells are capable of phagocytosis and antigen expression similar to mature macrophages, and are strongly CD163 and CD68 positive. Studies are ongoing on the roles of type-A and type-B intimal cells in normal synovial synthetic and immunologic activity, and particularly the contribution in inflammation and disease.

Subintima

Between the intimal lining and the joint capsule there is a variable depth of heterogenous connective tissue, the subintimal stroma. Normally, the predominant cell type is the fibroblast, with some macrophages. The cellularity and vascularity vary according to location. For example, at the lateral joint margin of the knee, it is cellular and well vascularized, but as it blends with the joint capsule, it becomes increasingly fibrous. Capillary density is greatest in adipose and areolar subintima, and much less in fibrous areas.

Vasculature

Normal synovium has a rich vascular supply.[16] There are extensive anastomoses of the arterial, venous, and lymphatic systems of the synovium with vessels of the joint capsule, ligaments, tendons, periosteum, and adjacent bone. In the synovial subintima a lymphatic plexus drains along the vessels to the regional deep lymph nodes. Joints receive their blood supply from periarticular arterial plexuses. The rami pierce the joint capsule and form subsynovial vascular plexuses. Some of the synovial vessels end near the articular margin in an anastomotic fringe, the circulus articuli vasculosus, which sends arcades of capillaries into the synovial villi and folds. Hunter[9] described this plexus of communicating arteries and veins around the neck of a bone, likening it to the mesentry. Close to the surface of the synovium there is a plexus of arterioles and venules forming a quadrilateral array, which sends capillary loops to immediately below or through the synovial intimal cells. These surface capillaries are fenestrated, allowing rapid exchange of solutes, water, and mediators of inflammation and immunity.

Synovial vasculature is capable of considerable plasticity. In inflammation, considerable angiogenesis is seen, whereas in animal models of joint immobilization, the capillary plexuses and blood flow decline.[17]

Innervation

Afferent joint innervation is by primary nerves, which are branches of adjacent peripheral nerves, and accessory nerves, which are branches of intramuscular nerves crossing the joint capsule. Some joints are also supplied by cutaneous nerves in the overlying skin, for example, ankle and knee. The articular nerves enter the spinal cord via several dorsal roots and therefore project to several spinal segments, which may contribute to the poor localization and referral of joint pain. Approximately 20 percent of articular afferents are myelinated fibers. The majority are finely myelinated Aδ fibers (conduction velocity 2.5 to 20 ms^{-1}) nociceptors, with a smaller number of large-diameter myelinated Aβ fibers (conduction velocity 20 to 65 ms^{-1}), which are important for proprioception and detection of joint movement. The remaining 80 percent are unmyelinated fibers, approximately half of which are C-fibers (conduction velocity < 2.5 ms^{-1}) and the others efferent sympathetic neurons.[18] The C-fibers transmit pain, usually a dull, poorly localized quality often called "slow" pain, compared with the acute, intense, well-localized pain transmitted by Aδ fibers, or "fast" pain. Sympathetic efferents are involved in the control of articular blood flow.

Afferent C-fibers terminate in the dorsal horn of the spinal cord, in layers I and II of Rexed's laminae. The spinal dorsal horn neurons have receptive fields usually extending beyond the joint, and may respond to mechanical pressure from both deep tissue and skin. Neurons detecting mechanical stimuli are either nociceptive-specific (NS) or wide-dynamic-range (WDR) type. NS neurons respond to intense pressure and/or painful movement stimuli such as forceful supination or pronation or movements beyond the normal working range. WDR neurons respond to both innocuous and noxious pressure and may be weakly activated by movements within the working range. They respond much more intensely to painful movements and those beyond the working range.[19]

Neurons receiving afferent joint input are subject to diffuse noxious inhibitory controls (DNIC) by heterotopic stimuli such that painful stimulation at one site in the body may inhibit pain transmission from another part. This may be the mechanism by which folk remedies such as rubbing stinging nettles into painful osteoarthritic joints work. Descending inhibitory pain mechanisms also operate tonically and interruption of these can reduce excitation thresholds of dorsal horn neurons and cause them to expand their receptive fields, contributing to hyperalgesia.

In inflammatory and chronic painful joint disease, mechanisms such as central sensitization and neuroplastic cortical representational changes contribute to the chronic pain problem.[20] Nerve endings are sensitized by mediators of inflammation such as prostaglandins and bradykinin. In complex regional pain syndrome, sympathetic efferent fibers become involved in the pain pathways although the mechanism is not clear. Affected limbs may become chronically vasoconstricted or vasodilated as a result of their aberrant activity.

SYNOVIAL FLUID

Synovial fluid is present in small amounts in normal joints, approximately 2.5 ml in the normal knee. It functions as both a lubricant and source of nutrition for the avascular articular cartilage and adjacent tendons. Synovial fluid is an ultrafiltrate of plasma with added components generated by the type-II synovial lining cells. Of these, the major added protein is hyaluronate, a high molecular weight ($>10^6$ Da) linear repeating disaccharide of β-D-glucuronyl-β-D-N-acetylglucosamine. Hyaluronate forms the central axis of the proteoglycan aggregates that are required for the functional integrity of articular cartilage and other extracellular matrices, as well as the major macromolecular constituent of synovial fluid providing it with viscoeleastic properties. Another glycoprotein found in synovial fluid secreted by the type-II lining cells is lubricin.[21] As the name suggests, it functions as a highly efficient lubricant.

Synovial Fluid Formation

The difference between the intracapillary and intra-articular hydrostatic pressures and between the colloid osmotic pressures of capillary plasma and synovial tissue fluid drive flow of plasma ultrafiltrate across the fenestrated capillary endothelium. This is an example of the Starlings law.[22] Water and low molecular weight solutes pass freely, glucose is assisted by an active transport system, while larger molecules and proteins are limited by the filtration process. Proteins are therefore present in synovial fluid at a level inversely proportional to their molecular size. Albumin is the most common protein present, at concentrations of about 45 percent of that in plasma.[23]

Synovial Fluid Clearance

This is by bulk flow through the lymphatics of the synovium, assisted by joint movement. Molecular size does not have an influence on the rate of clearance.

Lubrication

Lubrication is a complicated subject with an extensive literature in the biological and engineering fields.[24] A brief review of its relevance to the human synovial joint follows.

When one surface slides upon another, friction results, which is often expressed in terms of a "coefficient of friction." A high value indicates a less efficient system in which more energy will be used as one surface moves over the other, which will be detracted from the energy available for work. In normal joints, the coefficient of friction is very low as the system is a remarkably efficient one.

There are two basic mechanisms of lubrication:

1. *Boundary lubrication:* A layer of lubricant is bound to the bearing surfaces facilitating slippage and protecting against wear. Lubricin appears to be involved in this mechanism, although other phospholipids may contribute.

2. *Fluid-film lubrication:* Joint motion generates an incompressible fluid film between the cartilage surfaces, separating and cushioning them.

Intra-Articular Pressure

The pressure within a normal joint ranges between -3 and -6 cmH$_2$O at rest or during weight bearing, which is sub atmospheric.[25] This should be distinguished from the pressure generated between cartilage surfaces during weight bearing.

TENDONS

Tendons are composed of longitudinal bundles of type-1 collagen, and function as linkages between muscles and their insertions into bone. A fine network of type-III collagen, blood vessels, lymphatics, and tendon fibroblasts run among the bundles.[26] Tendon fibroblasts produce matrix components such as proteoglycans and type-I collagen. They can generate metalloproteinases and their inhibitors, which are involved in tendon inflammation and degeneration and repair.

Many tendons run in tendon sheaths formed of collagen lined with mesenchymal cells that resemble synovium. These produce hyaluronic acid, aiding lubrication.

LIGAMENTS

Ligaments provide stability to joints. They may be ill defined and appear to blend with the joint capsule, or be clearly defined structures such as the cruciate ligaments of the knee. Structurally, they are similar to tendons but have a higher content of elastic fires compared with collagen (1:4 versus 1:50), and are often more vascularized and, thus, often recover from injury better.

BURSAE

In the same way that joints facilitate movement of bone over bone, bursae aid movement of one tissue over another. They are sacks lined with tissue similar to that of tendon sheaths. Many are formed concurrently with synovial joints during embryogenesis, but others may develop in later life after inflammation or trauma. These processes may also hypertrophy a bursa, or form an abnormal communication between a deep bursa and an adjacent synovial joint. This can be seen in rheumatoid arthritis, with, for example, communication between the semimembranosus or gastrocnemius bursae and the knee joint.

CIRCULATION

Synovial blood flow is regulated by the arterioles. They are sensitive to a variety of factors, autocrine and paracrine, and humoral and neural. Angiotensin-converting enzyme, which produces angiotensin II, a vasoconstrictor, is found predominantly in arteriolar and capillary endothelia.[27] Angiotensin receptors are plentiful on the capillaries with lower densities on nearby arterioles. Receptors for the neuropeptide substance P are also found in similar locations.[28]

The endothelium generates some factors locally, such as the vasoconstrictor peptides angiotensin II and endothelin-1 and the vasodilatory nitric oxide.[29] The synovial arterioles are innervated by sympathetic nerve fibers, which may release vasoconstrictors such as neuropeptide Y and noradrenalin, and by sensory fibers, which may release vasodilatory substances such as substance P and calcitonin gene-related peptide (CGRP).[30]

Intra-articular pressure affects synovial circulation. Acute joint effusions cause elevation of intra-articular pressure, and chronic elevation of pressure as seen with chronic inflammatory joint disease impede circulatory flow especially during weight bearing. Reduced synovial circulation may therefore contribute to synovial hypoxia, and chronic hypoxia may be one mechanism contributing to joint damage in chronic inflammatory disease.

JOINT STABILITY

The shape of the opposing bones forming the joint contribute to stability. The "ball and socket" design of the hip and shoulder are clear examples, but almost all joints demonstrate a close fit of the surfaces. The shape also aids distribution of load through the joint.

Ligaments and tendons contribute to stability as they cross the joint. Ligaments provide a passive restraint, whereas the muscular forces conveyed along the tendons serve to drive the joint components together conferring stability. A major factor contributing to the instability of the knee in osteoarthritis is often weakness and wasting of the quadriceps muscles such that this active "drive" force is greatly diminished.

Synovial fluid is viscous, an essential property for lubrication under pressure. This also confers a degree of adhesion within the joint. When a distracting force is applied to the third metacarpophalangeal joint, if the surface area is taken as $1\ cm^2$, then atmospheric pressure would be overcome at 1 kg. However, in a bioengineering study, a force equivalent of 10 kg is required to distract the joint, and a "knuckle crack" is heard, and a gas bubble appears within the synovial fluid of the joint, demonstrating the adhesiveness of synovial fluid.[31]

Aging and Repair of Joints

While the mechanical properties, structure, and biochemical composition of articular cartilage change with age, it is difficult but important to differentiate between aging and diseases, such as osteoarthritis, that are strongly associated with age. This is not as straightforward as it may sound, and research is ongoing.

The degeneration of normal articulate cartilage is not simply due to aging and mechanical wear. The synthesis and degradation of type-II collagen is associated with the pericellular matrix and is maintained at a steady state throughout life. With aging of intact articular cartilage, there is a significant reduction in the denaturation of type-II collagen relative to collagenase-mediated cleavage, distinguishing it from the molecular degenerative changes seen in osteoarthritis.[32] However, there are many other aging changes in articular cartilage that may increase the risk of degeneration. Changes are seen in the stiffness and elasticity of the cartilage-bone unit, with a steady decline in viscoelastic energy after 29 years of age.[33] There may be fibrillation of the articular surface, decrease in the size and aggregation of proteoglycan aggrecans, and increased collagen cross-linking.[34] Many of these alterations may be due to age-related decline in chondrocyte function and decrease in the ability to maintain tissue reflected by decreased mitotic and synthetic activity, decreased response to anabolic growth factors, synthesis of smaller less-uniform aggregates, and less functional link proteins. There is an increased expression of β-galactosidase, erosion of telomere length, and mitochondrial degeneration due to oxidative damage.[35] Another study looking at donor-matched pairs of intact and degenerate cartilage explants showed that oxidative stress can induce telomere genomic instability leading to chondrocyte senescence and cartilage aging, which may have a role in the development of osteoarthritis.[36]

MRI studies have demonstrated loss of articular cartilage thickness in both aging and osteoarthritis.[37] Other research has compared postmortem articular knee cartilage from lesion-free joints and lesions in osteoarthritic joints. Lesions in aging cartilage exhibited molecular changes in matrix turnover similar to that in osteoarthritic articular cartilage, but not in healthy normal aging cartilage. Collagenase activity and denaturation and decreased glycosaminoglycan content together with a loss of coordination of collagen synthesis and degradation were implicated in the development of lesions. These focal lesions may represent the development of early osteoarthritis.[38]

The role of subchondral bone in the maintenance, repair, and aging of the overlying articular cartilage is not fully understood. The blood supply is important in cartilage nutrition, and the cells of subchondral bone may produce peptides involved in chondrocyte regulation. Subchondral bone sclerosis is an early feature of osteoarthritis, and whether this is a cause of, or a result of, osteoarthritis is still debated. The relative roles of cartilage versus subchondral bone in osteoarthritis is still widely debated.

Modern approaches to the treatment of osteoarthritis include joint debridement, subchondral bone penetration, transplantation of chondrocytes and mesenchymal stem cells, use of periosteal and perichondral grafts, transplantation of osteochondral autologous grafts and allografts, synthetic matrices, and growth factors. None of these methods has yet been shown to predictably restore a durable articular surface to an osteoarthritic joint, and work is ongoing.[39]

SYNOVIUM AND INFLAMMATION

An inflamed joint is characterized by the following:

1. Inflammatory cell infiltrate
2. Hypertrophic, hyperplastic intimal layer

3. Vasculature and nervous supply are buried deeper in the synovium
4. Changes in synovial fluid composition and volume
5. Cytokines and other pro-inflammatory molecules

The net result is hypoxia and ischemia through the increased metabolic demand of the inflamed synovium but poor perfusion (see the following text), resulting in an inadequate oxygen delivery. This will shift cellular metabolism to anaerobic oxidation of glucose, resulting in elevation of lactate and lowering of glucose that correlate well with falls in pO_2 and pH. ATP availability is reduced in hypoxic synovium, and cytosolic calcium levels rise. Mitochondria are calcium accumulators, and when calcium overloaded, their function is impaired further depleting ATP and maintaining a calcium imbalance. Actin-binding proteins regulate the endothelial cytoskeleton and are calcium dependent, and so calcium imbalance may contribute to altered vascular permeability.

Resting intra-articular pressure is elevated in inflamed joints to slightly above atmospheric pressure, and rises further upon weight bearing. This is sufficient to occlude parts of the capillary bed, inducing acute ischemia in an already hypoxic environment. When the joint is rested, reperfusion may occur. The postischemic reperfusion of the synovium evokes the generation of reactive oxygen metabolites and oxidative stress.[40,41] Free radicals can attack the lipids of the cell membrane, causing damage. They may also attack proteins, causing denaturation, cross-linking, aggregation, and fragmentation. Fragmentation of glycosaminoglycans would contribute to a loss of viscosity. Free radicals may affect immunity through differential effects on T-lymphocytes.

Angiogenesis is a synovial response to chronic hypoxia.[42] In rheumatoid arthritis, the resulting proliferating, invading inflammatory pannus causes destruction of articular cartilage and joint structures, eroding bone and leading to joint deformity and loss of function.

The following is a short summary of a complicated area in which ongoing research is continuing to yield more questions as well as answers, and is helping to reveal potential targets for possible new drug therapies.

SUMMARY

In this chapter, we have provided an overview of the physiology and basic science of the normal human joint and bone. Much of the science is still expanding with ongoing research adding to our knowledge and understanding of normal mechanisms. In parallel with this, advances are continually being made into many pathological conditions affecting bone and joints, which in turn is giving rise to new treatments. This knowledge is essential to provide a framework upon which disease, and thereby resulting pain, can be approached, researched, understood, and treated.

REFERENCES

1. Hunter AGW, Thompson MW. Acromesomelic dwarfism: description of a patient and comparison with previously reported cases. *Hum Genet* 1976; 34: 107-113.

2. Terrig Thomas J, Lin K, Nandedkar M, Camargo M, Cervenka J, Luyten FP. A human chondrodysplasia due to a mutation in a TGF-β superfamily member. *Nat Genet* 1996; 12: 315-317.

3. Howship J. Microscopic observations on the structure of bone. *Medico-Chirurgical Transactions*, London, 1815.

4. Fathallah DM, Bejaoui M, Lepaslier D, Chater K, Sly WS, Dellagi K. Carbonic anhydrase II (CA II) deficiency in Maghrebian patients: Evidence for founder effect and genomic recombination at the CA II locus. *Hum Genet* 1997; 99: 634-637.

5. Winterpacht A, Hilbert M, Schwarze U, Mundlos S, Spranger J, Zabel BU. Kniest and Stickler dysplasia phenotypes caused by collagen type II gene (COL2A1) defect. *Nat Genet* 1993; 3: 323-326.

6. Bonnemann CG, Cox GF, Shapiro F, Wu JJ, Feener CA, Thompson TG, et al. A mutation in the alpha 3 chain of type IX collagen causes autosomal dominant multiple epiphyseal dysplasia with mild myopathy. *Proc Natl Acad Sci USA* 2000; 1: 1212-1217.

7. Warman ML, Abbott M, Apte SS, Hefferon T, McIntosh I, Cohn DH, et al. A type X collagen mutation causes Schmid metaphyseal chondrodysplasia. *Nat Genet* 1993; 5: 79-82.

8. Richards AJ, Yates JR, Williams R, Payne SJ, Pope FM, Scott JD, et al. A family with Stickler syndrome type 2 has a mutation in the COL11A1 gene resulting in the substitution of glycine 97 by valine in alpha 1 (XI) collagen. *Hum Mol Genet* 1996; 5: 1339-1343.

9. Hunter W. On the structure and diseases of articulating cartilage. *Philosophical Transactions of the Royal Society of London Biol* 1743; 42.

10. Moses MA, Sudhalter J, Langer R. Identification of an inhibitor of neovascularization from cartilage. *Science* 1990; 248: 1408.

11. Key JA. *Special Cytology.* New York: PB Hoeber; 1932.

12. Barland P, Novikoff AB, Hamerman D. Electron microscopy of the human synovial membrane. *J Cell Biol* 1962; 14: 207-216.

13. Ghadially F, Roy S. *Ultrastructure of Synovial Joints in Health and Disease.* London: Butterworths; 1969.

14. Wilkinson L, Pitsillides A, Worrall, et al. Light microscopic characterisation of the fibroblast-like synovial intimal cell synoviocyte. *Arthritis Rheum 1992; 35: 1179.*

15. Edwards JCW. Synovial intimal fibroblasts. *Ann Rheum Dis* 1995; 54: 395-397.

16. Stevens C, Blake DR, Kidd BL, Merry P, Revell PA, Levick JR. A comparative study by morphometry of the microvasculature in normal and rheumatoid synovium. *Arthritis Rheum* 1992; 35: 1540-1541.

17. Lindstrom J. Microvascular anatomy of synovial tissue. *Acta Rheumatologica Scand* 1963; Sup7: 1-52.

18. Grubb BD. Activation of sensory neurons in the arthritic joint. In: Chadwick DJ, Goode J, eds. *Osteoarthritic Joint Pain.* John Wiley and Sons Ltd; 2004: 28-48.

19. Schaible H. Spinal mechanisms contributing to joint pain. In: Chadwick DJ, Goode J, eds. *Osteoarthritic Joint Pain.* John Wiley and Sons Ltd; 2004: 4-27.

20. Maihöfner C, Handwerker HO, Neundörfer B, Birklein F. Patterns of cortical reorganization in complex regional pain syndrome. *Neurology* 2003; 61: 1707-1715.

21. Swann D. Structure and function of lubricin, the glycoprotein responsible for the boundary lubrication of articular cartilage. In: Franchimont P, ed. *Articular Synovium.* Basel: Karger; 1982: 45.

22. Starling EH. On the absorption of fluids from connective tissue spaces. *J Physiol* 1896; 19: 312-326.

23. Kushner I, Somerville J. Permeability of the human synovial membrane to plasma proteins. *Arthritis Rheum* 1971; 14: 560-570.

24. McCutchen C. Lubrication of joints. In: Sokoloff L, ed. *The Joints and Synovial Fluid.* New York: Academic Press; 1978: 437.

25. Dixon A, Hawkins C. Raised intra-articular pressure—clinical consequences. 1990. Bath Institute for Rheumatic Diseases, Bath.

26. Canoso J. Bursae, tendons and ligaments. *Clin of Rheum Dis* 1981; 7: 181-221.

27. Walsh DA, Suzuki T, Knock G, Blake DR, Polak JM, Wharton J. AT1 receptor characteristics of angiotensin binding analogue binding in human synovium. *Br J Pharmacol* 1994; 112: 435-442.

28. Walsh DA, Mapp PI, Wharton J, Polak JM, Blake DR. Neuropeptide degrading enzymes in normal and inflamed human synovium. *Am J Pathol* 1993; 142: 1610-1621.

29. Wharton J, Rutherford RA, Walsh DA, Mapp PI, Knock G, Blake DR, et al. Autoradiographic localisation of and analysis of endothelin-1 binding sites in rheumatoid synovial tissue. *Arthritis Rheum* 1992; 35: 894-899.

30. Walsh DA, Mapp PI, Wharton J, Rutherford RA, Kidd BL, Revell PA, et al. Localisation and characterisation of substance P binding to human synovium in rheumatoid arthritis. *Ann Rheum Dis* 1992; 51: 313-317.

31. Unsworth A, Dowson D, Wright V. Cracking joints: A bioengineering study of cavitation in the metacarpophalangeal joint. *Ann Rheum Dis* 1971; 30: 348-358.

32. Aurich M, Poole AR, Reiner A, Mollenhauer C, Margulis A, Kuettner KE et al. Matrix homeostasis in aging normal human ankle cartilage. *Arthritis Rheum* 2002; 46: 2903-2910.

33. Ding M, Dalstra M, Linde F, Hvid I. Mechanical properties of the normal human tibial cartilage-bone complex in relation to age. *Clin Biomech* (Bristol, Avon). 1998; 13: 351-358.

34. Martin JA, Buckwalter JA. Roles of articular cartilage aging and chondrocyte senescence in the pathogenesis of osteoarthritis. *Iowa Orthop J* 2001; 21: 1-7.

35. Martin JA, Buckwalter JA. Aging, articular cartilage chondrocyte senescence and osteoarthritis. *Biogerontology* 2002; 3: 257-264.

36. Yudoh K, van Trieu N, Nakamura H, Hongo-Masuko K, Kato T, Nishioka K. Potential involvement of oxidative stress in cartilage senescence and development of osteoarthritis: oxidative stress induces chondrocyte telomere instability and down regulation of chondrocyte function. *Arthritis Res Ther* 2005; 7: R380-R391.

37. Karvonen RL, Negendank WG, Teitge RA, Reed AH, Miller PR, Fernandez-Madrid F. Factors affecting articular cartilage thickness in osteoarthritis and aging. *J Rheumatol* 1994; 21: 1310-1318.

38. Squires GR, Okouneff S, Ionescu M, Poole AR. The pathobiology of focal lesion development in aging human articular cartilage and molecular matrix changes characteristic of osteoarthritis. *Arthritis Rheum* 2003; 48: 1261-1270.

39. Buckwalter JA, Mankin HJ. Articular cartilage: degeneration and osteoarthritis, repair, regeneration, and transplantation. *Instr Course Lect* 1998; 47: 487-504.

40. Henrotin YE, Bruckner P, Pujol JP. The role of reactive oxygen species in homeostasis and degradation of cartilage. *Osteoarthritis Cartilage* 2003; 11: 747-755.

41. Winyard PG, Evans CH, Blake DR. Free radicals and inflammation. In: Parnham MJ, ed. *Progress in Inflammation Research.* Springer, New York; 2000.

42. Firestein GS. Starving the synovium: Angiogenesis and inflammation in rheumatoid arthritis. *J Clin Invest* 1999; 103: 3-4.

PART II

Chapter 3

NSAIDs for Painful Bone and Joint Conditions

Jennifer A. Elliott
Howard S. Smith

INTRODUCTION

Nonsteroidal anti-inflammatory drugs (NSAIDs) are among the most commonly used drugs in the world. It is suspected that NSAIDs and cyclo-oxygenase-2 (COX-2) inhibitors are the most common agents utilized and prescribed for musculoskeletal, bone, or joint pains. Many of us will use NSAIDs on at least an occasional basis during our lifetimes. As the population ages, and arthritic conditions become more prevalent, use of NSAIDs will likely continue to increase. Unfortunately, though they are often perceived to be very safe drugs, especially since some forms are available over the counter, NSAIDs have been associated with significant morbidity and mortality. Such conditions may include congestive heart failure, renal dysfunction, hypertension, and use of various pharmacologic agents that may negatively interact with NSAIDs. Adverse events related to NSAID use that may be of clinical concern include gastrointestinal bleeding, acute renal failure, and precipitation of congestive heart failure, cognitive impairment, and hypertension.

Clinical Management of Bone and Joint Pain
© 2007 by The Haworth Press, Inc. All rights reserved.
doi:10.1300/5771_04

MECHANISMS OF ACTION OF NSAIDS

Despite the explosion of novel analgesic agents, NSAIDs remain among the most widely prescribed and utilized agents for pain relief. This holds even truer of inflammatory pain, or painful conditions involving bones and or joints. NSAIDs are thought to modulate inflammation and pain largely via reversible inhibition of the membrane-bound enzyme COX, although NSAIDs may have many other effects, some of which affect immune cells in a COX-independent fashion. The inhibition of the COX enzyme leads to an inhibition of some of the proinflammatory, pronociceptive eicosanoid mediators involved.

Secreted phospholipase A (2) s generate arachidonic acid from cell membranes, which are further processed to yield various eicosanoids. The COX activity of prostaglandin (PG) endoperoxide synthase then catalyzes the incorporation of two molecules of oxygen into arachidonic acid to yield the hydroperoxy endoperoxide, prostaglandin G_2 (PGG_2), at the cyclo-oxygenase-active site (CAS). PGG_2 subsequently diffuses from the CAS and binds at the peroxidose-active site, where it is reduced from the hydroxyl endoperoxide to prostaglandins (PGs), thromboxane, and prostacyclin. COX structure is characterized by a membrane-binding domain (MBD) made up of amphipathic helices forming the entrance to a long hydrophobic tunnel leading deep into the protein. The CAS is separated from the opening near the MBD by a constriction formed predominantly from the amino acids Arg-120, Tyr-355, and Glu-524.

Investigations including X-ray crystallography have revealed that acetylsalicylic acid irreversible acetylates a serine (Ser-53) in COX-1 in the substrate channel leading to the COX-active site (Loll et al., 1995). NSAIDs with COX-1 activity are able to block this acetylation since they occupy this channel as well.

A high level of COX-2 inhibitor selectivity and a low level of COX-1 inhibitor activity are associated with a reduced interference of platelet cyclooxygenase-1 inactivation by aspirin (Ouellet et al., 2001).

It appears that three distinct anchoring sites and or conformations contribute to substrate and inhibitor binding in the CAS (Rowlinson et al., 2003). Proper anchoring and substrate orientation seems to be crucial for optimal enzymatic functioning, and mutations in the amino acids at the anchoring sites may lead to significant enzymatic dysfunction. The first anchoring site lies at the junction of Arg-120 and Tyr-355 near the membrane interface (e.g., which may affect indomethacin). The second major anchor point is the side pocket, defined by residues Tyr-355, Val-523, His-90, Gln-192, and Arg 513 (which may affect phenyl sulfonamides). The third anchoring conformation appears to involve a chelation/association with Tyr-385 and Ser-530 (which may affect diclofenac).

The type and possible degree of stimulus (e.g., inflammation, infection, tissue/trauma, cytokines, and growth factors) may also contribute to the various concentrations of specific eicosanoids that are generated. Furthermore, eicosanoid-mediated pathways may interact with nitrergic and multiple other pathways in contributing to chronic joint inflammation/pain (Day et al., 2004).

The major involvement of PGs in peripheral sensitization appears to be via PGE_2 binding to EP2 and thereby activating the PKA pathway (Aley and Levine, 1999). PKA subsequently phosphorylates (e.g., activates tetrodotoxin-resistant sodium channels, or TTX-R Na^+Ch) as well as inhibits voltages-gated potassium currents. PGs also possess indirect effects via enhancement of the sensitivity of sensory neurons to bradykinin (e.g., by acting on the B2 receptor) and to capsaicin (by acting TRPVI receptors).

NSAIDs act predominantly via inhibition of COX, an enzyme required for PG synthesis. PGs are active in many tissues and have also been associated with the production of fever, inflammation, and pain. Two forms of the COX enzyme known to serve significant functions have been identified. COX-1 is mostly constitutively expressed in many tissues and plays an important role in the regulation of several important physiologic processes, such as regulation of renal blood flow, maintenance of gastrointestinal mucosal integrity, and platelet aggregation. COX-2 appears to be predominantly an inducible enzyme that becomes upregulated in the setting of inflammation. Most traditional NSAIDs lack selectivity in their inhibition of COX isoenzymes. In the past few years, a new generation of NSAIDs with COX-2 selectivity has become available for clinical use. These newer agents may provide some advantage over the nonselective NSAIDs with regard to potential undesired effects. However, some adverse effects seen with the use of traditional NSAIDs have not been eliminated through the use of COX-2 inhibitors (e.g., nephrotoxicity). NSAIDs undergo hepatic metabolism and are renally excreted. Age-related declines renal function or hepatic impairment associated with such conditions as congestive heart failure may result in drug accumulation and thereby may increase the risk of development of a variety of adverse effects from these agents.

GASTROINTESTINAL EFFECTS OF NSAIDS

PGs play an important role in maintenance of gastrointestinal mucosal integrity. When NSAIDs are administered, homeostatic mechanisms in the gastrointestinal mucosa may be disrupted, resulting in the development of ulcerations or frank perforations in some patients. A significant number of people suffer fatal gastrointestinal hemorrhage every year as a consequence. Unfortunately, many significant gastrointestinal bleeding episodes (up to 80 percent) occur in the absence of premonitory warning signs of abdominal pain or dyspepsia, making prediction of such events difficult. The elderly may have lower baseline levels of PGs in the gastrointestinal mucosa and are at higher risk for gastrointestinal bleeding as compared with younger populations in general, making them potentially more susceptible to adverse gastrointestinal effects of NSAIDs. Other factors that may increase risk of gastrointestinal hemorrhage in the elderly using NSAIDs include concurrent use of aspirin (commonly used for prophylaxis against acute coronary events in the elderly) and concomitant anticoagulant therapy, which might exacerbate gastrointestinal hemorrhage. Some of these effects may be mitigated by the use of gastroprotective agents in conjunction with NSAID therapy. Such treatments might include the use of misprostol, proton pump inhibitors, and H_2 receptor antagonists. Use of COX-2 inhibitors appears to result in a lower incidence of significant gastrointestinal adverse effects as compared with traditional NSAIDs.

RENAL EFFECTS OF NSAIDS

NSAIDs may cause a variety of changes in renal physiology. This is a n important consideration when NSAIDs are selected for use inelderly patients, as many elderly patients suffer from comorbid conditions that can increase the risk of adverse renal effects from NSAIDs, or may experience exacerbation of underlying disease states as a result of the renal effects of NSAIDs. PGs play a role in the regulation of renal blood flow. In patients with such diseases as congestive heart failure, significant hepatic dysfunction, renal insufficiency, and intravascular volume depletion, use of NSAIDs may precipitate acute renal failure due to changes in renal blood flow related to PG inhibition. Renal PGs also play an important role in the regulation of sodium reabsorption in loop of Henle. Inhibition of these PGs by NSAIDs may result in increased sodium reabsorption, which consequently may cause excess fluid retention. This may be of particular importance when NSAIDs are administered to patients with preexisting heart failure, renal insufficiency, or hypertension, which may be worsened under these circumstances. Such effects may be seen relatively quickly after NSAID therapy is initiated. Another important consideration with regards to NSAID use in the hypertensive patient is the decreased efficacy of several antihypertensives when used in conjunction with NSAIDs. In particular, the activity of β-blockers, angiotensin-converting enzyme inhibitors and diuretics may be affected. It should be noted that, while the incidence of adverse gastrointestinal events appears to be lower when COX-2 inhibitors are used (as compared with traditional NSAIDs), the incidence of adverse renal and cardiovascular events remains significant even when COX-2 inhibitors are chosen.

PLATELET EFFECTS OF NSAIDS

Many NSAIDs affect platelet aggregation and may thereby increase the potential for bleeding complications in patients taking NSAIDs. Aspirin is particularly well known for this effect, and is used for this very property in the management of patients at risk for myocardial infarction or stroke. Aspirin permanently acetylates platelets, causing platelet dysfunction that lasts the duration of the life span of the platelet, typically 7 to 14 days. Most nonselective NSAIDs also create platelet dysfunction, but this effect is reversible and platelet aggregation will return to normal within four to five drug half-lives after these drugs are discontinued. COX-2-specific inhibitors do not impact platelet aggregation in doses used in clinical practice. NSAID use in patients may lead to bleeding complications particularly when combined with coumadin. This drug combination may increase the risk of bleeding due to both the antiplatelet effects of NSAIDs and the anticoagulant effects of coumadin, resulting in impairment of the two primary clotting mechanisms of the body. In addition, displacement of coumadin from serum-protein-binding sites by some NSAIDs may enhance the effective anticoagulant activity of coumadin. Therefore, caution and monitoring is warranted when these classes of drugs are to be coprescribed.

CENTRAL NERVOUS SYSTEM EFFECTS OF NSAIDS

Central nervous system side effects are commonly seen with analgesics such as opioids, and are not widely appreciated as a potential consequence of NSAID use. However, NSAIDs are not devoid of central nervous system effects. NSAIDs may manifest central nervous system toxicity with sedation, confusion, cognitive dysfunction, psychosis, and personality changes. Such side effects may be construed as signs of developing dementia in the elderly, but will abate with discontinuation of the drug. Dizziness and tinnitus have also been described with NSAID use. In particular, indomethacin has been associated with complaints of headache.

OTHER NSAID EFFECTS

NSAIDs have potentially beneficial effects in the prevention of cancer and Alzheimer's disease. Currently, COX-2 inhibitors (particularly celecoxib) are being used in treatment of patients with familial adenomatous polyposis, a genetic condition that predisposes individuals to the development of colon cancer. It appears that the development of polyps in these patients can be substantially diminished when COX-2 inhibitors are used. This finding may have relevance to other forms of cancer as well, although thus far COX-2 inhibitors are not being used for prophylaxis against cancer at this point. Further studies may help to further elucidate a potential role for chronic COX-2 inhibitor therapy in individuals who are at risk for the development of cancer. If a clear benefit can be established for the use of COX-2 inhibitors for this purpose, there will undoubtedly be a large population of individuals taking these drugs for prolonged periods of time. With regard to Alzheimer's disease, it has been speculated that NSAIDs may delay the onset of dementia in this disease. It has been theorized that Alzheimer's disease may involve an inflammatory process in the brain that leads the development of dementia.

CLASSIFICATION OF NSAIDS

NSAIDs are classified according to their chemical structure into various groups. The following is a breakdown of NSAIDs in current clinical use:

Nonselective COX Inhibitors (NSAIDs)	Salicylates	Aspirin
		Nonacetylated salicylates
		  Choline magnesium
		    trisalicylate (Trilisate)
		  Diflunisal (Dolobid)

	Propionic Acid Derivatives	Naproxen (Naprosyn, Aleve, Anaprox) Ketorolac (Toradol) Oxaprozin (Daypro) Ketoprofen (Orudis, Oruvail) Ibuprofen (Advil, Motrin) Flurbiprofen (Ansaid)
	Indoleacetic Acids	Etodolac (Lodine) Indomethacin (Indocin) Sulindac (Clinoril)
	Phenylacetic Acids	Diclofenac (Cataflam, Voltaren, and Arthrotec, which consists of Diclofenac in combination with Misprostol)
	Naphthylalkanones	Nabumetone (Relafen)
	Pyrroleacetic Acids	Tolmetin (Tolectin)
COX-2 Partially Selective Inhibitors (CPSI)	Oxicams	Piroxicam (Feldene) Meloxicam (Mobic)
COX-2 Selective Inhibitors (CSI)		Celecoxib (Celebrex) Rofecoxib (Vioxx), currently not available in the United States Valdecoxib (Bextra), currently not available in the United States

With regard to selection of a particular agent for any particular patient, duration of action, the potential for organ specific side effects, comorbid conditions, and potential for drug interactions may play a role in the choice of NSAID to be used. Specific areas of concern will be addressed as certain individual NSAIDs are further described in the following text.

Aspirin

Aspirin is the prototypical NSAID and has been used clinically for well over a century. It is widely used as it is available over the counter and is present in many combination analgesic preparations. For this reason, patients may be unaware that they are consuming substantial amounts of aspirin on a regular basis, and may not consider it important to inform their physicians about using such products. This situation can lead to problems, as physicians may prescribe NSAID therapy, unaware of concurrent aspirin therapy, which could increase the potential for adverse effects. Patients may also be taking aspirin as a means of preventive therapy for myocardial infarction and stroke, which should also be taken into consideration. Gastrointestinal toxicity is a concern when aspirin is used, and selection of an enteric-coated aspirin product may be advisable. A single dose of aspirin can irreversibly acetylate platelets, rendering them permanently dysfunctional. This property may be of significant concern in patients on anticoagulant therapy.

Nonacetylated Salicylates

Nonacetylated salicylates in clinical use for arthritic conditions include choline magnesium trisalicylate (Trilisate) and diflunisal (Dolobid). Trilisate is usually dosed between 2000 and 3000 mg daily, while diflunisal is usually given in doses of 500 to 1000 mg daily. These agents are typically dosed two to three times per day and appear to have lower potential for gastrointestinal toxicity as compared with aspirin. Antiplatelet effects are less intense as well, which may make these agents more desirable than other NSAIDs in certain populations.

Propionic Acid Derivatives

Commonly used propionic acid derivative NSAIDs include naproxen (Naprosyn, Aleve, and Anaprox), ketorolac (Toradol), oxaprozin (Daypro), ketoprofen (Orudis and Oruvail), ibuprofen (Advil and

Motrin), and flurbiprofen (Ansaid). Typical daily doses for naproxen are 500 to 1000 mg. Ketorolac is given in doses of up to 120 mg per day parenterally and 40 mg per day orally. Oxaprozin dosing is usually 1200 mg daily, while ketoprofen is dosed at 200 to 300 mg daily. Ibuprofen is given in a dose range of 1200 to 3200 mg daily and flurbiprofen in a dose of 200 to 300 mg per day. These drugs are typically administered two to four times per day, but oxaprozin may be administered once daily. Naproxen and ibuprofen are available over the counter and are generally inexpensive as compared with other NSAIDs. Ketorolac is unique in that it is available for parenteral use. However, it also has significant potential for toxicity, and it is therefore recommended that its use (both parenteral and enteral) be limited to a total of 5 days. It is typically used in acute settings, especially those in which a patient has restriction of oral intake such as the perioperative period. Dose reduction is recommended in the elderly.

Indoleacetic Acid Derivatives

Sulindac (Clinoril) is a prodrug that is converted in the liver to its active metabolite. It is dosed in the range of 300 to 400 mg daily. It should be dose reduced in the elderly and in the presence of significant renal or hepatic disease. Indomethacin (Indocin) is unique among NSAIDs in its ability to penetrate the blood-brain barrier to a significant extent. This property has made indomethacin useful in the management of certain headache syndromes (ironically, headache is also a frequently occurring side effect of indomethacin that may result in termination of its use). It may also explain a relatively higher incidence of adverse central nervous system effects with this drug as compared with other NSAIDs, particularly in patients with pre-existing central nervous system disorders such as depression, psychosis, and Parkinsonism. Indomethacin is also available in suppository form for patients incapable of taking the drug orally. Its utility is limited, however, due to significant gastrointestinal toxicity with relatively high potential for ulcer formation with repeated use. Dosing of indomethacin is typically 150 to 200 mg daily. Etodolac (Lodine) is more COX-2 selective than most traditional NSAIDs, and accordingly appears to have a lower incidence of adverse gastrointestinal side effects relative to many other NSAIDs. It has an extended release preparation available that allows for once-a-day dosing. Etodolac is dosed at 400 to 1200 mg daily with dosage varying depending on the formulation chosen (Lodine versus Lodine XL).

Phenylacetic Acids

Diclofenac is available in an immediate-release (Cataflam), a delayed-release enteric-coated (Voltaren), and an extended-release (Voltaren-XR) formulation. It is also available in combination with misprostol (a PGE_1 analog) for enhanced gastrointestinal protection (Arthrotec). The typical adult daily dose of diclofenac is 100 to 200 mg daily. This may de administered in divided doses, or as a single dose when the Voltaren XR formulation is chosen.

Naphthylalkanones

Nabumetone (Relafen), like sulindac, is a prodrug that is converted to its active metabolite in the liver. This property may decrease the risk of gastrointestinal ulceration as the gastrointestinal mucosa is not directly exposed to active drug. Nabumetone is typically dosed between 1000 and 2000 mg daily in single or divided doses. Dose reduction may be advisable in the elderly.

Oxicams

Piroxicam (Feldene) is a long-acting NSAID that can be dosed once daily. The recommended daily dose of piroxicam is 20 mg, which may be divided. Steady state blood levels of piroxicam may not be achieved for 1 to 2 weeks after initiation of therapy due to its prolonged half-life. Meloxicam (Mobic) may have relative COX-2 selectivity when used in low doses (7.5 mg per day). Typical daily dosing of meloxicam is in the range of 7.5 to 15 mg.

Pyrroleacetic Acids

Tolmetin (Tolectin) is usually dosed between 600 and 1800 mg daily, with typical adult dosing being 400 mg three times daily.

COX-2-Selective Inhibitors (CSI)

These drugs are relatively new among the NSAIDs. They have become widely used due to their lower levels of gastrointestinal toxicity as compared with traditional NSAIDs. These agents also do not exhibit significant antiplatelet effects, making them attractive for use in patients on anticoagulant therapy who need to use anti-inflammatory medication. Unfortunately, there still does appear to be potential for renal adverse effects with use of these drugs, and so at-risk patients with renal disease may still be prohibited from using them. Use of Celecoxib and Valdecoxib is contraindicated in patients with sulfonamide allergy because of the presence of a sulfa moiety on these compounds. Celecoxib is typically dosed as 100 to 400 mg daily in single- or twice-daily doses. Dose reduction is not necessary in the elderly. Rofecoxib is typically dosed once a day with doses of 12.5 to 25 mg. As with nonselective NSAIDs, it is recommended that the lowest effective dose be used. Valdecoxib is typically initially dosed as 10 mg daily. Celecoxib is currently the only CSI available in the United States.

POTENTIAL ADVERSE DRUG INTERACTIONS WITH NSAIDS

The administration of medications for concomitant diseases in conjunction with NSAIDs may lead to potential complications as interactions between these drugs may render them more or less effective or may increase the potential for NSAID associated toxicity.

Antihypertensives

NSAIDs may interact with β-blockers, calcium channel blockers, and angiotensin-converting enzyme inhibitors, resulting in diminished antihypertensive effects of these agents. This is possibly related to antagonism of synthesis of vasodilatory PGs by NSAIDs as well as fluid and salt retention.

Diuretics

NSAIDs may disrupt the natriutetic and diuretic effects of thiazides and furosemide via inhibition of formation of PGE_2, which affects sodium resorption in the kidney and acts to antagonize the antidiuretic effect of vasopressin. This may lead to fluid and salt retention with edema formation and hypertension, and possibly congestive heart failure in susceptible individuals. It has also been reported that there may be a significant risk for the development of frank renal failure when indomethacin is used in combination with triamterene, and therefore combined use of these drugs is contraindicated.

Digoxin

The half-life of digoxin may be increased in the presence of NSAIDs. This could result in the accumulation of digoxin and subsequent digoxin toxicity. Caution is warranted when NSAIDs are used in patients on digoxin therapy.

Anticoagulants

NSAIDs may cause displacement of anticoagulants such as warfarin from protein-binding sites resulting in increased effective serum anticoagulant concentration and subsequent overanticoagulation. This is of particular concern with the potential for development of gastrointestinal bleeding from NSAID-associated gastropathy, which could be complicated in the presence of anticoagulation. In addition, antiplatelet effects that many traditional NSAIDs exhibit may enhance the risk of bleeding when added to anticoagulants.

Lithium

NSAIDs can cause decreased renal clearance of lithium, and thereby increase serum lithium levels in patients taking this drug, potentially increasing the risk for lithium toxicity.

Oral Hypoglycemics

Hyper- or hypoglycemia may result when NSAIDs are used in combination with oral hypoglycemic agents. Careful monitoring of blood glucose levels is warranted when diabetics taking these drugs are prescribed concurrent NSAID therapy.

Immunosuppressants

The clearance of methotrexate may be decreased in the presence of NSAIDs, increasing the potential for methotrexate toxicity. Likewise, there may be increased potential for cyclosporine nephrotoxicity when combined with NSAIDs. Caution is warranted when these agents are given simultaneously, as each agent may produce renal toxicity, which can be compounded when they are coadministered.

CONCLUSION

NSAIDs are effective in the management of painful conditions especially those involving musculoskeletal conditions and/or with bone/joint "pain generators" (e.g., osteoarthritis and rheumatoid arthritis) and may significantly improve the quality of life of patients suffering from these disease entities. It is important for clinicians employing these agents to keep in mind the potential for serious adverse effects that may be associated with these drugs. These adverse effects may include effects on the gastrointestinal system, kidneys, central nervous system, and on platelet aggregation. In addition, hypertension and congestive heart failure may occasionally occur when NSAIDs are administered to certain patients taking antihypertensives or diuretics. Other potential drug interactions of concern with NSAIDs include potential adverse effects when coadministered with anticoagulants, oral hypoglycemics, lithium, digoxin, and immunosuppressants. An appreciation for the potential adverse effects as well as the benefits of NSAIDs are necessary when utilizing these agents for the pain associated with various bone and joint conditions.

BIBLIOGRAPHY

Aley KO, Levine JD. Role of protein kinase A in the maintenance of inflammatory pain. *J Neurosci* 1999; 19:2181-2186.

Bell GM, Schnitzer TJ. COX-2 Inhibitors and other nonsteroidal anti-inflammatory drugs in the treatment of pain in the elderly. *Clin Geriatr Med* 2001; 17:489-502.

Buffum M, Buffum JC. Nonsteroidal anti-inflammatory drugs in the elderly. *Pain Manag Nurs* 2000; 1:40-50.

Day SM, Lockhart JC, Ferrell WR, et al. Divergent roles of nitrergic and prostanoid pathways in chronic joint inflammation. *Ann Rheum Dis* 2004; 63:1564-1570.

Heerdinnk ER, Leufkens HG, Herings RM, et al. NSAIDS associated with increased risk of congestive heart failure in elderly patients taking diuretics. *Arch Intern Med* 1998; 158:1108-1112.

Johnson AG. NSAIDS and blood pressure: Clinical importance for older patients. *Drugs Aging* 1998; 12:17-27.

Loll PJ, Picot D, Garavito RM. The structural basis of aspirin activity inferred from the crystal structure of inactivated prostaglandin H_2 synthase. *Nat Struct Biol* 1995; 2:637-643.

Mamdani M, Rochon PA, Juurlink, DN, et al. Observational study of upper gastrointestinal haemmorhage in elderly patients given selective cyclo-oxygenase-2 inhibitors or conventional non-steroidal anti-inflammatory drugs. *BMJ* 2002; 325:624-627.

Mulkerrin EC, Clark BA, Epstein FH. Increased salt retention and hypertension from non-steroidal agents in the elderly. *Q J Med* 1997; 90:411-415.

Ouellet M, Riendeau D, Percival MD. A high level of cyclooxygenase-2 inhibitor selectivity is associated with a reduced interference of platelet cyclooxygenase-1 inactivation by aspirin. *Proc Natl Acad Sci USA* 2001; 98:14583-14588.

Page J, Henry D. Consumption of NSAIDS and the development of congestive heart failure in elderly patients: An underrecognized public health problem. *Arch Intern Med* 2000; 160:777-784.

Pertusi RM, Godwin KS, House JK, et al. Gastropathy induced by nonsteroidal anti-inflammatory drugs: Prescribing patterns among geriatric practitioners. *JAOA* 1999; 99:305-310.

Phillips AC, Polisson RP, Simon LS. NSAIDS and the elderly: Toxicity and economic implications. *Drugs Aging* 1997; 10:119-130.

Pilotto A, Franceschi M, Leandro G, et al. NSAID and aspirin use by the elderly in general practice. *Drugs Aging* 2003; 20:701-710.

Roberts LJ, Morrow JD. Analgesic-antipyretic and anti-inflammatory agents and drugs employed in the treatment of gout. In: Hardman JG, Limbird LE, eds. *Goodman & Gilman's The Pharmacological Basis of Therapeutics*, 10th ed. McGraw-Hill, New York, 2001.

Rowlinson SW, Kiefer JR, Prusakiewicz JJ, et al. A novel mechanism of cyclooxygenase-2 inhibition involving interactions with Ser-530 and Tyr-385. *J Biol Chem* 2003; 278:45763-45769.

Samad T, Abdi S. A Basic science aspect of COX-2 inhibitors. In: Smith HS. *Drugs for Pain*. Hanley & Belfus, Philadelphia, 2003.

Simon LS. Nonsteroidal anti-inflammatory drugs and cyclooxygenase-2 selective inhibitors. In: Smith HS. *Drugs for Pain*. Hanley & Belfus, Philadelphia, 2003.

Smith HS. Nonsteroidal anti-inflammatory drugs: Bedside. In: Smith HS. *Drugs for Pain*. Hanley & Belfus, Philadelphia, 2003.

Whelton A, Fort JG, Puma JA, et al. Cyclooxygenase-2-specific inhibitors and cardiorenal function: A randomized, controlled trial of celecoxib and rofecoxib in older hypertensive osteoarthritis patients. *Am J Therapeut* 2001; 8:85-95.

Chapter 4

Capsaicin

Gary McCleane

The pain-relieving effects of derivatives of the chilli pepper have been known for over one-and-a-half centuries. We now know that among the most potent extract from these peppers is capsaicin. While capsaicin can hardly be described as the most effective analgesic treatment, it represents a simple, low-risk option to which many patients are attracted because of its topical application and the perception that, being "plant" based, it must be safe.

When capsaicin is used at high strengths, it has a neurotoxic effect. It is only when used at lower strengths that the reversible pain-relieving effect is apparent. Currently two strengths are available commercially: 0.025 percent and 0.075 percent capsaicin, both as cream-based formulations.

It is suggested that capsaicin achieves its pain-relieving effects in a number of ways. It has long been held that its primary effect is a reversible depletion of substance P from nociceptive nerve endings. This substance P has an important role in pain transmission, and is found both peripherally and in the central nervous system. When capsaicin is administered systemically in animals, both the peripheral and central effects may be apparent. In human practice, capsaicin is administered topically so that its major effect is peripheral.

More recently it has been suggested that, in fact, the effect of capsaicin in humans may be to reduce, again reversibly, the density of epidermal nerve fibers. With this decrease in nerve fibers a "desensitization" occurs.

Clinical Management of Bone and Joint Pain
© 2007 by The Haworth Press, Inc. All rights reserved.
doi:10.1300/5771_05

CLINICAL USE OF CAPSAICIN

Osteoarthritis

Both pain and stiffness are common accompaniments in patients with osteoarthritis (OA). Many of the joints commonly affected by oa are superficial and therefore potentially amenable to application of therapeutic substances that have a localized effect. Several studies have confirmed that repeated application of capsaicin does in fact reduce the pain, stiffness, and joint tenderness frequently seen in patients with OA. That said, total relief of pain is uncommon. Rather, what is observed is a reduction of pain to a more manageable level.

As capsaicin use requires sustained application of the cream, patients need to concentrate on one or a small number of joints. Therefore, capsaicin use is more suitable for those with monoarticular OA, or for those with polyarticular arthritis but in whom one or a few joints are significantly sorer than others.

Rheumatoid Arthritis

Very few studies have investigated the effect of capsaicin application in rheumatoid arthritis sufferers. One shows no effect, while the other, larger study indicates that just over 50 percent of rheumatoid suffers obtained at least some relief with capsaicin use.

Neck Pain

A single open-label study suggests that the use of 0.025 percent capsaicin can reduce "neck pain." It could be argued that it would be better to identify which neck structure was giving rise to pain, for example, muscle, joint, enthesis, and so on, but even when the less descriptive approach is taken of giving the broad diagnosis of "neck pain," capsaicin can have a useful effect.

Tendinitis

To date there are no studies confirming a pain-relieving effect when capsaicin is used in patients with tendinitis. However, logically one would expect that repeated application of capsaicin to the skin overlying a painful structure that itself is often superficial would produce pain relief. Clinical experience confirms this hypothesis.

Enthetic Pain

In a similar vein, evidence for an effect when capsaicin is used for enthetic pain is lacking, but experience points to a useful effect. Conventional treatment of conditions such as tennis elbow includes physiotherapy, nonsteroidal anti-inflammatory drugs (NSAIDs), and steroid injection. Unfortunately such approaches are not always successful, and in these circumstances treatments such as capsaicin are worth remembering.

When pain relief is achieved with frequent, regular application of capsaicin, many patients report that the pain relief can be maintained by less frequent application of the substance. Therefore, patients should use the capsaicin three to four times daily to assess its effectiveness and hopefully derive pain relief, which, if apparent, can be maintained by application once to twice daily. In those with, for example, polyarticular arthritis, this can allow them to move on and concentrate use in another painful joint.

SIDE EFFECTS OF TOPICAL CAPSAICIN APPLICATION

The primary side effect of capsaicin application is a burning, tingling sensation in the area of application. This is not infrequently of a severity to discourage the patient from further use of the cream. Usually this discomfort diminishes with sustained use, although, even with repeated use, discomfort still occurs if the cream is applied outside the margins of previous use.

Of course, it is not just in the area of intended application that this burning discomfort can occur. When the cream is applied to the painful area, the finger used for application may be used to rub an eye, nose, or elsewhere, with the creation of intense discomfort in those areas. Similarly, mothers using capsaicin may accidentally transfer the cream to the skin of their babies with obvious results. Accidental contamination can be reduced if gloves are used for application, with these being disposed of after application.

The discomfort of application is more pronounced when capsaicin is applied to a moist area. Therefore, caution should be used with areas of the body that are naturally moist. Similarly, if sweating is predicted after, for example, exercise, then the cream should be used after exercise rather than before. In the same vein, cream application is likely to be less unpleasant if it occurs after bathing, and thorough drying, rather than before.

Localized discomfort can be reduced by pretreatment of the area with a local anesthetic cream such as EMLA (eutectic mixture of local anesthetic, containing lidocaine and prilocaine) or Ametop (topical amethocaine).

An alternate approach is the addition of glyceryl trinitrate (GTN) to capsaicin. When this is done, the discomfort of application is reduced, as is the allodynia (pain created by a normally nonpainful stimulus) that is associated with capsaicin use. This reduction in the discomfort of application is often substantial. GTN itself has an analgesic effect, as outlined in Chapter 5, which is achieved through its action as a nitric oxide donor. When it is used with capsaicin, the analgesic effect achieved with both components of the mixture is additive. Therefore, when GTN is added to capsaicin, the use of capsaicin is more tolerable and the result of treatment more extensive than if either component is used alone. However, the principle side effect of GTN use is headache. When patch versions of GTN are used, a measured amount can be administered. When the ointment variety is used, it is very difficult to apply a measured amount. GTN ointment is available as 2 percent strength and is also used in a 0.2 percent concentration for the treatment of anal fissure. Some dilution of the GTN may be needed to minimize the risk of nitrate headache, although it is not yet established what concentration of GTN is required to produce analgesia, nor which concentration is optimal in the reduction of capsaicin associated discomfort.

When capsaicin is repeatedly applied, the discomfort of application usually decreases in the area of application. However, if accidental application occurs outside the usually area, then discomfort is expected. To minimize this risk, the area surrounding the usual site of application can be protected by preapplication of petroleum jelly to form a barrier impervious to the capsaicin.

Other side effects associated with capsaicin use are infrequent. Some individuals experience bouts of sneezing after topical capsaicin use. When this occurs, it is usually associated with overgenerous application. When this excess cream dries, a dust of dried cream can be raised, which, when breathed in, can cause nasal irritation, hence the sneezing. This sneezing can affect not only the patient but family members living in close proximity to the patient.

UNANSWERED QUESTIONS REGARDING USE OF CAPSAICIN

Despite many human studies demonstrating a pain-relieving effect associated with capsaicin use in variety of disorders where pain is prominent, it is yet to be established what the optimal concentration of capsaicin is to achieve maximum pain relief. In some countries capsaicin 0.025 percent is licensed for use in patients with osteoarthritis, while the 0.075 percent strength is licensed for use in postherpetic neuralgia and painful diabetic neuropathy. What is not clear is whether either strength is more effective than the other for their individual indications or whether any enhancement of analgesia is achieved by using the higher-strength preparation.

Work in animal models demonstrates that high-strength capsaicin has a neurotoxic effect, and that the reversible effect is seen when lower strengths are used. Emerging work now suggests that single applications of capsaicin at a concentration above what is currently licensed can achieve pain relief that persists for weeks and even months, but even this use is at a strength well below that associated with neurotoxicity.

In the same way that it is unknown what concentration of capsaicin is associated with the most extensive pain relief, it is also unclear as to which concentration produces the most rapid onset of pain relief and the most rapid reduction of the discomfort associated with application. Similarly, we have seen that the addition of GTN to capsaicin both enhances the quality of pain relief and minimizes the discomfort associated with capsaicin use, but it is still unknown what concentration of GTN optimilizes these effects.

SUGGESTED CLINICAL USE OF CAPSAICIN

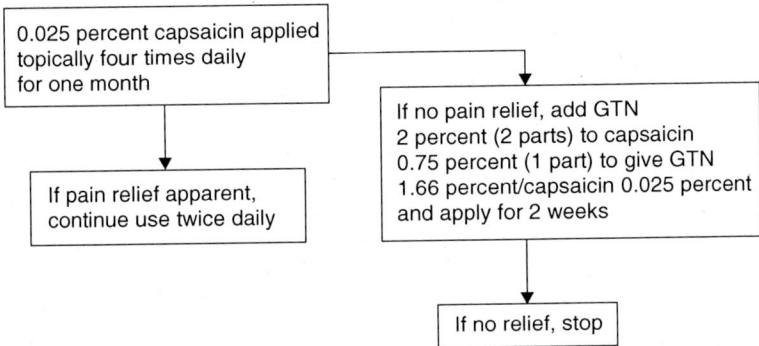

```
┌─────────────────────────────┐
│ 0.025 percent capsaicin applied │
│ topically four times daily   │─────────────┐
│ for one month                │             │
└─────────────────────────────┘             ▼
             │              ┌──────────────────────────────────────────┐
             │              │ If no pain relief, add GTN               │
             │              │ 2 percent (2 parts) to capsaicin         │
             ▼              │ 0.75 percent (1 part) to give GTN        │
┌─────────────────────────┐ │ 1.66 percent/capsaicin 0.025 percent     │
│ If pain relief apparent,│ │ and apply for 2 weeks                    │
│ continue use twice daily│ └──────────────────────────────────────────┘
└─────────────────────────┘             │
                                        ▼
                            ┌──────────────────┐
                            │ If no relief, stop │
                            └──────────────────┘
```

STRATEGIES TO REDUCE DISCOMFORT OF APPLICATION OF CAPSAICIN

- Use disposable gloves when applying capsaicin
- Apply only to dry areas
- Avoid area of application becoming moist
- When applying to areas normally covered by clothing, do not dress that area until cream dries
- Surround area of application with petroleum jelly
- Pretreat area of application with EMLA cream or Ametop jelly
- Mix GTN ointment with capsaicin

BIBLIOGRAPHY

Historical Use

Turnbull A. Tincture of capsicum as a remedy for chilblains and toothache. *Dublin Medical Press* 1850: 95-96.

Reviews

Fitzgerald M. Capsaicin and sensory neurones. *Pain* 1983; 15: 109-130.
Rains C, Bryson HM. Topical capsaicin. A review of its pharmacological properties and therapeutic potential in post herpetic neuralgia, diabetic neuropathy and osteoarthritis. *Drugs Aging* 1995; 7: 317-328.

Mode of Action

Nolano M, Simone DA, Wendelschafer-Crabb G, Johnson T, Hazen E, Kennedy WR. Topical capsaicin in humans: Parallel loss of epidermal nerve fibers and pain sensation. *Pain* 1999; 81: 135-145.

Osteoarthritis

Altman RD, Aven A, Holmburg CE, Pfeifer LM, Sack M, Young GT. Capsaicin cream 0.025% as monotherapy for osteoarthritis: A double-blind study. *Sem Arth Rheum* 1994; 23S: 25-33.

Deal CL. The use of topical capsaicin in managing arthritis pain: A clinician's perspective. *Sem Arth Rheum* 1994; 23S: 48-52.

Deal CL, Schnitzer TJ, Lipstein E, et al. Treatment of arthritis with topical capsaicin: A double-blind trial. *Clin Ther* 1991; 13: 383-395.

McCarthy GM, McCarty DJ. Effect of topical capsaicin in the therapy of painful osteoarthritis of the hands. *J Rheumatol* 1992; 19: 604-607.

McCleane GJ. The analgesic efficacy of topical capsaicin is enhanced by glyceryl trinitrate in painful osteoarthritis: A randomized, double-blind, placebo controlled study. *Eur J Pain* 2000; 4: 355-360.

Schnitzer T, Morton C, Coker S. Topical capsaicin therapy for osteoarthritis pain: Achieving a maintenance regimen. *Sem Arth Rheum* 1994; 23S: 34-40.

Neck Pain

Mathias BJ, Dillingham TR, Zeigler DN, Chang AS, Belandres PV. Topical capsaicin for chronic neck pain. A pilot study. *Am J Phys Med Rehabil* 1995; 74: 39-44.

Strategies to Reduce the Discomfort Associated with Capsaicin Application

McCleane GJ, McLaughlin M. The addition of GTN to capsaicin cream reduces the discomfort associated with application of capsaicin alone. A volunteer study. *Pain* 1998; 78: 149-151.

Walker RA, McCleane GJ. The addition of glyceryl trinitrate to capsaicin cream reduces the thermal allodynia associated with the use of capsaicin alone in humans. *Neuroscience Letters* 2002; 323: 78-80.

Yosipovitch G, Mailbach HI, Rowbotham MC. Effect of EMLA pre-treatment on capsaicin-induced burning and hyperalgesia. *Acta Derm Venereol* 1999; 79: 118-121.

Chapter 5

Topical Nitrates

Gary McCleane

Extensive clinical experience suggests that both corticosteroids and the nonsteroidal anti-inflammatory agents (NSAIDs) can reduce inflammatory and other types of joint pain and that a similar effect is observed when NSAIDs are used in patients with pain emanating from bone. That said, neither is universally effective nor devoid of potential side effects. The danger of serious gastric side effects when NSAIDs are used is well known, while the risk of fluid retention and renal impairment, platelet dysfunction, and even allergy can be associated with their use. Of recent times anxiety has arisen that the more recently introduced selective COX-2 inhibitors may be associated with cardiovascular side effects. On the other hand, corticosteroids and NSAIDs can both be remarkably effective when used to reduce pain.

The topical application of glyceryl trinitrate (GTN) may offer an alternative to the use of NSAIDs and, in some circumstances, to the use of corticosteroids. GTN lacks the potential for gastric, renal, and hematological upset, while its cardiovascular effect of vasodilatation may be of coincidental benefit. Allied to this, many patients like the concept of application of pain relief directly to the area of discomfort. Topical application of GTN may, therefore, represent an alternative to the use of NSAIDs when the latter's use proves ineffective or whose use is contraindicated. Indeed the primary use of topical GTN before NSAIDs are considered has much appeal.

In this chapter some insight into the proposed mode of action of the nitrates will be given, the evidence that they can be of use in musculoskeletal pain reviewed, and guidance on practical use given.

Clinical Management of Bone and Joint Pain
© 2007 by The Haworth Press, Inc. All rights reserved.
doi:10.1300/5771_06

MODE OF ACTION OF TOPICAL NITRATES
WHEN USED AS ANALGESICS

It is known that exogenous nitrates stimulate the release of nitric oxide (NO). This substance is known to be a potent mediator in a wide variety of different cellular systems such as the endothelium and both the central and peripheral nervous systems. It is released from the endothelium and from neutrophils and macrophages, all known to be intimately involved in the inflammatory process. It appears that NO exerts its effect by stimulating increases in guanylate cyclase, thereby increasing the levels of 3′,5′cyclic guanidine monophosphate (cGMP). Cholinergic drugs, such as acetylcholine, produce analgesia in a similar fashion by releasing NO and increasing NO at nociceptor level.

In addition to this action, NO may activate adenosine triphosphate (ATP)-sensitive potassium channels and activate peripheral antinociception. Endogenous NO levels may be increased if glutamate levels are raised. Glutamate is known to be an excitatory amino-acid-activating N-methyl-D-aspartate (NMDA) receptors, thereby initiating sensitization and protracting the pain process.

HUMAN EXPERIMENTAL PAIN

Since a number of animal studies suggest that nitric oxide plays a role in the peripheral and central modulation of nociception, and GTN acts as a nitric oxide donor, one would expect GTN to have some effect on pain thresholds. Thomsen and colleagues (1996) studied human volunteers in a double-blind, placebo-controlled crossover study. Subjects received infusions of GTN and placebo. They found that GTN infusion was associated with an effect on nociceptive thresholds as measured using a pressure algometer.

STUDIES SUGGESTING AN ANALGESIC EFFECT
WHEN NITRATES ARE USED TOPICALLY

Isolated studies have examined the effect of topical application of GTN in a variety of musculoskeletal conditions. Clinical use would suggest that the results of these studies have wider application and that pain associated with conditions not examined in these studies may respond in a similar fashion to those described in the literature.

Supraspinatus Tendonitis

Berrazueta and colleagues (1996) studied 20 patients with this painful shoulder condition. The subjects were randomized to receive either a GTN patch (5 mg/24 hours) or a placebo patch. Within 48 hours of commencement of treatment, those patients receiving GTN patch treatment recorded a fall of just over 2.5 points on a 10 cm visual analog score of pain. Those in the placebo group recorded no change in pain. Two patients in the GTN group reported headache.

Achilles Tendinopathy

Paoloni and colleagues (2004) report a randomized, double-blind, placebo-controlled study of 65 patients with either unilateral or bilateral noninsertional Achilles' tendinopathy. Subjects were randomized to receive either GTN patch (1.25 mg/24 hours) or placebo. Those receiving GTN patch were significantly more likely to report pain relief, and after 6 months 78 percent of those receiving GTN were symptom free compared with 49 percent in the placebo group.

Tennis Elbow (Extensor Tendinosis)

This degenerative overuse tendinopathy affects the wrist extensors at the attachment to the lateral humeral epicondyle. Paolini and colleagues (2003) studied 86 patients with this condition, randomizing them to receive either GTN or placebo patches. Pain relief was again more common in the GTN group. After 6 months, 81 percent of those in the GTN group were asymptomatic as compared with 60 percent in the control group.

Musculoskeletal Pain

McCleane (2000a) reports 200 patients with chronic musculoskeletal pain. Patients were divided into 4 groups of equal size. They were treated with topical 2.5 percent piroxicam, 1 percent GTN ointment, placebo, or a combination of piroxicam and GTN. Neither placebo nor piroxicam reduced pain scores, while GTN alone and in combination with piroxicam demonstrated an analgesic effect. That said, after 4 weeks' use, pain scores in the GTN group reverted toward baseline levels, suggesting that tachyphylaxis to the analgesic effect of GTN was occurring. Tachyphylaxis is also associated with the use of GTN when used to treat angina.

Osteoarthritis

It is not only in those with pain arising from tendons or soft tissue that can get pain relief with topical GTN. McCleane (2000b) reports the use of topical GTN in patients with painful osteoarthritis. In his study results were compared with those achieved with use of placebo, capsaicin, and a mixture of capsaicin and GTN. The nitrate was applied in a 1 percent ointment formulation. Pain relief achieved with GTN use was of a similar magnitude to that observed with capsaicin use. The duration of this study was 6 weeks, and over this time period tachyphylaxis was not observed. The secondary objective of this study was to measure the effect of addition of GTN on the discomfort associated with application of capsaicin. When capsaicin is used alone, a burning, tingling sensation is often experienced, and in some this is of an intensity to reduce compliance. It was found that addition of GTN to capsaicin significantly reduced the discomfort of application and that the analgesic effect achieved by the use of a combination of GTN and capsaicin was additive.

EFFECT OF TOPICAL GLYCERYL TRINITRATE ON INFLAMMATION

Evidence of an anti-inflammatory effect when GTN is applied transdermally is revealed in a study examining the effect on inflammation and pain of transdermal GTN in patients undergoing sclerosis of leg varicose veins undertaken by Berrazueta and colleges (1994).

They selected patients undergoing sclerotherapy in both legs. On one leg GTN ointment was applied around the sclerotherapy site, while on the other placebo was applied. Erythema, local warmth, and edema each was graded on a 0 to 10 scale, the composite result being presented as an overall score. Pain was measured on a 0 to 10 analog scale. Within 15 min of ointment application, inflammation was significantly less pronounce on the side of GTN application when compared with the placebo side (GTN score 10.4, placebo score 24.6). No sign of inflammation was recorded by 48 hours on the GTN side, whereas by the end of the observation period of 72 hours, evidence of inflammation was still present on the placebo leg.

EFFECT OF TOPICAL NITRATE ON ANALGESIC EFFECT OF OPIOIDS

We have seen some evidence that the topical application of GTN can reduce pain arising at sites close to the area of application. But it seems that topically applied GTN can also have an effect on the analgesic action of systemic opioids.

It has been suggested that endogenous nitric oxide has a part to play in the development of analgesic tolerance with sustained use of opioids. Therefore, it is suggested, a synthetic nitric oxide donor such as GTN may have an effect on opioid derived analgesia. Lauretti and colleagues (2002) report a randomized, double-blind study of 36 patients suffering from cancer pain. Patients received morphine in doses up to 90 mg daily to achieve pain scores, as measured on a 10 cm linear visual analog scale (VAS) of 4 or less. Patients were divided into two equal groups, one of which received topical GTN, 5 mg/24 hours, the other an inactive, placebo patch. Patients were free to adjust their morphine dose to maintain their VAS pain score at 4 or less. Those patients in the GTN-treated group required significantly less morphine to maintain adequate pain relief (Figure 5.1), while those in the placebo group reported more somnolence than the GTN group.

The same group report (Lauretti, 1999) that, when sufentanil is used as a spinal anaesthetic, the time to first request for additional analgesia was significantly longer in a group receiving transdermal GTN at a dose of 5 mg/24 hours.

While these reports suggest that transdermal GTN may usefully augment the analgesia derived from opioids, clearly much work is needed to define the role of transdermal GTN in this role. However, it is reassuring to think that, when transdermal GTN is used for a

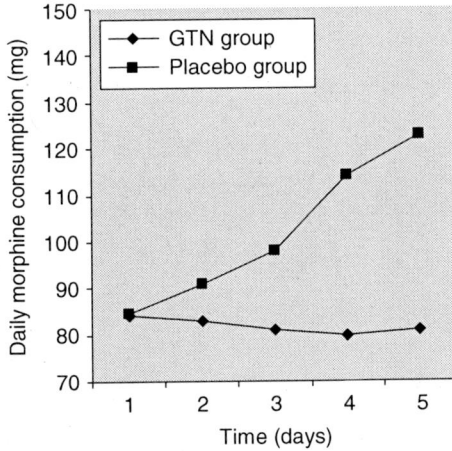

FIGURE 5.1. Daily consumption of oral morphine to keep visual analog score <4/10 cm in patients receiving transdermal GTN 5 mg/24 hours or placebo. *Source:* Reprinted from *International Journal of Clinical Anesthesia,* 14, GR Lauretti, MV Perez, MP Reis, and ML Pereira, Double-blind evaluation of transdermal nitroglycerine as adjuvant to oral morphine for cancer pain management, 83-86, (2002), with permission from the Society for Education in Anesthesia.

localized pain, it may also have a positive influence on opioids prescribed for pain elsewhere.

ISSUES WITH THE USE
OF TRANSDERMAL NITRATES

- Is the effect described earlier in a small number of defined conditions have a wider application across the broad range of conditions that give rise to localized pain?
- What is the optimal dose of GTN necessary to achieve maximum analgesia and minimum side effects?
- Does transdermal application of GTN augment opioid derived analgesia routinely?
- Does the oral use of nitrates replicate the effect on opioid analgesics exhibited by transdermal GTN?
- Do nitrates other than GTN exhibit analgesic and anti-inflammatory properties?

GLYCERYL TRINITRATE FORMULATIONS

Two main formulations of GTN can be used in treatment of localized pain. Transdermal patches are available either as a drug-impregnated membrane or as a reservoir of GTN in the form of a cream covered by a semipermeable membrane. In both cases a known amount is released. It is conventional for this amount to be recorded as milligrams per 24 hours, so patches are available that deliver 5, 10, and 15 mg over 24 hours. As the major dose-limiting side effect is headache, a side effect that is directly dose related, use of larger delivery patches is frequently associated with headache. In practice, less than 5 mg/24 hours is required to reduce inflammation and pain, and so, if the impregnated membrane patches are used, these can be cut into segments that may release less GTN. This enables less GTN to be used for an isolated area of pain or multiple segments of patch to be used for polyarticular pain conditions or indeed to surround a larger single area of pain.

GTN is also presented as an ointment formulation containing 2 percent GTN. As with any ointment or cream, measurement of dose is difficult, and as the major dose-limiting side effect, headache, is dose related, which may limit the utility of the ointment formulation. A further problem with GTN ointment is its oily nature, which some patients find unpleasant and which has a tendency to stain clothing.

SIDE EFFECTS OF TOPICAL
GLYCERYL TRINITRATE

As with all nitrates, headache is the most frequent accompaniment of the use of topical GTN. This headache is dose related and is often of a severity to compromise compliance. Local erythema and skin irritation can complicate prolonged use. These areas of erythema can be unsightly, particularly over visible areas of the body. Systemic side effects such as postural hypotension and dizziness are occasional complications of use, particularly if the patient is receiving oral vasodilators for the treatment of hypertension or ischemic heart disease.

Tachyphylaxis, described as a side effect of use in the management of angina, rarely seems to occur when GTN is used for pain treatment.

SUGGESTED CLINICAL USE

Topical application of GTN has much to commend it. GTN appears to exert both an analgesic and anti-inflammatory effect, and yet is devoid of the complications on gastric, renal, and hematological systems that can occur with the use of NSAIDs. In addition, as GTN appears to exert its effects via a different mechanism than NSAIDs, it is worth trying when a NSAID fails to provide pain relief. Alternatively, both can be used together.

Use of topical GTN is worth considering whenever the area of pain is localized. Therefore, it may be considered for use in any condition producing joint pain or localized bone pain. While transdermal application of GTN is unlikely to be sufficient to remove the pain from a bone fracture in the absence of stabilization, it certainly can be used with effect to reduce fracture pain when other steps have been implemented to stabilize that fracture. When the stabilization involves surgical intervention, topical GTN can reduce both residual fracture pain and that coming from the surgical wound.

Where pain is more widespread, patients can target their worst area of pain with their GTN patch. Alternatively, multiple segments of patches can be used over a number of painful areas provided nitrate headache does not complicate use (see Figure 5.2).

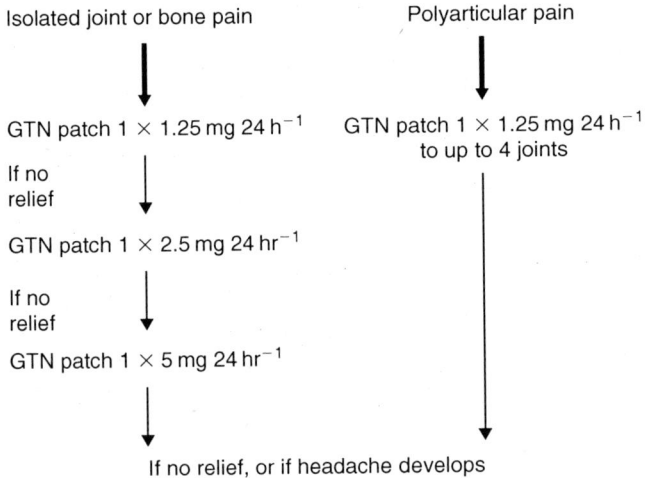

Isolated joint or bone pain   Polyarticular pain

GTN patch 1×1.25 mg 24 h^{-1} GTN patch 1×1.25 mg 24 h^{-1}
to up to 4 joints

If no relief

GTN patch 1×2.5 mg 24 hr^{-1}

If no relief

GTN patch 1×5 mg 24 hr^{-1}

If no relief, or if headache develops

FIGURE 5.2. Suggested clinical use of topical Glyceryl Trinitrate in bone and joint pain.

BIBLIOGRAPHY

Mode of Action

Devulder JE. Could nitric oxide be an important mediator in opioid tolerance and morphine side effects? *J Clin Anaesth* 2002; 14: 81-82.

Duarte ID, Lorenzetti BB, Ferreira SH. Acetylcholine induces peripheral analgesia by the release of nitric oxide. In: Moncada S, Higgs A (Eds), Nitric oxide from L-arginine. A bioregulatory System. Elsevier, Amsterdam, 1990; 165-170.

Feelisch M, Noack EA. Correlation between nitric oxide formation during degradation of organic nitrates and activation of guanylate cyclase. *Eur J Pharmacol* 1987; 139: 19-30.

Knowles RG, Palacios M, Palmer RM, Moncada S. Formation of nitric oxide from L-arginine in the central nervous system: a transduction mechanism for stimulation of the soluble guanylate cyclase. *Proc Natl Acad Sci USA* 1989; 86: 5159-5162.

Okuda K, Sakurada C, Takahashi M, Yamada T, Sakurada T. Characterization of nociceptive responses and spinal releases of nitric oxide metabolites and glutamate evoked by different concentrations of formalin in rats. *Pain* 2001; 92: 107-115.

Soares A, Leite R, Tatsuo M, Duarte I. Activation of ATP sensitive K channels: mechanisms of peripheral antinociceptive action of the nitric oxide donor, sodium nitroprusside. *Eur J Pharmacol* 2000; 14: 67-71.

Thomsen LL, Brennum J, Iversen HK, Olesen J. Effect of a nitric oxide donor (glyceryl trinitrate) on nociceptive thresholds in man. *Cephalgia* 1996; 16: 169-174.

Musculoskeletal Pain

Berrazueta JR, Losada A, Poveda J, Ochoteco A, Riestra A, Salas E, Amado JA. Successful treatment of shoulder pain syndrome due to supraspinatus tendonitis with transdermal nitroglycerin. A double blind study. *Pain* 1996; 66: 63-67.

McCleane GJ. The addition of piroxicam to topically applied glyceryl trinitrate enhances its analgesic effect in musculoskeletal pain: a randomised, double-blind, placebo-controlled study. *Pain Clinic* 2000a; 12: 113-116.

McCleane GJ. The analgesic efficacy of topical capsaicin is enhanced by glyceryl trinitrate in painful osteoarthritis: a randomized, double-blind, placebo controlled study. *Eur J Pain* 2000b; 4: 355-360.

Paoloni JA, Appleyard RC, Nelson J, Murell GA. Topical glyceryl trinitrate treatment of chronic noninsertional Achilles tendinopathy. A randomized double-blind, placebo-controlled trial. *J Bone Joint Surg Am* 2004; 86: 916-922.

Paoloni JA, Appleyard RC, Nelson RC, Murrell GA. Topical nitric oxide application in the treatment of chronic extensor tendinosis at the elbow: a randomized, double-blinded, placebo-controlled clinical trial. *Am J Sports Med* 2003; 31: 915-920.

Anti-Inflammatory Effect of GTN

Berrazueta JR, Fleitas M, Salas E, et al. Local transdermal glyceryl trinitrate has an ani-inflammatory action on thrombophlebitis induced by sclerosis of leg varicose veins. *Angiology* 1994; 45: 347-351.

Augmentation of Systemic Analgesics by Topical Nitrates

Lauretti GR, de Oliveira R, Reis MP, Mattos AL, Pereira NL. Transdermal nitroglycerine enhances spinal sufentanil postoperative analgesia following orthopaedic surgery. *Anesthesiology* 1999; 90: 734-739.

Lauretti GR, Lima IC, Reis MP, Prado WA, Pereira NL. Oral ketamine and transdermal nitroglycerin as analgesic adjuvant to oral morphine therapy for cancer pain management. *Anesthesiology* 1999; 90: 1528-1533.

Lauretti GR, Perez MV, Reis MP, Pereira NL. Double-blind evaluation of transdermal nitroglycerine as adjuvant to oral morphine for cancer pain management. *J Clin Anesth* 2002; 14: 83-86.

Chapter 6

Topical Analgesic Options

Charles Argoff

TOPICAL VERSUS TRANSDERMAL

Topical analgesics exert their analgesic activity locally and without significant systemic absorption. This is in contrast to transdermal analgesics in which systemic absorption is required for clinical benefit. Five percent lidocaine patch (Lidoderm) is an example of a topical agent, and the transdermal fentanyl patch (Durogesic) is an example of a transdermal analgesic. Each topical analgesic's mechanism of action is unique to the specific drugs contained within the topical analgesic. Topical analgesics are being studied in an increasing number of painful states and the results of some of these studies are summarized in the following text.

We all recognize that the experience known as pain can occur without the involvement of the brain. The role of the central nervous system including the spinal cord and especially the brain in the experience of pain therefore cannot be emphasized enough. Yet, topical analgesics are believed to exert their principle analgesic activity within the peripheral nervous system. Certain specific painful conditions such as central poststroke pain or spinal cord injury pain are believed to be associated with mechanisms that lie entirely within the brain and/or central nervous system; however, many commonly treated pain syndromes including chronic low back pain and osteoarthritis and even a neuropathic pain state such as postherpetic neuralgia (PHN) likely result from a combination of both peripheral as well as central nervous system mechanisms. The term topical analgesic has

Clinical Management of Bone and Joint Pain
© 2007 by The Haworth Press, Inc. All rights reserved.
doi:10.1300/5771_07

been used to describe analgesics that are applied locally and directly to painful areas and whose site of action is local to the site of analgesic application. One must be careful to avoid using the term topical analgesic except in situations in which formal completed studies have in fact demonstrated a lack of systemic activity of that preparation. One must also keep in mind that, although the mechanism of action of a topical analgesic may largely be within the peripheral nervous system, its effect on peripheral processing of pain transmission may actually and ultimately lead to a reduction of central pain mechanisms as well. Thus, and in other words, if pain is not pain until such information reaches the brain, or if less pain-producing information comes in from the periphery for central processing, it is likely that fewer central mechanisms will be activated and thus less pain experienced. This article will review the use of topical analgesics in the treatment of various painful conditions including those affecting bones and joints, and provides an update to previously published similar reviews.[1,2]

Side Effects

Several important factors in choosing an analgesic agent include its efficacy, side-effect profile, ease of administration, and cost. The efficacy of many analgesic agents has been undermined by the analgesic's side-effect profile, toxicities, and drug-drug interactions. An ideal analgesic agent would be effective in relieving pain and at the same time be well tolerated, easy to use, and not too costly. In general, the risk and severity of significant adverse effects as well as of drug-drug interactions are less with a topical agent than with a similar agent given systemically.[3] Localized reactions such as rash or unpleasant skin sensations may occur when using a topical agent, but certainly are not commonly experienced.[4] There are, in fact, few currently commercially available United States Food and Drug Administration (USFDA)-approved topical analgesics, and of the USFDA-approved topical agents, the 5 percent lidocaine patch has been the most extensively studied. Noting the aforementioned guiding principles, the tolerability and safety of daily 24 hours/day use of four lidocaine 5 percent patches was studied. With this regimen, significant systemic side effects were not experienced and measured plasma lidocaine levels remained below those associated with cardiac adverse effects. Safety and tolerability were similar in this study regardless of whether or not the patch was used for 12 or 24 hours each day.[5] In a separate study, patients, with chronic low back pain were treated safely with four lidocaine 5 percent patches every 24 hours for extended periods.[6] No significant dermal reactions were experienced in either study.[5,6,7] In my clinical practice, patients infrequently complain of erythema and less frequently a rash at the site of application.

Adverse effects including dermal sensitivity, which may be associated with the use of a topical analgesic, are, in general, unique to the specific analgesic. As an example consider the use of capsaicin. After applying topical capsaicin, severe burning of the skin at the site of application has been reported to occur in almost 80 percent of treated patients. This drug when applied topically in its currently available forms does not result in significant systemic accumulation or in any life-threatening outcomes, and the incidence of burning may decrease with repeated use; however, for some patients the occurrence of this side effect may impact negatively upon patient compliance and, as a result, may hinder a patient's ability to benefit from that treatment.[8] Other instances of dermal sensitivity may occur as the result of the vehicle within which the topical agent is contained.

Reducing the likelihood of drug-drug interactions when using topical analgesics may be of great practical value for an individual who is also actively using systemic medications for other medical disorders. Consider a 69-year-old patient who suffers from hypertension, hyperlipidemia, and diabetes mellitus. This person now requires analgesic treatment for his osteoarthritis (OA). She is already using a number of medications for her different medical conditions and her physician is concerned about prescribing any analgesics including nonsteroidal anti-inflammatory medications (NSAIDs) because of their potential to adversely affect these other conditions. Assuming that acceptable pain relief is experienced with the patient's use of a topical analgesic in this setting, using a topical agent here may offer several advantages over a systemic agent due to the lack of drug-drug interactions. Another advantage of the use of a topical analgesic may be that the use of a topical analgesic does not often, if ever, require dose titration: this property of topical analgesics makes these relatively simple drugs to use. Yet, since many available agents come as "fixed doses," this property also makes it less helpful if a "higher" dose would have been potentially more helpful.

The prescriber must keep in mind that not all "topical" analgesics are commercially available agents. The prescriber must be aware of the differences between those topical analgesics that are USFDA approved and commercially available from those that may be manufactured on an individualized basis by a specialized compounding pharmacy. Certainly not all of the topical analgesics currently in use and/or prescribed by health care providers are commercially available products, and for many years many health care providers have utilized compounding pharmacies to obtain custom-made agents through other means. This article will only review the use of those topical agents that are commercially available or for which there is clear evidence that they were manufactured in a consistent and reliable manner. Although for many compounding pharmacies there is no proof of such quality control or consistency from one batch to another, one should realize that compounded, noncommercially available agents are often prescribed as topical preparations by pain practitioners. For example, in one recent survey of members of the American Society of Regional Anesthesia and Pain Medicine, 27 percent of the respondents indicated that they prescribed such a compounded topical agent and 47 percent of the responders indicated that they felt that their patient responded favorably to the agent prescribed.[9] These are merely retrospective survey data and a prospective study was not done. From a commercial viewpoint, there seems to be great interest in the development of new topical analgesics. Among the agents being developed or being considered for development as topical analgesics are NSAIDs, opioids, capsaicin, local anesthetics, antidepressants, glutamate receptor antagonists, α-adrenergic receptor agonists, adenosine, cannabinoids, cholinergic receptor agonists, gaba agonists, prostanoids, bradykinin, ATP, biogenic amines, and nerve growth factor.[10]

Modes of Action

As noted previously, the mechanism of action of each topical analgesic depends on the specific analgesic. Capsaicin-containing topical analgesics, for example, appear to achieve their action through their agonist activity at the transient receptor potential vanilloid receptor 1

(TRPV1).[11,12] This activity results in the release of substance P as well as calcitonin gene-related peptide (CGRP). With currently available topical agents, a therapeutic response to capsaicin is generally achieved only with repeated topical application. It has been hypothesized that reduced peripheral as well as central excitability with resulting less pain through reduced afferent input results form the depletion of substance P in C-fibers.[8,11,12] Histopathological examination results of human nerve biopsies as well as animal experiments have suggested that application of capsaicin may lead to the degeneration of nerve fibers in the skin underneath the application site. This neurodegenerative effect of capsaicin has been hypothesized to be one of its mechanisms of pain relief.[13] In contrast, the mechanism of action of an NSAID has been hypothesized to be related to its inhibition of prostaglandin synthesis and reduction of inflammation; however, because it has been observed that the anti-inflammatory effect of these types of medications is not always proportional to the amount of pain relief experienced, other mechanisms of action might also be relevant.[14] Combinations of different agents may lead to synergy of these agents, and as an example, the antinociceptive effects of topical morphine have been shown to be enhanced by a topical cannabinoid in a recent study.[15]

While other mechanisms of action of local anesthetics are under active investigation, the analgesic action of local anesthetic agents based on currently available date appears to be related to the ability of these agents to suppress the activity of peripheral sodium channels within sensory afferents and thus reduce pain transmission. Reduced expression of mRNA for specific sodium channel subtypes following local anesthetic use has been reported as well.[1,4] Several local anesthetic containing analgesics that may be considered topical agents are currently commercially available. Although the lidocaine 5 percent patch is able to have an analgesic effect without creating anesthetic skin, the use of EMLA cream (eutectic mixture of local anesthetics, 2.5 percent lidocaine/2.5 percent prilocaine), in contrast, creates both analgesia as well as anesthesia when applied topically. Depending on the clinical setting, this property may or may not be desirable.[4] The clinical setting should help the prescriber to determine which topical analgesic to use. For example, if the goal of using a topical agent was to create anesthetic skin before venipuncture, the use of EMLA would be more appropriate than the lidocaine 5 percent patch. A mechanism of action of the lidocaine 5 percent patch as a topical agent that is unrelated to the active medication is that the patch itself may help to reduce the allodynia seen especially with neuropathic pain states such as PHN through the patch's ability to protect the skin.[1]

Of great interest is the current development of tricyclic antidepressants as topical analgesics. The tricyclic antidepressants as a group are known to have multiple mechanisms of action, and of these, the potential clinical benefit of their ability to block sodium channels when applied topically is under active investigation at this time.[16,17] In my informal polling of health care practitioners, many in the United States did not recognize that there was currently one USFDA-approved commercially available topical antidepressant, Zanalon (doxepin hydrochloride) cream. While it is indicated for use by the USFDA for the treatment of eczema-associated pruritus, there have been anecdotal reports of use of this agent in an "off-label" manner as a topical analgesic.[18] Other topical agents including topical opioids, glutamate receptor antagonists, and cannabinoids have stirred great interest among basic and clinical scientists in their potential as topical analgesics. Several of the more recent studies of some of these agents will be considered int he following text.

CHOICE OF AGENTS

I will now summarize many of the clinical uses of topical agents as analgesics, based on the painful disorder for which they are being used.

Neuropathic Pain

There is evidence from clinical trial data to support the use of certain topical analgesics in the treatment of certain neuropathic pain disorders.[19]

Local Anesthetics

The lidocaine 5 percent patch is USFDA approved for the treatment of PHN. Completed clinical trials patients with PHN, which led to its USFDA approval, demonstrated that use of the lidocaine

5 percent patch compared with placebo patches resulted in statistically significant more pain reduction and was in addition safe and well tolerated.[20,21] Postapproval open-label studies have demonstrated improvement in various quality-of-life measures for patients with PHN who are using this preparation.[22] The use of the lidocaine 5 percent patch has been studied as well in patients with neuropathic pain states other than PHN. A randomized, double-blind, placebo-controlled trial completed in Europe studied the efficacy of the lidocaine 5 percent patch in the treatment of "focal" neuropathic pain syndromes such as mononeuropathies, intercostal neuralgia, and ilioinguinal neuralgia. This study demonstrated that, when the lidocaine 5 percent patch is added to other analgesic regimens, the 5 percent lidocaine patch can reduce ongoing pain as well as allodynia as quickly as in the first 8 hours of use and over a period of 7 days.[23] Prior to this study, the results of a smaller open-label study of 16 patients with various chronic neuropathic pain conditions (post-thoracotomy pain, complex regional pain syndrome, postamputation pain, painful diabetic neuropathy, meralgia parasthetica, postmastectomy pain, and neuroma pain) suggested that the lidocaine 5 percent patch may be able to provide pain relief without significant side effects in 81 percent of these patients.[24] A few other noncontrolled studies, each enrolling patients with painful diabetic neuropathy who were treated with the lidocaine 5 percent patch, have been completed. Patients in each of these studies were told that they could apply as many as four lidocaine 5 percent patches for as long as 18 hours/day. The results of these studies overall reported pain relief for the majority of patients with an acceptable adverse effect profile with this agent.[25-28] In another study, changes in the quality of the pain of patients with PHN treated with the lidocaine 5 percent patch compared with placebo was examined.[29]

EMLA cream, another local anesthetic preparation (the eutectic mixture of 2.5 percent lidocaine and 2.5 percent prilocaine), is not USFDA approved for any neuropathic pain disorder; nevertheless, several studies of the use of EMLA cream in the treatment of PHN have been completed. In the only randomized, controlled study of PHN patients in which EMLA has been studied, treatment with EMLA resulted in similar efficacy as did treatment with placebo.[30] Two uncontrolled studies have suggested that use of EMLA cream might relieve the pain associated with PHN.[31,32] In another open-label study, the potential benefit of a combination of topical amitriptyline and ketamine for neuropathic pain has yielded encouraging results, but the one controlled study was not as encouraging.[33-35] Additional non-controlled studies, one in patients with PHN and the other in patients with complex regional pain syndrome type 1 have suggested that topical ketamine may be an effective topical analgesics; however, serum ketamine levels were not measured in either study.[36] Another report has suggested that the topical application of geranium oil may be helpful in providing temporary relief from PHN.[37]

Capsaicin

Although there has been great interest in using capsaicin in a number of neuropathic pain disorders such as diabetic neuropathy, PHN, and postmastectomy pain, currently available strengths of capsaicin, for example, 0.025 and 0.075 percent, yielded disappointing results with the treatment being poorly tolerated, regimens poorly adhered to, and insufficient pain relief experienced.[38] Yet, use of this agent remains of great interest to many, and in contrast, in an early study examining the results of a capsaicin preparation in clinical development notable analgesia was reported by patients with painful HIV neuropathy who were receiving a 7.5 percent topical capsaicin cream. While this is certainly appears to be an exciting result, in order for the patients to tolerate this medication concurrent epidural anesthesia was required for these patients in at least this one study.[39] However, new studies have not shown this requirement, and at the 2004 Annual Scientific Meeting of the American Academy of Neurology, two open-label studies, one in patients with PHN and the other in patients with painful HIV-associated distal symmetrical polyneuropathy reported notable pain relief for the majority of patients following the single application of a high-concentration (8 percent) *trans*-capsaicin patch. The duration of pain relief seen was as long as 48 weeks (PHN).[40,41] A recently published review of the published randomized trials involving the use of topical capsaicin in the treatment of either neuropathic or musculoskeletal pain syndromes concluded that "although topically applied capsaicin has moderate to poor efficacy in the treatment of chronic musculoskeletal or neuropathic pain, it may be useful as an adjunct or sole therapy for a small number of patients who are unresponsive to, or intolerant of, other treatments."[42]

In a novel and fascinating study that compared the analgesic effect of a topical preparation containing either 3.3 percent doxepin alone or 3.3 percent doxepin combined with 0.075 percent capsaicin and placebo in patients with various different chronic neuropathic pain problems, it was demonstrated that each treatment resulted in equal degrees of analgesia and each was superior to placebo.[43]

Other Agents

As suggested previously in this chapter, there has been increasing interest in the use of topical tricyclic antidepressants in the treatment of neuropathic pain. Two recently published studies by a similar group of investigators have yielded some information regarding the development of such. In each of these studies, the preparation tested was a combination of 2 percent amitriptyline/1 percent ketamine. The results of one of these studies, a double blind randomized placebo controlled study of 92 patients with neuropathic pain (diabetic neuropathy/PHN/postsurgical/post-traumatic) concluded that there was no difference in pain relief among the four treatment groups (placebo, amitriptyline 2 percent alone, ketamine 1 percent alone, or the combination amitriptyline 2 percent/ketamine 1 percent).[34] Of interest is that a similar group of investigators studied 28 patients with neuropathic pain for 6 to 12 months in an open-label study of the combination topical analgesic 2 percent amitryptyline/1 percent ketamine, and concluded that on average patients experienced 34 percent pain reduction.[35] In another open-label study by the same investigators, assessing the potential benefit of a combination of topical amitriptyline and ketamine for neuropathic pain has yielded encouraging results, but again no positive controlled study has yet been published.[33]

Soft Tissue Injuries and Osteoarthritis

Soft tissue injuries and osteoarthritis are each commonly experienced musculoskeletal pain states. The use of topical analgesics for these heterogeneous conditions is being studied. While various systemic analgesics and various injection therapies have been utilized in this setting, they are used again not without the risk of significant side effects especially with long-term and repeated use. The successful development of topical analgesics for these conditions therefore could be of great value and importance to both the patient as well as the treatment provider. A number of studies completed outside of the United States for the most part provide us with whatever evidence exists for their use in this setting as use of these in the United States in quite limited.

NSAIDs

In a 14-day randomized, placebo-controlled study completed in France of 163 patients with an ankle sprain, the use of a topical ketoprofen patch (100 mg) was superior to placebo in reducing pain after 1 week of treatment.[44] A similar group of investigators studied a similar ketoprofen preparation in patients with tendonitis. The results of this randomized, double-blind, placebo-controlled study were also positive, and the treatment was in general, except for skin irritation, well tolerated.[45] In a randomized controlled study of a diclofenac patch in 120 individuals experiencing acute pain following a "blunt" injury, use of the patch was well tolerated and was significantly better as an analgesic than placebo in reducing the pain associated with this injury.[46] In one open-label study of patients generally described as suffering, in general, from "soft tissue pain," the investigators concluded that topical flurbiprofen was associated with greater pain reduction than oral diclofenac with fewer adverse effects reported.[47] In two other reported investigations, each of which was performed separately by different investigators, one an open-label study and the other a multicenter, randomized, controlled 2-week study of pain associated with acute sports injuries, a diclofenac patch was found to be effective in providing pain relief, and in each study, the treatment was well tolerated. The average patient experienced 60 percent pain relief in the open-label study.[48,49] Another controlled study examined the use of topical ibuprofen cream in the management of acute ankle sprains. Ibuprofen cream was found, in this study, to be more effective than placebo in reducing pain.[50] In a controlled study of the use of ketoprofen gel in the management of acute soft tissue pain, the gel was also found to be more effective than placebo in providing pain relief.[51] The potential efficacy of a topical formulation of ibuprofen

5 percent gel was examined in a placebo-controlled study in patients with painful soft tissue injuries. Patients received either the ibuprofen 5 percent gel (n = 40) or placebo gel (n = 41) for a maximum of 7 days. Pain intensity levels as well as limitations of physical activity were assessed daily using visual analogue and other scales. There was a significant difference ($p < 0.001$) in pain reduction as well as improvement in physical activities for those patients who received the active gel compared with placebo recipients.[52] In a second study performed by the same group of investigators involving similar types of patients, 50 patients were studied with similar outcomes seen.[53]

It is certainly not surprising that there has also been interest in studying the use of topical analgesics in the treatment of osteoarthritis. A diclofenac patch preparation has been studied in a randomized, double-blind controlled study assessing the potential benefits of such an agent in patients with osteoarthritis of the knee. This study has demonstrated that this patch may be safe and effective for this condition.[54] A separate randomized controlled study comparing the efficacy and side effects of a topical diclofenac solution and oral diclofenac in the treatment of osteoarthritis of the knee concluded that use of this topical diclofenac solution in patients with osteoarthritis of the knee produced symptom relief that was equivalent to oral diclofenac with significantly reduced incidence of diclofenac-related gastrointestinal complaints.[55] In a study of patients with pain in the temporo-mandibular joint, one group of patients received diclofenac solution applied topically several times daily and a second group received oral diclofenac. Although there was no significant difference seen from an analgesic viewpoint, there were significantly fewer gastrointestinal side effects experienced by the patients receiving the diclofenac topical solution.[56] A meta-analysis examining the use of topical NSAIDs in the treatment of osteoarthritis concluded that there was evidence that topical NSAIDs are superior to placebo during the first 2 weeks of treatment but not afterwards. In addition, this meta-analysis also concluded that available evidence suggested that topical NSAIDs were inferior to oral NSAIDs during the first week of treatment.[57] A separate meta-analysis examining the evidence for the use of topical NSAIDs for chronic musculoskeletal pain concluded that topical NSAIDs are effective and safe in treating chronic musculoskeletal conditions for 2 weeks. The investigators suggested that larger and longer trials must be completed to fully understand the practical role of topical NSAIDs in clinical settings.[58] Commonly, topical salicylates are used by patients in nonprescription preparations. A meta-analysis examining the potential benefit of topical salicylates in acute and chronic pain concluded that, based on the few studies that could be reviewed, topically applied rubefacients containing salicylates might be helpful in the treatment of acute pain but that available trials of musculoskeletal and arthritic pain resulted in moderate to poor efficacy. Adverse events were rare in studies of acute pain and poorly reported in those of chronic pain. The authors emphasized that efficacy estimates for rubefacients were at present unreliable since there is a lack of appropriate clinical trials.[59]

A randomized controlled study completed in Germany examined the effect of topical eltenac, another NSAID, compared with placebo in 237 patients with osteoarthritis of the knee. Demonstrated efficacy and safety of the use of topical eltenac in the treatment of osteoarthritis of the knee compared with placebo were concluded by the authors.[60] In a separate study, topical eltenac gel was compared with oral diclofenac and placebo in patients with osteoarthritis of the knee. While both therapies were found to be superior to placebo with respect to analgesia, as reported in the aforementioned meta-analysis, the incidence of gastrointestinal side effects was notably lower in the group treated with topical eltenac gel compared with those treated with oral diclofenac.[61] Three additional studies have demonstrated that topical diclofenac may be effective in reducing the pain associated with various types of degenerative joint disease.[62-64]

Other topical agents have been studied in these conditions as well. There was no benefit of 0.025 percent capsaicin crème over inactive cream in a randomized, double-blind study of 30 patients with pain in the temporo-mandibular joint.[65] A randomized controlled study of a topical crème containing glucosamine sulfate, chondroitin sulfate, and camphor for osteoarthritis of the knee showed a significant reduction of pain in the treatment group after 8 weeks compared with the placebo group.[66] There are no formal published reports of formal clinical trials exploring the use of a topical local anesthetic agent in the treatment of an acute soft tissue injury or in the treatment of osteoarthritis; however, two anecdotal reports of the use of the lidocaine 5 percent patch for an acute sports injury. As a basketball fan,

I am particularly interested in the following! A professional basketball player with a ligamentous strain in his left fifth toe was advised by the team doctor to use the lidocaine 5 percent patch for pain relief with a good outcome, and a professional football player with chronic acromioclavicular joint pain due to a dislocation was anecdotally reported to experience pain relief with use of the lidocaine 5 percent patch as well. The basis for using such an agent in this setting is under active investigation.

Case Report

Consider an 84-year-old male with osteoarthritis of both knees who cannot tolerate any NSAID due to esophageal reflux, has had no response to short-acting opiates, injection therapy, and/or physical therapy, and is not a candidate for knee replacement; he might be an excellent candidate for the use of a topical analgesic.

Low Back and Myofascial Pain

Very few published studies of any topical analgesic in chronic low back or myofascial pain have been published. A double-blind, placebo-controlled study comparing topical capsaicin to placebo in 154 patients with chronic low back pain did report that 60.8 percent of capsaicin-treated patients compared with 42.1 percent of placebo patients experienced 30 percent pain relief after 3 weeks of treatment ($p < 0.02$), without any deleterious side effects experienced in either group.[67] Other studies have been presented in an abstract form only and will be reviewed briefly. For example, an open-label study of 120 patients with acute (<6 weeks), subacute (<3 months), short-term chronic (3 to 12 months), or long-term chronic (>12 months) low back pain was completed at eight sites in the United States. During the 6 week study period, participants applied four lidocaine 5 percent patches to areas of maximal low back pain every 24 hours. Analysis of the first 2 weeks of data was presented at the 10th World Congress on Pain, and the data suggested that majority of the patients experienced moderate or greater degree of pain relief. A more complete analysis of these data as well as additional studies are expected soon.[6] In a double-blind study comparing topical capsaicin with placebo in 154 patients with chronic low back pain, 60.8 percent of capsaicin-treated patients compared with 42.1 percent of placebo patients experienced

30 percent pain relief after 3 weeks of treatment ($p < 0.02$). Fifteen of the capsaicin-treated and nine of the placebo-treated patients experienced adverse effects none of which were believed to be harmful.[67]

An open-label study of patients with chronic myofascial pain in which 16 patients with chronic myofascial pain were treated with the lidocaine 5 percent patch was presented at the 2002 Scientific Meeting of the American Pain Society. After 28 days of treatment, statistically significant improvements were noted for average pain, general activity level, ability to walk, ability to work, relationships, sleep, and overall enjoyment of life in approximately 50 percent of the patients studied.[68]

OTHER USES OF TOPICAL ANALGESICS

Based on the results of a number of small studies, mostly case reports, topical analgesic of various types including opiates may be very helpful in reducing the pain associated with pressure ulcers or dressing changes.[69-73] The purpose of including the studies here is to make the reader aware of these other novel uses. In theory, patients undergoing a procedure might benefit from the use of a topical analgesic to treat postprocedure pain and reduce the need for systemic analgesics. Controlled studies have demonstrated the benefit of EMLA cream in the reduction of pain associated with circumcision and venipuncture as well as for the pain associated with breast cancer surgery.[4,74] Several other studies have suggested that either ketamine or morphine may be used topically for mucositis-associated pain following chemotherapy or radiation therapy in patients with head and neck carcinomas.[75,76] There is also a recent report of two children with epidermolysis bullosa who were treated successfully with topical opiates.[77] A rather interest recent report suggests that the analgesic effect of menthol, an ingredient common to many over-the-counter analgesic preparations, may be exerted partially through the activation of κ-opioid receptors.[78]

In a single case report, a patient with a condition know as "central neuropathic itch" has been treated apparently successfully with the lidocaine 5 percent patch.[79] Several studies recently presented at professional association meetings are worthy of mention as well. At the 2004 joint meeting of the American Pain Society/Canadian Pain

Society, two new studies of new topical analgesic preparations were reported. The results of an enriched enrollment study, in which an open-label initial study led to the randomization of responders in a placeb-controlled study of the use of either a 4 percent amitriptyline/ 2 percent ketamine cream and 2 percent amitriptyline/1 percent keta-mine cream or placebo for patients with PHN, demonstrated that after 3 weeks of treatment the average daily pain intensity was lowest in patients receiving the higher-concentration combination cream compared with the lower-concentration combination or placebo ($p = 0.026$ high-concentration cream versus placebo). Plasma levels of either drug were detected in fewer than 10 percent of those patients receiving active treatment.[80] An open-label study of the use of a 0.25 percent capsaicin topical agent in a lidocaine-containing vehicle in 25 patients with painful diabetic polyneuropathy and 7 patients with PHN demonstrated pain relief in majority of the patients who were studied.[81]

There is clearly interest in the use of these types of agents with a need for larger and better-designed trials to be completed. Although formal evidence is lacking, there is more than a sense that topical analgesics may provide pain relief in various painful conditions. Studies involving the "off-label" use of a number of agents suggest a potential role for new topical therapies in the management of a diverse group of painful conditions. This is of great importance since use of a topical agent is generally associated with a better side-effect profile than orally, transdermally, parenterally, or spinally administered analgesics.

REFERENCES

1. Argoff CE. New analgesics for neuropathic pain: The lidocaine patch. *Clin J Pain* 2000;Suppl 16(2):S62-S65.

2. Argoff CE. Topical treatments for pain. *Current Pain and Headache Reports* 2004;8:261-267.

3. Argoff CE. Targeted topical peripheral analgesics in the management of pain. *Curr Pain Headache Rep* 2002;7:34-38.

4. Galer BS. Topical medications. In: Loeser JD, ed. Bonica's Management of Pain. Philadelphia: Lippincott-Williams & Wilkins; 2001:1736-1741.

5. Gammaitoni AR, Alvarez NA. 24-hour application of the lidocaine patch 5% for 3 consecutive days is safe and well tolerated in healthy adult men and women. Abstract PO6.20. Presented at the 54th Annual American Academy of Neurology Meeting, April 13-20, 2002, Denver, CO.

6. Argoff C, Nicholson B, Moskowitz M, et al. Effectiveness of lidocaine patch 5% (Lidoderm®) in the treatment of low back pain. Presented at the 10th World Congress on Pain, August 17-22, 2002, San Diego, CA.

7. Gammaitoni AR, Davis MW. Pharmacokinetics and tolerability of lidocaine 5% patch with extended dosing. *Ann Pharmacother* 2002;36:236-240.

8. Watson CPN. Topical capsaicin as an adjuvant analgesic. *J Pain Symptom Manage* 1994;9:425-433.

9. Ness TJ, Jones L, Smith H. Use of compounded topical analgesics- results of an Internet survey. *Reg Anesth Pain Med* 2002;27:309-312.

10. Sawynok J. Topical and peripherally acting analgesics. *Pharmacol Rev* 2003; 55:1-20.

11. Robbins W. Clinical applications of capsaicinoids. *Clin J Pain* 2000;Suppl 16:S86-S89.

12. Bley KR. Recent developments in transient receptor potential vanilloid receptor 1 agonist based therapy. *Expert Opin Investig Drugs* 2004;13:1445-1456.

13. Rowbotham MC. Topical analgesic agents. In: Fields HL, Liebeskind JC, eds. Pharmacologic Approaches to the Treatment of Chronic Pain: New Concepts and Critical Issues. Seattle: IASP Press; 1994:211-227.

14. Cashman JN. The mechanism of action of NSAIDs in analgesia. *Drugs* 1996;52 (Suppl 5):13-23.

15. Yesilyurt O, Dogrul A, Gul H, et al. Topical cannabinoid enhances topical morphine antinociception. *Pain* 2003 Sep;105:303-308.

16. Sawynok J, Esser MJ, Reid AR. Antidepressants as analgesics: An overview of central and peripheral mechanisms of action. *J Psychiatry Neurosci* 2001;26:21-29.

17. Gerner P, Kao G, Srinivasa V, et al. Topical amitriptyline in health volunteers. *Reg Anesth Pain Med* 2003 Jul-Aug;28:289-293.

18. *Physicians Desk Reference*, 55th ed. Montvale, NJ: Medical Economics Company; 2002.

19. Sawynok J. Topical analgesics in neuropathic pain. *Curr Pharm Des* 2005; 11: 2995-3004.

20. Rowbotham MC, Davies PS, Verkempinck, et al. Lidocaine patch: Double-blind controlled study of a new treatment method for post-herpetic neuralgia. *Pain* 1996;65:39-44.

21. Galer BS, Rowbotham MC, Perander J, et al. Topical lidocaine patch relieves post-herpetic neuralgia more effectively than vehicle patch: Results of an enriched enrollment study. *Pain* 1999;80:533-538.

22. Katz NP, Davis MW, Dworkin RH. Topical lidocaine patch produces a significant improvement in mean pain scores and pain relief in treated PHN patients: results of a multicenter open-label trial. *J Pain* 2001;2:9-18.

23. Meier T, Wasner G, Faust M, et al. Efficacy of lidocaine patch 5% in the treatment of focal peripheral neuropathic pain syndromes: A randomized, double-blind, placebo-controlled study. *Pain* 2003;106:151-158.

24. Devers A, Galer BS. Topical lidocaine patch relieves a variety of neuropathic pain conditions: An open-label study. *Clin J Pain* 2000;16:205-208.

25. Data on file. Endo Pharmaceuticals, Inc. Chadds Ford, PA.

26. Hart-Gouleau S, Gammaitoni A, Galer BS, et al. Open-label study of the effectiveness and safety of the lidocaine patch 5% (Lidoderm®) in patients with painful diabetic neuropathy. Presented at the 10th World Congress on Pain, August 17-22, 2002, San Diego, CA.

27. Galer BS, Jensen MP. Development and preliminary validation of a pain measure specific to neuropathic pain: The Neuropathic Pain Scale. *Neurology* 1997; 48:332-338.

28. Barbano RL, Herrmann DN, Hart-Gouleau S, et al. Effectiveness, tolerability and impact on quality of life of lidocaine patch 5% in diabetic polyneuropathy. Accepted for publication in *Archives of Neurology*.

29. Galer BS, Jensen MP, Ma T, et al. The lidocaine patch 5% effectively treats all Neuropathic Pain Qualities: Results of a randomized, double-blind, vehicle-controlled, 3-week efficacy study with use of the Neuropathic Pain Scale. *Clinical J Pain* 2002;18:297-301.

30. Lycka BA, Watson CP, Nevin K, et al. EMLA cream for the treatment of pain caused by post-herpetic neuralgia: A double-blind, placebo-controlled study. In: Proceedings of the annual meeting of the American Pain Society. 1996:A111 (abstract).

31. Attal N, Brasseur L, Chauvin M, et al. Effects of single and repeated applications of a eutectic mixture of local anesthetics (EMLA®) cream on spontaneous and evoked pain in post-herpetic neuralgia. *Pain* 1999;81:203-209.

32. Litman SJ, Vitkun SA, Poppers PJ. Use of EMLA® cream in the treatment of post-herpetic neuralgia. *J Clin Anesth* 1996;8:54-57.

33. Lynch ME, Clark AJ, Sawynok J. A pilot study examining topical amitriptyline, ketamine, and a combination of both in the treatment of neuropathic pain. *Clin J Pain* 2003;19:323-328.

34. Lynch ME, Clark AJ, Sawynok J, et al. Topical 2% amitriptyline and 1% ketamine in neuropathic pain syndromes: A randomized, double-blind, placebo-controlled trial. *Anesthesiology* 2005;103:140-146.

35. Lynch ME, Clark AJ, Sawynok J, et al. Topical amitriptyline and ketamine in neuropathic pain syndromes: an open-label study. *J Pain* 2005;6:644-649.

36. Quan D, Wellish M, Gilden DH. Topical ketamine treatment of postherpetic neuralgia. *Neurology* 2003;60:1391-1392.

37. Greenway FL, Frome BM, Engels TM, et al. Temporary relief of postherpetic neuralgia pain with topical geranium oil. *Am J Med* 2003;115:586-587.

38. Rains C, Bryson HM. Topical capsaicin: A review of its pharmacological properties and therapeutic potential in post-herpetic neuralgia, diabetic neuropathy, and osteoarthritis. *Drugs Aging* 1995;7:317-328.

39. Robbins WR, Staats PS, Levine J, et al. Treatment of intractable pain with topical large-dose capsaicin: Preliminary report. *Anesth Analg* 1998;86:579-583.

40. Backonja M, Malan P, Brady S, et al. One-hour high concentration trans-capsaicin applications provide durable pain relief in initial and repeat treatment of postherpetic neuralgia. Presented at the 2004 Annual Scientific Meeting of the American Academy of Neurology, San Francisco, CA.

41. Simpson D, Brown S, Sampson J, et al. A Single application of high-concentration trans-capsaicin leads to 12 weeks of pain relief in HIV-associated distal symmetrical polyneuropathy: Results of an open label trial. Presented at the

2004 Annual Scientific Meeting of the American Academy of Neurology, San Francisco, CA.

42. Mason L, Moore RA, Derry S, et al. Systematic review of topical capsaicin for the treatment of chronic pain. *BMJ* 2004;328(7446):991-996.

43. McCleane G. Topical application of doxepin hydrochloride, capsaicin and a combination of both produces analgesia in chronic neuropathic pain: A randomized, double-blind, placebo-controlled study. *Br J Clin Pharmacol* 2000;49:574-579.

44. Mazieres B, Rouanet S, Velicy J, et al. Topical ketoprofen patch (100 mg) for the treatment of ankle sprain: A randomized, double-blind, placebo-controlled study. *Am J Sports Med* 2005;33:515-523.

45. Mazieres B, Rouanet S, Guillon Y, et al. Topical ketoprofen patch in the treatment of tendonitis: A randomized, double blind, placebo controlled study. *J Rheumatol* 2005;32:1563-1570.

46. Predel HG, Koll R, Pabst H, et al. Diclofenac patch for topical treatment of acute impact injuries: A randomized, double blind, placebo controlled, multicenter study. *Br J Sports Med* 2004;38:318-323.

47. Marten M. Efficacy and tolerability of a topical NSAID patch (local action transcutaneous flurbiprofen) and oral diclofenac in the treatment of soft-tissue rheumatism. *Clin Rheumatol* 1997;16:25-31.

48. Galer BS, Rowbotham MC, Perander J, et al. Topical diclofenac patch significantly reduces pain associated with minor sports injuries: Results of a randomized, double-blind, placebo-controlled, multicenter study. *J Pain Symptom Manage* 2000; 19:287-294.

49. Jenoure P, Segesser B, Luhti U, et al. A trial with diclofenac HEP plaster as topical treatment in minor sports injuries. *Drugs Exp Clin Res* 1993;19:125-131.

50. Campbell J, Dunn T. Evaluation of topical ibuprofen cream in the treatment of acute ankle sprains. *J Accidental Emerg Med* 1994;11:178-182.

51. Airaksinen O, Venalainen J, Pietilainen T. Ketoprofen 2.5% gel versus placebo gel in the treatment of acute soft tissue injuries. *Int J Clin Pharmacol Ther Toxicol* 1993;31:561-563.

52. Machen J, Whitefield M. Efficacy of a proprietary ibuprofen gel in soft tissue injuries: A randomized, double-blind, placebo-controlled study. *Intl J Clin Prac* 2002 March;56:102-106.

53. Whitefield M, O'Kane CJ, Anderson S. Comparative efficacy of a proprietary topical ibuprofen gel and oral ibuprofen in acute soft tissue injuries: A randomized, double-blind study. *J Clin Pharm Ther* 2002;27:409-417.

54. Bruhlmann P, Michel BA. Topical diclofenac patch in patients with knee osteoarthritis: A randomized, double-blind, controlled clinical trial. *Clin Exp Rheumatol* 2003;21:193-198.

55. Tugwell PS, Wells GA, Shainhouse JZ. Equivalence study of a topical diclofenac solution (pennsaid) compared with oral diclofenac in symptomatic treatment of osteoarthritis of the knee: A randomized, controlled trial. *J Rheumatol* 2004;31:2002-2012.

56. Di Rienzo BL, Di Rienzo BA, D'Emilia E, et al. Topical versus systemic diclofenac in the treatment of temporo-mandibular joint dysfunction symptoms. *Acta Otorhinolaryngol Ital* 2004;24:279-283.

57. Lin J, Zhang W, Jones A, et al. Efficacy of topical non-steroidal anti-inflammatory drugs in the treatment of osteoarthritis: Meta-analysis of randomized controlled trials. *BMJ* 2004 August;329:324-328.

58. Mason L, Moore RA, Edwards JE, et al. Topical NSAIDS for chronic musculoskeletal pain: A systematic review and meta-analysis. *BMC Musculoskelet Disord* 2004;5:28.

59. Mason L, Moore RA, Edwards JE, et al. Systematic review of topical rubefacients containing salicylates for the treatment of acute and chronic pain. *BMJ* 2004;328:995.

60. Ottillinger B, Gomor B, Michel BA, et al. Efficacy and safety of eltenac gel in the treatment of knee osteoarthritis. *Osteoarthritis Cartilage* 2001;9:273-280.

61. Sandelin J, Harilainen A, Crone H, et al. Local NSAID gel (eltenac) in the treatment of osteoarthritis of the knee. A double-blind study comparing eltenac with oral diclofenac and placebo gel. *Scand J Rheumatol* 1997;26:287-292.

62. Dreiser RL, Tisne-Camus M. DHEP plasters as a topical treatment of knee osteoarthritis: A double-blind placebo-controlled study. *Drugs Exp Clin Res* 1993;19:107-115.

63. Galeazzi M, Marcolongo R. A placebo-controlled study of the efficacy and tolerability of a nonsteroidal anti-inflammatory drug, DHEP plaster in inflammatory peri- and extra-articular rheumatological diseases. *Drugs Exp Clin Res* 1993; 19:107-115.

64. Gallachia G, Marcolongo R. Pharmacokinetics of diclofenac hydroxyethylpyrrolidine (DHEP) plasters in patients with monolateral knee joint effusion. *Drugs Exp Clin Res* 1993;19:95-97.

65. Winocur E, Gavish A, Halachmi M, et al. Topical application of capsaicin for the treatment of localized pain in the temporomandibular joint area. *J Orofac Pain* 2000;14:31-36.

66. Cohen M, Wolfe R, Mai T, et al. A randomized, double blind placebo-controlled trial of a topical crème containing glucosamine sulfate, chondroitin sulfate and camphor for osteoarthritis of the knee. *J Rheumatol* 2003;30:523-528.

67. Keitel W, Frerick H, Kuhn U, et al. Capsicum pain plaster in chronic non-specific low back pain. *Arzneimittelforschung* 2001;51:896-903.

68. Lipman AG, Dalpiaz AS, London SP. Topical lidocaine patch therapy for myofascial pain. Abstract 782. Presented at the Annual Scientific Meeting of the American Pain Society, March 14-17, 2002, Baltimore, MD.

69. Briggs M, Nelson EA. Topical agents or dressings for pain in venous leg ulcers. *Cochrane Database Syst Rev* 2003;1:CD001177.

70. Flock P. Pilot study to determine the effectiveness of diamorphine gel to control pressure ulcer pain. *J Pain Symptom Manage* 2003;25:547-554.

71. Zeppetella G, Ribeiro PJ. Analgesic efficacy of morphine applied topically to painful ulcers. *J Pain Symptom Manage* 2003;25:555-558.

72. Gallagher RE, Arndt DR, Hunt KL. Analgesic effects of topical methadone: a report of four cases. *Clin J Pain* 2005;21:190-192.

73. Vernassiere C, Cornet C, Trechot P, et al. Study to determine the efficacy of topical morphine on painful chronic skin ulcers. *J Wound Care* 2005;14:289-293.

74. Fassoulaki A, Sarantopoulos C, Melemeni A, et al. EMLA reduces acute and chronic pain after breast surgery for cancer. *Reg Anesth Pain Med* 2000;25:35-355.

75. Cerchietti LC, Navigante AH, Bonomi MR, et al. Effect of topical morphine for mucositis-associated pain following concomitant chemoradiotherapy for head and neck carcinoma. *Cancer* 2002;95:2230-2236.

76. Slatkin NE, Rhiner M. Topical ketamine in the treatment of mucositis pain. *Pain Med* 2003;4:298-303.

77. Watterson G, Howard R, Goldman A. Peripheral opiates in inflammatory pain. *Arch Dis Child* 2004;89:679-681.

78. Galeotti N, DeCesare Mannelli L, Mazzanti G, et al. Menthol: A natural analgesic compound. *Neurosci Lett* 2002;322:145-148.

79. Sandroni P. Central neuropathic itch: A new treatment option? *Neurology* 2002;59:778-779.

80. Lockhart E. Topical combination of amitriptyline and ketamine for post herpetic neuralgia. *J Pain* 2004;5(Suppl 1):S82.

81. Bernstein J, Phillips S, Group T. A new topical medication for the adjunctive relief of painful diabetic neuropathy and postherpetic neuralgia. *J Pain* 2004;3 (Suppl 1):S82.

Chapter 7A

Intra-Articular Injections

William Lavelle
Elizabeth Demers
Lori Lavelle

Intra-articular injections are one of a multitude of methods physicians treating joint pain employ. The first material to be commonly injected in the intra-articular space was corticosteroids. This mode of treatment became widely accepted in the 1950s.[1] Early on, corticosteroids were found to lower intra-articular leukocyte count and other indicators of the inflammatory response.[1,2] In over 50 years of common clinical practice, physicians continue to debate the effectiveness and indications for intra-articular steroid injections. More recently, viscosupplementation has gained popularity. This topic is extensively discussed in the Chapter 12 on Hyaluronic Acid within this text. Anesthesiologists as well as orthopedic surgeons have begun exploring the use of intra-articular opiates as a method of postoperative pain control.

HISTORY OF INTRA-ARTICULAR
STEROID INJECTIONS

In the 1930s, arthrocentesis was first described in a U.S. textbook. Formalin and glycerin, lipodol, lactic acid, and petroleum jelly were among the first intra-articular injections.[3,4] These injections yielded little clinical benefit. Hollander attempted joint injections with hydrocortisone acetate and found his patients, in a series of more than

Clinical Management of Bone and Joint Pain
© 2007 by The Haworth Press, Inc. All rights reserved.
doi:10.1300/5771_08

100,000 injections in 4,000 patients, had a much better clinical response.[5,6] From the 1950s to the present, many physicians have utilized corticosteroid injections as an adjunctive treatment for joint pain.

MECHANISM OF ACTION
OF INTRA-ARTICULAR STEROID INJECTIONS

Steroids have long been believed to possess anti-inflammatory properties. On the cellular level, steroids are highly lipophylic and are thought to bind to the cell nuclei. It is believed that steroids act on the level of genetic expression, altering transcription. The pathway by which this occurs is not completely understood. Intra-articular steroids do appear to reduce the number of lymphocytes, macrophages, and mast cells.[7,8] This, in turn, reduces phagocytosis, lysosomal enzyme release, and the release of inflammatory mediators,[1] particularly interleukin-1, leukotrienes, and prostaglandins.[9,10] With the reduction of these inflammatory mediators, pain symptoms are often improved.

It would seem that intra-articular steroid injections avoid most of the systemic effects of oral steroids such as muscle weakness, skin thinning, resulting in easy bruising, peptic ulceration, and aggravation of diabetes.

Adverse Reactions

The most obvious concern about intra-articular injections is infection; however, only 12.6 percent of respondents to a recent survey of orthopedists and rheumatologists have ever encountered a case of poststeroid septic arthritis.[11] Avoidance of this complication entails strict adherence to sterile technique. Suspicion of either an indolent intra-articular infection or an overlying soft tissue infection contraindicates the injection of a joint with corticosteroid. Other contraindications include a local fracture of total joint. In one of the earliest reports on over 100,000 injections, Hollander reported an infection rate of 1:10,000.[6] More recent reports have found similar statistics with incidence between 1:3,000 and 1:50,000.[11] The most common infecting organism is *Staphylococcus aureus.*[11,12]

Mild local reactions do occur after injection. Postinjection flares occur in about 2 percent to 6 percent of patients and are believed to result from chemical synovitis in response to the injected crystals.[11] Facial flushing may be seen in up to 15 percent of patients, mostly in women.[7] At the actual site of needle entry, skin or fat atrophy may be observed.[7,13] Steroid induced osteoporosis and myopathy are not reported as a common finding after intra-articular steroid injection.[14,15] In fact, a study of intra-articular triamcinolone acetonide found no net change in the markers of bone metabolism.[7,16] There is some concern in the medical community regarding the use of intra-articular steroid injections in the diabetic population. Transient increases in blood glucose may be seen in patients receiving corticosteroid injections. However, in a study of diabetic patients who received soft tissue injections of methylprednisolone acetate, there was no detectable effect on blood glucose levels in the 14 days after injection.[17] Intra-articular steroids also transiently affect the hypothalamic-pituitary-adrenal axis. These changes, which include a 21.5 percent reduction in serum cortisol levels, typically normalize within 3 days,[18] but an episode of Cushing's syndrome has been reported.[7,19]

A common concern in the orthopedic surgery and rheumatology communities is joint destruction after repetitive injections. Animal studies have been suggestive of damage to articular cartilage as a result of intra-articular steroid injections; however, to date there is no human data corroborating this claim.[9,20] In 1958, Chandler and Wright reported on hip joint destruction after monthly hip joint injections.[21,22] A Charcot-like arthropathy has also been speculated and reported;[11] however, no evidence of increased loss of joint space was observed in patients receiving triamcinolone acetonide injections every 3 months for up to 2 years for osteoarthritis of the knee.[11] As a testament to this fact, a study that followed the rate of total joint replacements in rheumatoid patients treated with intra-articular steroid injections did not find an increased rate in this population.[7,23] Still, many physicians recommend 3 months between injections of the same joint for fear of possible joint destruction.[21,24] The growth and development of the pediatric joint was also not found to be altered by therapeutic steroid injections. In a study involving 21 children who received intra-articular corticosteroid injections into the knee, ankle, or elbow, there was no effect on cartilage integrity or statural growth.[11]

Skin Preparation

Skin preparation is as individualized as that seen for surgical site preparation. In a survey of orthopedists and rheumatologists, 57.6 percent used alcohol swabs, with the remaining using either chlorhexidine or Betadine. Only 16.3 percent used sterile towels to isolate the injection site and only 32.5 percent of respondents used sterile gloves.[11] The authors of this chapter recommend preparation with alcohol followed by preparation with Betadine and the use of sterile gloves.

Choice of Steroid

Based strictly on chemical structure, duration of effect is inversely proportional to solubility. Triamcinolone hexacetonide is the least soluble and should be the longest-lasting steroid. Supporting this fact is a review of 300 patients receiving hydrocortisone succinate, triamcinolone hexacetide, and triamcinolone acetonide who found longer-lasting relief in a population treated with triamcinolone hexacetide.[21,25] However, another large study illustrated quite the opposite. Fifty-seven patients were treated with either triamcinolone hexacetide or methylprednisolone acetate. Patients reported improved pain scores and functional testing for both agents at 3 weeks; however, triamcinolone hexacetide failed to show a significant improvement in pain scores and functional testing at 8 weeks, while treatment with methylprednisolone acetate, an agent with a higher solubility, resulted in clinical improvement[26] (Table 7A.1). Little data exist touting the true efficacy of one agent over another. It seems that the choice of steroid used by physicians is more related to personal preference rather than true science. In a survey performed on members of the 1994 American

TABLE 7A.1. Steroid solubility.

Name of steroid	Solubility (percentage weight/volume)
Hydrocortisone acetate	0.002
Methylprednisolone acetate	0.001
Prednisolone tebutate	0.001
Triamcinolone acetate	0.004
Triamcinolone hexacetonide	0.0002

College of Rheumatology, 34.6 percent favored methylprednisolone, 31.2 percent triamcinolone hexacetide, and 21.7 percent triamcinolone acetonide.[21,27]

Use of Local Anesthetic

Local anesthetics such as lidocaine are at times combined with steroid. Some hold the contention that the local agent acts to dilute the steroid crystals, but whether this process has any impact on the effect of the steroid is unclear. Lidocaine itself may have a transient anti-inflammatory effect.[28,29]

Clinical Trials

No report of the clinical efficacy of intra-articular steroid injections is complete without mention of the early series by Hollander in the 1950s. Hydrocortisone injections of 1,034 knees ridden with osteoarthritis revealed an 80 percent success rate.[5,6] Time has proven the short-term effects (1 to 4 weeks) of injected corticosteroids.[24] Longer-term results have not been as promising; however, short-term pain relief may allow this patient population the ability to begin enough physical activity to aide in their convalescence.

Illustrating this fact is a large meta-analysis that examined the literature for randomized placebo-control trials and systematic reviews that investigated intra-articular steroid injections for osteoarthritis of the knee. The authors specifically sought newer agents that were felt to be longer-lasting agents. These agents included triamcinolone hexacetonide, methylprednisolone, betamethasone, and cortivazol (not currently an approved steroid in the United States).[7] Five articles satisfied their inclusion criteria. The reviewers examined whether the target levels of pain reduction that were set by each of the five studies were achieved. At 1 week, treated patients were more likely to achieve a clinically significant pain reduction based both on the target set in the individual studies and on their visual analog pain scores. At 3 to 4 weeks, pain symptoms were improved according to the target set in the individual studies, but visual analog pain scores did not reach statistical significance. At 6 to 8 weeks, there was no reduction of pain symptoms by either the target set in the individual studies or by visual analog scores.[30] These authors felt that pain relief was likely to last a week and quite possibly for a month, but longer durations are questionable.

A second large meta-analysis also examined randomized placebo-control trials and included studies in which the efficacy of intra-articular corticosteroids for osteoarthritis of the knee. Ten studies met their inclusion criteria. Six of these studies provided data on improvement of symptoms of osteoarthritis of the knee after intra-articular steroid as compared with placebo. These studies illustrated symptom improvement at 2 weeks. Two studies adequately examined treated patients at 16 to 24 weeks and did find improvement in pain symptoms. The authors proposed that a dose of 50 mg of prednisone may be required to statistically prove this benefit.[31]

As a component of both of these meta-analysis was a double-blind, placebo-controlled, crossover study involving 59 patients with symptomatic osteoarthritis of the knee. The data from this study were analyzed to determine if predictors of response could be identified using logistic regression. Unfortunately, despite reporting a significant reduction in pain symptoms based on a visual analog pain scale, no predictors of patients who would respond to treatment could be identified.[32]

An adjunct to the success of steroid treatment in the patient with an effusion may be the aspiration of that effusion. Eighty-four patients with osteoarthritis were randomized to receive either triamcinolone hexacetonide or placebo. Patients receiving the steroid reported a statistically significant improvement in pain, distance walked in 1 min, and Health Assessment Questionnaire. Subgroup analysis of steroid-treated patients revealed greater improvement among those with an effusion ($p < 0.05$) and those whose effusion was successfully aspirated at the time of steroid injection.[33] Similar results have been reported for patients who underwent joint lavage at the time of steroid injection.[34]

Intra-articular steroids are not the only materials injected intra-articular in the treatment of osteoarthritis. A randomized placebo-controlled study compared hyaluronic acid, corticosteroid (Depo-medrol), and isotonic saline. Over 100 patients with osteoarthritis of the hip were enrolled randomly receive one of the three agents. These injections were placed with the aide of ultrasound. Injections were administered at 14 day intervals with each patient receiving three injections.

The primary outcome measure was pain on walking as measured on a visual analog scale. Significant improvement was seen at 3 months in the population treated with corticosteroid compared with patients treated with saline ($p = 0.006$ at 14 days, $p = 0.006$ at 28 days, and $p = 0.58$ at 3 months), while the group treated with hyaluronic acid failed to reach statistical significance ($p = 0.069$ at 14 days, $p = 0.14$ at 28 days, and $p = 0.57$ at 3 months). Statistically, there was no significant difference between hyaluronic acid and corticosteroid at any time point ($p > 0.21$).[35]

Clinical efficacy has also been examined for treatment of rheumatoid arthritis. Sixty-nine rheumatoid arthritis patients were randomized to either receive intra-articular injections of triamcinolone hexacetonide in a multitude of their affected joints (six to eight swollen joints) or intramuscular minipulse therapy with triamcinolone acetonide in an equivalent dose. Patients were assessed by blinded examiners at baseline, 1, 4, 12, and 24 weeks, and American College of Rheumatology improvement criteria were recorded. This scale includes components for tender and swollen joint counts, global pain by visual analog pain scale, patient and physician evaluation of disease activity, function by the Stanford Health Assessment Questionnaire, and erythrocyte sedimentation rate (ESR). A separate visual analog scale for pain was used for each of the twelve joints studied. A range of motion scale was also included. All patients also completed a Brazilian version of the Medical Outcome Study Short Form-36 (SF-36). Significantly better results were seen for the patients treated with intra-articular injections than those treated with minipulse systemic steroids. ACR 20 percent (61.7 percent versus 28.5 percent at 1 week; 73.5 percent versus 42.8 percent at 4 weeks), ACR 50 percent (29.4 percent versus 5.7 percent at 1 week; 44.1 percent versus 20 percent at 4 weeks), ACR 70 percent (11.7 percent versus 0 percent at 1 week). Patient evaluation of disease activity, tender joint count, lower blood pressure, lower side effects, calls to the physician, and hospital visits were all significantly better ($p < 0.05$) for those treated with intra-articular steroids.[36]

Postoperative Intra-Articular Analgesia

The analgesic effects of intra-articular agents in the postoperative period are controversial; however, their use is becoming ever more common in the outpatient orthopedic setting.[37] Peripheral nerve blocks are also useful for extremity surgery but require greater skill in placement and have a greater potential for significant complications.[38-41] Intra-articular analgesia techniques are most commonly used for knee and shoulder surgery, such as for arthroscopies. The advent of arthroscopy has been touted in the orthopedic community as a method of decreased morbidity, but not one of decreased pain.[38] Poor pain control may make the difference in a procedure being acceptable in an outpatient setting. With some debate, intra-articular administration of local agents has proven effective for knee arthroscopy;[42-50] however, pain control for the shoulder has proven a greater task. Severe pain scores have been reported for even the most minor of shoulder procedures despite multimodal pain controlling techniques.[51]

Local Agents

Most anesthesiologists and orthopedic surgeons select bupivacaine because of its long duration of action. This does not preclude the use of other local agents. In one study comparing ropivacaine 0.75 percent with bupivacaine 0.50 percent for intra-articular injection after knee arthroscopy, investigators found significantly improved visual analog pain scores for the group treated with ropivacaine 0.75 percent.[52]

The literature on the use of intra-articular local anesthetics holds numerous studies, but is difficult to interpret due to confounding agents used in these studies such as intra-articular opiates, clonidine, and nonsteroidals. A large number of these studies are also flawed with regard to their study design, data collection, and reporting. A systematic review of double-blind, randomized, controlled trials that compared intra-articular local with either placebo or no intervention was completed in 1999. Outcome measures were pain scores, supplementary analgesia such as intravenous patient-controlled analgesia (PCA), and time to first analgesic request. Twenty studies were identified in this review as appropriate. Data from the 895 patients involved in these studies was pooled. Twelve of the 20 studies showed statistically significant improved pain after intra-articular local in one of the three recorder outcomes measures. In 10 of the 12 studies that showed improvement, pain scores were significantly lower in the treatment groups compared with the controls. In nine of the original 20 studies, the consumption of supplemental analgesics was reduced by 10 to 50 percent with most cased requiring only a small amount of supplemental analgesia. With respect to the parameter of time to first analgesic, only 6 of the original 20 studies utilized this parameter. Only two of these six studies showed a significant improvement.[53] The authors of this review speculate that the lack of uniform dosing and other confounding variables cited here may be responsible for the weak data supporting the efficacy of intra-articular local agents. One such study found that 75 mg of intra-articular bupivacaine provided better postoperative pain relief than either 25 or 50 mg.[53,54] Another factor that may alter the activity of intra-articular local analgesia is the presence of hemarthrosis, which can increase the level of pain and decrease the concentration of local agent.[49] Even though the data from this review would seem that intra-articular local is only mildly effective, the use of local in the outpatient orthopedic setting is popular and a relatively safe adjuvant in this setting.[55]

A continuous infusion of intra-articular analgesia has also been examined. In a prospective randomized trial involving 50 subjects undergoing acromioplasty and rotator cuff repair received a multiorifice placed in the subachromial space. Twenty of the subjects received 0.25 percent bupivacaine, while 22 received saline. The outcome measure was the amount of PCA consumed by the patient as well as pain scores recorded with a visual analog scale for the first 48 hours. No statistically significant difference in pain scores or PCA use was detected.[56]

Opiates

The presence of opiate receptors in the peripheral nervous system has recently been discovered. The first descriptions entailed a rat model where the effects were seen in inflamed tissue. Mu, delta, and kappa receptors have been all been found on peripheral nerves.[49,57] This association with effectiveness of opiates in inflamed tissues has been explained by a disruption in the perineurium, allowing for easier access of opioids to neuronal receptors. This may also be associated with an unmasking or upregulation of inactive opiate receptors.[49,58] Stein and colleagues first demonstrated this fact in humans when the effects of morphine injected peripherally could be reversed by injection of intra-articular naloxone.[59,60] It has been proposed that effects seen from intra-articular morphine may be simple due to systemic absorption; however, the plasma concentration achieved from an intra-articular injection would be far too low for a systemic effect to be observed.[49] Within the joint itself, the relative concentration is quite high. The lowest effective dose of 1 mg in a 20 ml injection would have a concentration of 200 μmol/l (50 mcg/ml). Typical blood levels after effective systemic injections are quantified in nmol/l, a 1000 times lower concentration.[61] Opiate receptors in the joint would be well saturated at this level.

In a review by Kalso et al., 36 randomized controlled trials were reviewed. Six of these studies involved both a local anesthetic arm and a placebo arm. Four of these studies found efficacy of intra-articular morphine against placebo. Six of the 36 studies compared intra-articular morphine with intravenous or intramuscular morphine or with intra-articular saline. Four of the six studies showed greater efficacy for intra-articular morphine. No dose response was detected in the literature reviewed. Specifically, the minimum dose tested (0.5 mg) did not show efficacy, but a dose of 1 mg did. No greater effect was found when a dose of 1 mg was compared with a dose of 2 mg.[61,62] This review did not complete an analysis of pooled data. The reviewers felt that intra-articular morphine may have some effect in reducing postoperative pain; however, the reviewers felt the studies were flawed with difficulties in data design, data collection, statistical analysis, and reporting.[61]

A later review by Gupta and colleagues analyzed the same topic. A meta-analysis was completed on the pooled data of 19 prospective, placebo controlled, randomized studies in which intra-articular morphine was utilized. Within these studies, visual analog scores were colleted at the early phase (0 to 2 hours), the intermediate phase (2 to 6 hours), and the late phase (6 to 24 hours). This analysis concluded that although no clear dose-response effect was seen, a definite but mild analgesic effect was present.[59]

Another recent review is a bit more skeptical. In 2005, Rosseland and colleagues reviewed randomized controlled trials involving intra-articular morphine. Forty-three publications were included. Rosseland and colleagues were very critical of the literature, which included many of the studies examined be Gupta and colleagues and Kalso and colleagues. Twenty-three were thought to be of low scientific quality with poor randomization and blinding or unsound statistics. Thirteen were thought to have usable information; however, four of the positive outcomes were believed to be due to uneven distribution of patients whose natural course was low postoperative pain. The only randomized control trial Rosseland and colleagues felt adequate found no statistically significance in the use of morphine in intra-articular injections. Small sample size for positive studies was also raised as a concern.[63]

Timing for the placement of intra-articular local and morphine is also an issue discussed in the literature. One prospective, double-blind, randomized trial reviewed two groups—one was injected with morphine and bupivacaine 10 min before tourniquet release, while the second received the same injection after the tourniquet was released. Pain scores were recorded with a visual analog scale at 10 min, 30 min, and 1, 2, 4, 8, 12, and 24 hours. The only statistically significant difference in pain scores between the two groups was at 30 min. The trial also recorded the timing and amount of PCA required. The first analgesic requirement as well as the total analgesic requirement was significantly lower in the group receiving the injection after tourniquet release, indicating that perhaps it is better to administer the intra-articular analgesia after tourniquet release.[64]

Intra-articular clonidine has also been investigated. Clonidine is an α-agonist that has been shown to prolong the duration of local anesthetics.[49] This was demonstrated in a study in which 40 patients who were undergoing knee arthroscopy were randomized in a controlled study involving intra-articular clonidine in combination with 1 mg of morphine. Patients receiving clonidine had significantly longer analgesia durations.[49,65] It has also been proposed that clonidine may also produce analgesia by releasing enkephalin-like substances.[49]

Combinations of various intra-articular agents have also been investigated. A study involving 60 patients undergoing arthroscopic meniscus repair saw patients randomized into four groups One received 30 ml of 0.25 percent bupivacaine, a second received 30 ml of 0.25 percent bupivacaine and 1 μg/kg of clonidine, a third received 30 ml of 0.25 percent bupivacaine and 3 mg of morphine, and a final group receiving 30 ml of 0.25 percent bupivacaine, 1 μg/kg of clonidine, and 3 mg of morphine. The study found significant improvement in pain with the group receiving 0.25 percent bupivacaine, 1 μg/kg of clonidine, and 3 mg of morphine as compared with all the other groups.[66]

Currently, many physicians who participate in outpatient orthopedic surgery recommend a multimodal approach consisting of intra-articular agents including local, an opiate, and an adjunct such as clonidine.[49] The specifics of this cocktail are left to the individual to decide. Local analgesia would appear to be helpful early on in the postoperative period (2 to 4 hours), preventing a deleterious physiologic pain response. Intra-articular morphine may be more helpful in the hours after surgery.[49] The use of nonsteroidal agents is not covered in this chapter, but may play a role in the postoperative management of these patients. In general, the use of pre-emptive and multimodal analgesia is important to abate postoperative pain with an emphasis on minimizing systemic narcotic analgesia, which has the deleterious effects of respiratory depression, sedation, nausea, purities, and delayed discharge.[49]

Techniques to Improve Placement

Image guidance with the aide of either ultrasound or fluoroscopic guidance is a valuable tool to help access difficult joints such as the hip. Fluoroscopy and a radio-opaque tracer also allow for the documented delivery of an agent into a joint; however, these methods are often unavailable in the office setting. One method that may allow for improved accuracy is the aspiration of synovial fluid prior to injection of a steroid. One study examined this question. One hundred and ninety-one knees in 147 patients with rheumatoid arthritis were randomly assigned to undergo either arthrocentesis prior to injection of 20 mg of triamcinolone hexacetonide or injection of the steroid without arthrocentesis. A statistically significant relapse reduction was seen in the group that had undergone arthrocentesis prior to injection of the steroid.[67] This method does, however, require the presence of a mild effusion.

A recent article assessed the accuracy of needle placement in the intra-articular space of the knee using three commonly employed knee joint sites. The authors documented the location of the injected fluid by fluoroscopic imaging of the injected material. The authors of this study found far more success with a lateral midpatellar injection than any of the other injection sites.[68]

Whichever method is chosen, careful attention to the anatomic landmarks and experience are critical to the successful placement of an intra-articular injection. The following section outlines techniques for injection into the more common joints treated in the office setting.

SELECTED INJECTION TECHNIQUES

Knee

Anterior. With the patient seated, the knee joint may be entered either just medial or lateral to the patellar tendon. Upon entering, the needle should be directed toward the center of the knee. To place the needle through the lateral portal, palpate the depression above Gerdy's tubercle and place the needle just above it. The inferior pole of the patella is commonly used as the upper landmark for this injection site. One detriment of this approach is placing the injection in the anterior fat pad of the knee. See Figure 7A.1. (See also color gallery.)

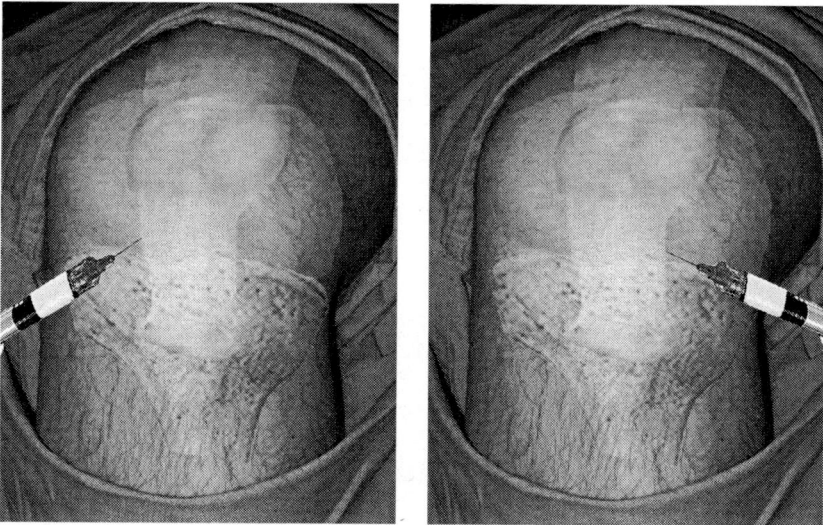

FIGURE 7A.1. Injection technique for knee, anterior.

Lateral. With the knee fully extended, the needle is placed beneath either the superior and medial or lateral knee. This position avoids entering the anterior fat pad of the knee. Care should be taken not to impact the articular cartilage. See Figure 7A.2. (See also color gallery.)

Shoulder

Glenohumeral

Anterior Approach. Position the needle just medial to the head of the humerus and 1 cm lateral to the coracoid process. The needle is directed posteriorly and slightly superiorly and laterally. See Figure 7A.3. (See also color gallery.)

Posterior Approach. The needle should be inserted 2 to 3 cm inferior to the poster lateral corner of the acromion. Palpate the coracoid as you insert the needle. Direct the needle anteriorly toward the coracoid process. See Figure 7A.4. (See also color gallery.)

Acromioclavicular

Patients are placed in the supine or seated position with the affected arm resting comfortably at their side. The acromioclavicular (AC)

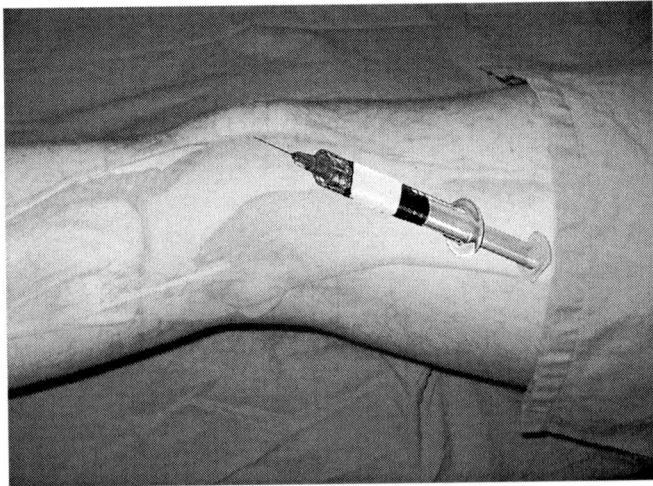

FIGURE 7A.2. Injection technique for knee, lateral.

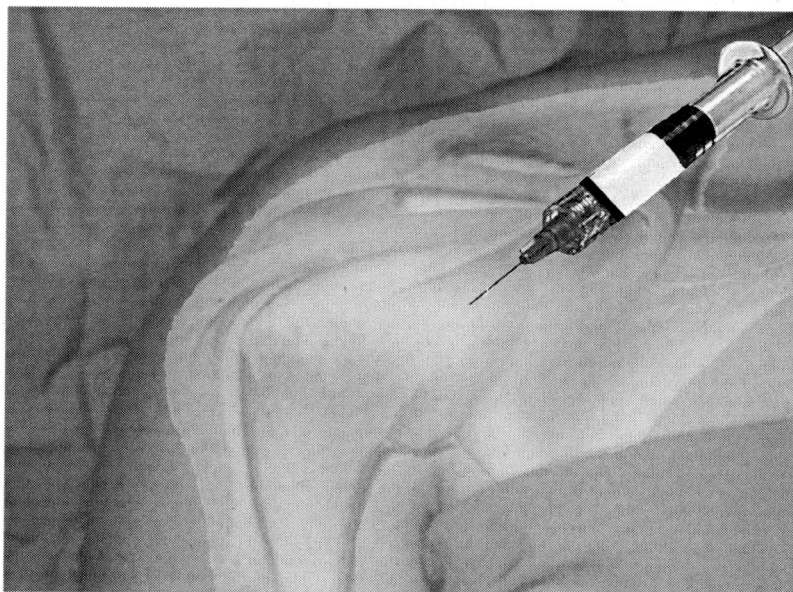

FIGURE 7A.3. Injection technique for shoulder, glenohumeral, anterior approach.

joint is identified by palpating the clavicle from medial to lateral. At its most lateral point a slight depression will be felt at the joint articulation. The needle is inserted from a superior and anterior position into the AC joint. See Figure 7A.5. (See also color gallery.)

Subachromial Injection

This injection is best performed in a seated position so as to allow gravity to pull the arm and humeral head away from the acromion. The distal, lateral, and posterior edges of the acromion are palpated. It is sometimes helpful to mark these with a skin marker. The needle is inserted just inferior to the posterolateral edge of the acromion. See Figure 7A.6. (See also color gallery.)

First Carpometacarpal Joint

Move the thumb up and down while palpating the base of the metacarpal. The needle is placed just proximal to the first metacarpal on

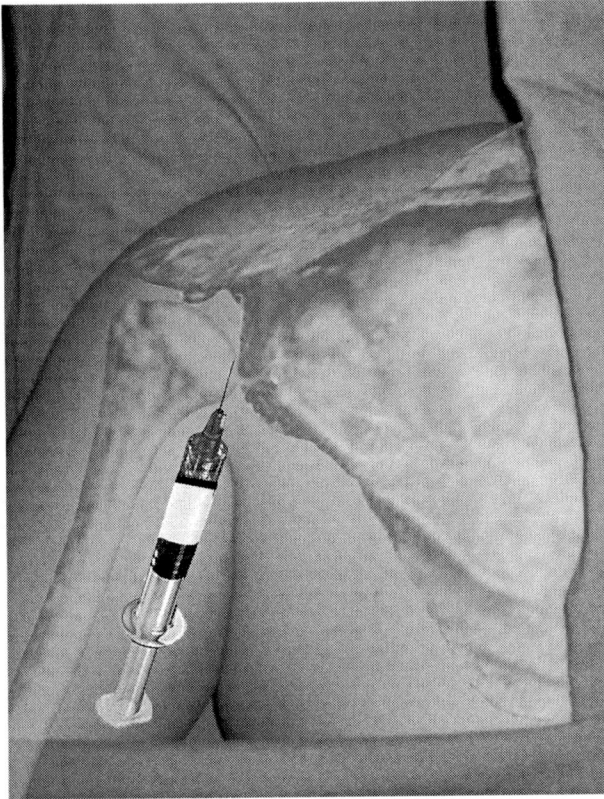

FIGURE 7A.4. Injection technique for shoulder, glenohumeral, posterior approach.

the extensor surface. Be sure to avoid the radial artery and the extensor pollicis tendons. See Figure 7A.7. (See also color gallery.)

Ankle

Palpate between the dorsum of the foot between the medial border of the tibialis anterior tendon and the anterior border of the medial malleolus. Feel for the distal edge of the tibia and insert the needle within these landmarks. Advance the needle in a posterolateral direction. See Figure 7A.8. (See also color gallery.)

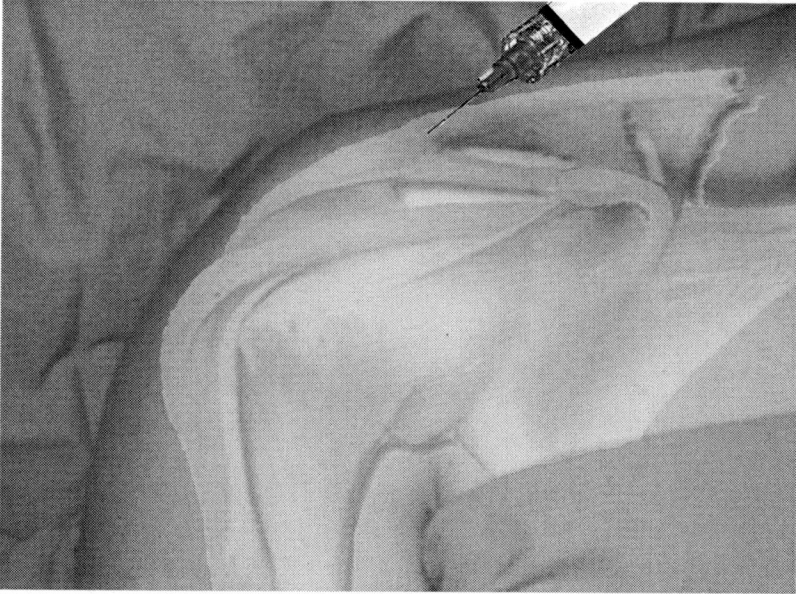

FIGURE 7A.5. Injection technique for shoulder, acromioclavicular.

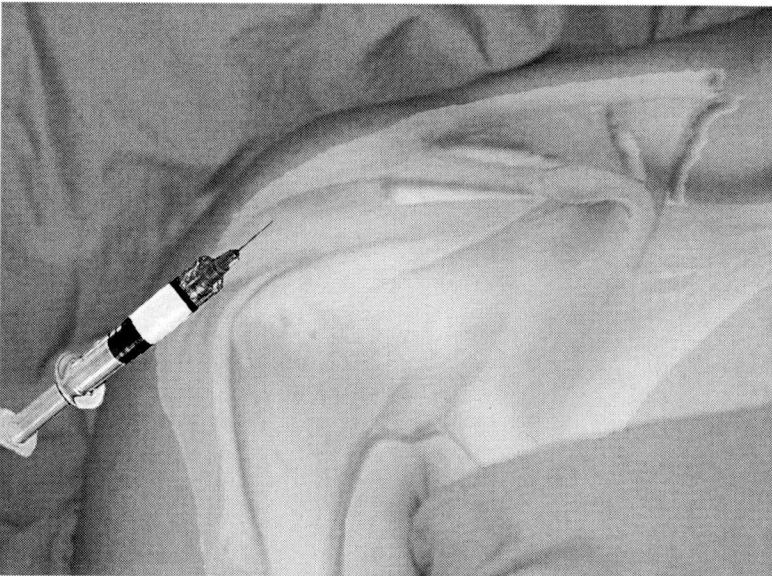

FIGURE 7A.6. Injection technique for shoulder, subachromial injection.

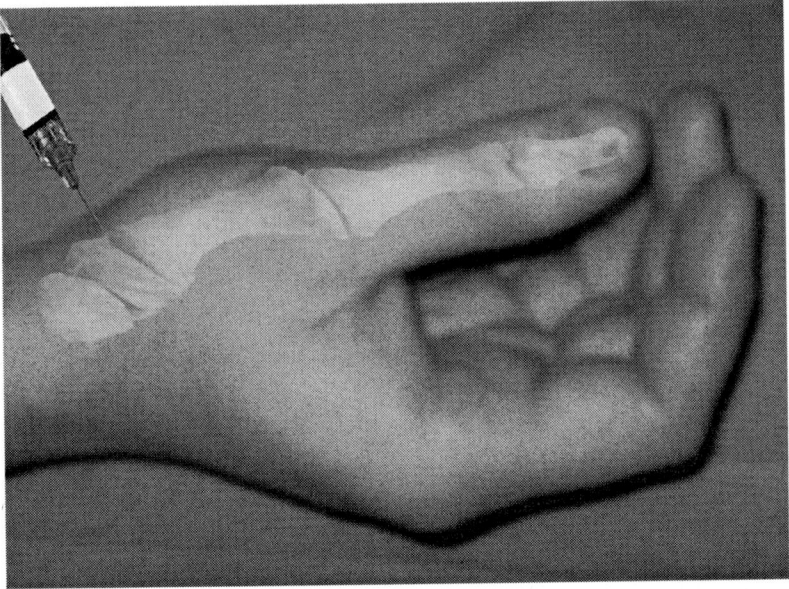

FIGURE 7A.7. Injection technique for first carpometacarpal joint.

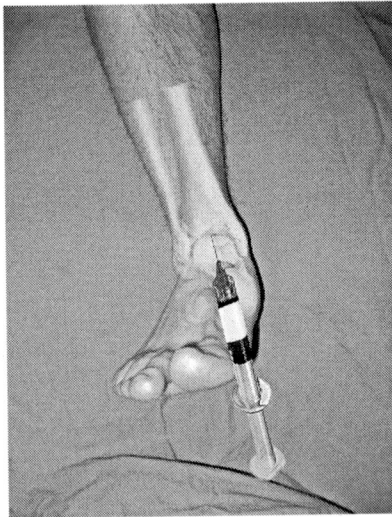

FIGURE 7A.8. Injection technique for ankle.

REFERENCES

1. Snibbe JC, Gambardella RA. Use of injections for osteoarthritis in joints and sports activity. *Clin Sports Med* 2005;24:83-91.

2. Hollander JL, Brown EM Jr, Jessar RA, Brown CY. Hydrocortisone and cortisone injected into arthritic joints; comparative effects of and use of hydrocortisone as a local antiarthritic agent. *JAMA* 1951;147:1629-1635.

3. Pemberton, R. *Arthritis and Rheumatoid Conditions. Their Nature and Treatment.* Philadelphia, PA: Lea and Febiger, 1935.

4. Ropes, MW, Bauer, W. *Synovial Fluid Changes in Joint Disease.* Cambridge, MA: Harvard University Press, 1953.

5. Hollander, JL. Hydrocortisone and cortisone injected into arthritic joints. Comparative effects of and use of hydrocortisone as a local antiarthritic agent. *JAMA* 1951;147:1629.

6. Hollander, JL. Intrasynovial corticosteroid therapy: A decade of use. *Bull Rheum Dis* 1961;11:239.

7. Cole BJ, Schumacher HR Jr. Injectable corticosteroids in modern practice. *J Am Acad Orthop Surg* 2005;13:37-46.

8. Centeno LM, Moore ME. Preferred intraarticular corticosteroids and associated practice: A survey of members of the American College of Rheumatology. *Arthritis Care Res* 1994;7:151-155.

9. Uthman I, Raynauld JP, Haraoui B. Intra-articular therapy in osteoarthritis. *Postgrad Med J* 2003;79:449-453.

10. Wilder RL. Corticosteroids. In: Klippel JH, Cornelia WM, Wortmann RL, eds. *Primer on Rheumatic Diseases.* Atlanta: Arthritis Foundation, 1997: 427-431.

11. Charalambous CP, Tryfonidis M, Sadiq S, Hirst P, Paul A. Septic arthritis following intra-articular steroid injection of the knee—A survey of current practice regarding antiseptic technique used during intra-articular steroid injection of the knee. *Clin Rheumatol* 2003;22:386-390.

12. von Essen R, Savolainen HA. Bacterial infection following intra-articular injection. A brief review. *Scand J Rheumatol* 1989;18:7-12.

13. Kumar N, Newman RJ. Complications of intra- and peri-articular steroid injections. *Br J Gen Pract* 1999;49:465-466.

14. Emkey RD, Lindsay R, Lyssy J, Weisberg JS, Dempster DW, Shen V. The systemic effect of intraarticular administration of corticosteroid on markers of bone formation and bone resorption in patients with rheumatoid arthritis. *Arthritis Rheum* 1996;39:277-282.

15. Dekhuijzen PN, Decramer M. Steroid-induced myopathy and its significance to respiratory disease: A known disease rediscovered. *Eur Respir J* 1992; 5:997-1003.

16. Emkey RD, Lindsay R, Lyssy J, Weisberg JS, Dempster DW, Shen V. The systemic effect of intraarticular administration of corticosteroid on markers of bone formation and bone resorption in patients with rheumatoid arthritis. *Arthritis Rheum* 1996;39:277-282.

17. Slotkoff A, Clauw D, Nashel D. Effect of soft tissue corticosteroid injection on glucose control in diabetics. *Arthritis Rheum* 1994;37(suppl 9):S347.

18. Lazarevic MB, Skosey JL, Djordjevic-Denic G, Swedler WI, Zgradic I, Myones BL. Reduction of cortisol levels after single intra-articular and intramuscular steroid injection. *Am J Med* 1995;99:370-373.

19. O'Sullivan MM, Rumfeld WR, Jones MK, Williams BD. Cushing's syndrome with suppression of the hypothalamic-pituitary-adrenal axis after intra-articular steroid injections. *Ann Rheum Dis* 1985;44:561-563.

20. Pelletier JP, Martel-Pelletier J. Protective effects of corticosteroids on cartilage lesions and osteophyte formation in the Pond-Nuki dog model of osteoarthritis. *Arthritis Rheum* 1989;32:181-193.

21. Rozental TD, Sculco TP. Intra-articular corticosteroids: An updated overview. *Am J Orthop* 2000;29:18-23.

22. Chandler GN, Wright V. Deleterious effect of intra-articular hydrocortisone. *Lancet* 1958;2:661-663.

23. Roberts WN, Babcock EA, Breitbach SA, Owen DS, Irby WR. Corticosteroid injection in rheumatoid arthritis does not increase rate of total joint arthroplasty. *J Rheumatol* 1996;23:1001-1004.

24. Chumacher HR, Chen LX. Injectable corticosteroids in treatment of arthritis of the knee. *Am J Med* 2005;118:1208-1214.

25. Blyth T, Hunter JA, Stirling A. Pain relief in the rheumatoid knee after steroid injection. A single-blind comparison of hydrocortisone succinate, and triamcinolone acetonide or hexacetonide. *Br J Rheumatol* 1994;33:461-463.

26. Pyne D, Ioannou Y, Mootoo R, Bhanji A. Intra-articular steroids in knee osteoarthritis: A comparative study of triamcinolone hexacetonide and methylprednisolone acetate. *Clin Rheumatol* 2004;23:116-120.

27. Centeno LM, Moore ME. Preferred intraarticular corticosteroids and associated practice: A survey of members of the American College of Rheumatology. *Arthritis Care Res* 1994;7:151-155.

28. Schumacher HR Jr. Aspiration and injection therapies for joints. *Arthritis Rheum* 2003;49:413-420.

29. Paul H, Clayburne G, Schumacher HR. Lidocaine inhibits leukocyte migration and phagocytosis in monosodium urate crystal-induced synovitis in dogs. *J Rheumatol* 1983;10:434-439.

30. Godwin M, Dawes M. Intra-articular steroid injections for painful knees. Systematic review with meta-analysis. *Can Fam Physician* 2004;50:241-248.

31. Arroll B, Goodyear-Smith F. Corticosteroid injections for painful shoulder: A meta-analysis. *Br J Gen Pract* 2005;55:224-228.

32. Jones A, Doherty M. Intra-articular corticosteroids are effective in osteoarthritis but there are no clinical predictors of response. *Ann Rheum Dis* 1996;55:829-832.

33. Gaffney K, Ledingham J, Perry JD. Intra-articular triamcinolone hexacetonide in knee osteoarthritis: Factors influencing the clinical response. *Ann Rheum Dis* 1995;54:379-381.

34. Ravaud P, Moulinier L, Giraudeau B, Ayral X, Guerin C, Noel E, Thomas P, Fautrel B, Mazieres B, Dougados M. Effects of joint lavage and steroid injection in

patients with osteoarthritis of the knee: results of a multicenter, randomized, controlled trial. *Arthritis Rheum* 1999;42:475-482.

35. Qvistgaard E, Christensen R, Torp-Pedersen S, Bliddal H. Intra-articular treatment of hip osteoarthritis: A randomized trial of hyaluronic acid, corticosteroid, and isotonic saline. *Osteoarthritis Cartilage* 2006;14:163-170.

36. Furtado RN, Oliveira LM, Natour J. Polyarticular corticosteroid injection versus systemic administration in treatment of rheumatoid arthritis patients: A randomized controlled study. *J Rheumatol* 2005;32:1691-1698.

37. Savoie FH, Field LD, Jenkins RN, Mallon WJ, Phelps RA 2nd. The pain control infusion pump for postoperative pain control in shoulder surgery. *Arthroscopy* 2000;16:339-342.

38. Rawal N. Incisional and intra-articular infusions. *Best Pract Res Clin Anaesthesiol* 2002;16:321-343.

39. Rosseland LA, Stubhaug A, Grevbo F, Reikeras O, Breivik H. Effective pain relief from intra-articular saline with or without morphine 2 mg in patients with moderate-to-severe pain after knee arthroscopy: A randomized, double-blind controlled clinical study. *Acta Anaesthesiol Scand* 2003;47:732-738.

40. Rosseland LA, Helgesen KG, Breivik H, Stubhaug A. Moderate-to-severe pain after knee arthroscopy is relieved by intraarticular saline: A randomized controlled trial. *Anesth Analg* 2004;98:1546-1551.

41. Rosseland LA, Stubhaug A, Skoglund A, Breivik H. Intra-articular morphine for pain relief after knee arthroscopy. *Acta Anaesthesiol Scand* 1999;43:252-257.

42. Geutjens G, Hambidge JE. Analgesic effects of intraarticular bupivacaine after day-case arthroscopy. *Arthroscopy* 1994;10:299-300.

43. Morrow BC, Milligan KR, Murthy BV. Analgesia following day-case knee arthroscopy—The effect of piroxicam with or without bupivacaine infiltration. *Anesthesia* 1995;50:461-463.

44. Vranken JH, Vissers K, de Jongh R, HeylenR. Intraarticular sufentanil administration facilitates recovery after day-case knee arthroscopy. *Anesth Analg* 2001;92:625-628.

45. Henderson RC, Campion ER, DeMasi RA, Taft TN. Post arthroscopy analgesia with bupivacaine. A prospective, randomized, blinded evaluation. *Am J Sports Med* 1990;18:614-617.

46. Osborne D, Keene G. Pain relief after arthroscopic surgery of the knee: A prospective, randomized, and blinded assessment of bupivacaine and bupivacaine with adrenaline. *Arthroscopy* 1993;9:177-180.

47. Aasbo V, Raeder JC, Grogaard B, Roise O. No additional analgesic effect of intra-articular morphine or bupivacaine compared with placebo after elective knee arthroscopy. *Acta Anaesthesiol Scand* 1996;40:585-588.

48. Highgenboten CL, Jackson AW, Meske NB. Arthroscopy of the knee. Ten-day pain profiles and corticosteroids. *Am J Sports Med* 1993;21:503-506.

49. Reuben SS, Sklar J. Pain management in patients who undergo outpatient arthroscopic surgery of the knee. *J Bone Joint Surg Am* 2000;82:1754-1766.

50. Dye SF, Vaupel GL, Dye CC. Conscious neurosensory mapping of the internal structures of the human knee without intraarticular anesthesia. *Am J Sports Med* 1998;26:773-777.

51. Ritchie ED, Tong D, Chung F, Norris AM, Miniaci A, Vairavanathan SD. Suprascapular nerve block for postoperative pain relief in arthroscopic shoulder surgery: a new modality? *Anesth Analg* 1997;84:1306-1312.

52. Marret E, Gentili M, Bonnet MP, Bonnet F. Intra-articular ropivacaine 0.75% and bupivacaine 0.50% for analgesia after arthroscopic knee surgery: A randomized prospective study. *Arthroscopy* 2005;21:313-316.

53. Moiniche S, Mikkelsen S, Wetterslev J, Dahl JB. A systematic review of intra-articular local anesthesia for postoperative pain relief after arthroscopic knee surgery. *Reg Anesth Pain Med* 1999;24:430-437.

54. Gyrn JP, Olsen KS, Appelquist E, Chraemmer-Jorgensen B, Duus B, Berner Hansen L. Intra-articular bupivacaine plus adrenaline for arthroscopic surgery of the knee. *Acta Anaesthesiol Scand* 1992;36:643-646.

55. Meinig RP, Holtgrewe JL, Wiedel JD, Christie DB, Kestin KJ. Plasma bupivacaine levels following single dose intraarticular instillation for arthroscopy. *Am J Sports Med* 1988;16:295-300.

56. Boss AP, Maurer T, Seiler S, Aeschbach A, Hintermann B, Strebel S. Continuous subachromial bupivacaine infusion for postoperative analgesia after open acromioplasty and rotator cuff repair: Preliminary results. *J Shoulder Elbow Surg* 2004;13:630-634.

57. Stein C, Millan MJ, Shippenberg TS, Peter K, Herz A. Peripheral opioid receptors mediating antinociception in inflammation. Evidence for involvement of mu, delta and kappa receptors. *J Pharmacol Exp Ther* 1989;248:1269-1275.

58. Stein C, Yassouridis A. Peripheral morphine analgesia. *Pain* 1997;71:119-121.

59. Gupta A, Bodin L, Holmstrom B, Berggren L. A systematic review of the peripheral analgesic effects of intraarticular morphine. *Anesth Analg* 2001;93:761-770.

60. Stein C, Comisel K, Haimerl E, Yassouridis A, Lehrberger K, Herz A, Peter K. Analgesic effect of intraarticular morphine after arthroscopic knee surgery. *N Engl J Med* 1991;325:1123-1126.

61. Kalso E, Tramer MR, Carroll D, McQuay HJ, Moore RA. Pain relief from intra-articular morphine after knee surgery: A qualitative systematic review. *Pain* 1997;71:127-134.

62. Allen GC, St Amand MA, Lui AC, Johnson DH, Lindsay MP. Post arthroscopy analgesia with intraarticular bupivacaine/morphine. A randomized clinical trial. *Anesthesiology* 1993;79:475-480.

63. Rosseland LA. No evidence for analgesic effect of intra-articular morphine after knee arthroscopy: A qualitative systematic review. *Reg Anesth Pain Med* 2005;30:83-98.

64. Guler G, Karaoglu S, Akin A, Dogru K, Demir L, Madenoglu H, Boyaci A. When to inject analgesic agents intra-articularly in anterior cruciate ligament reconstruction: before or after tourniquet releasing. *Arthroscopy* 2004;20:918-921.

65. Gentili M, Juhel A, Bonnet F. Peripheral analgesic effect of intra-articular clonidine. *Pain* 1996;64:593-596.

66. Joshi W, Reuben SS, Kilaru PR, Sklar J, Maciolek H. Postoperative analgesia for outpatient arthroscopic knee surgery with intraarticular clonidine and/or morphine. *Anesth Analg* 2000;90:1102-1106.

67. Weitoft T, Uddenfeldt P. Importance of synovial fluid aspiration when injecting intra-articular corticosteroids. *Ann Rheum Dis* 2000;59:233-235.

68. Jackson DW, Evans NA, Thomas BM. Accuracy of needle placement into the intra-articular space of the knee. *J Bone Joint Surg Am* 2002;84:1522-1527.

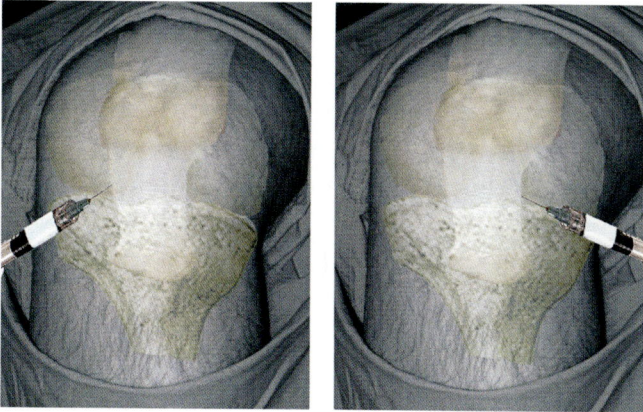

FIGURE 7A.1. Injection technique for knee, anterior. With the patient seated, the knee joint may be entered either just medial or lateral to the patellar tendon. Upon entering, the needle should be directed toward the center of the knee. To place the needle through the lateral portal, palpate the depression above Gerdy's tubercle and place the needle just above it. The inferior pole of the patella is commonly used as the upper landmark for this injection site. One detriment of this approach is placing the injection in the anterior fat pad of the knee.

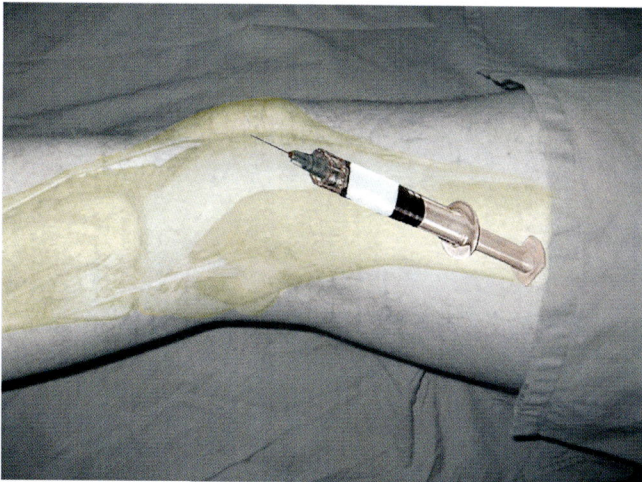

FIGURE 7A.2. Injection technique for knee, lateral. With the knee fully extended, the needle is placed beneath either the superior and medial or lateral knee. This position avoids entering the anterior fat pad of the knee. Care should be taken not to impact the articular cartilage.

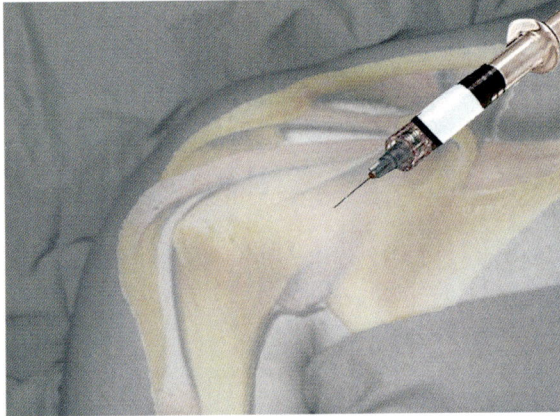

FIGURE 7A.3. Injection technique for shoulder, glenohumeral, anterior approach. Position the needle just medial to the head of the humerus and 1 cm lateral to the coracoid process. The needle is directed posteriorly and slightly superiorly and laterally.

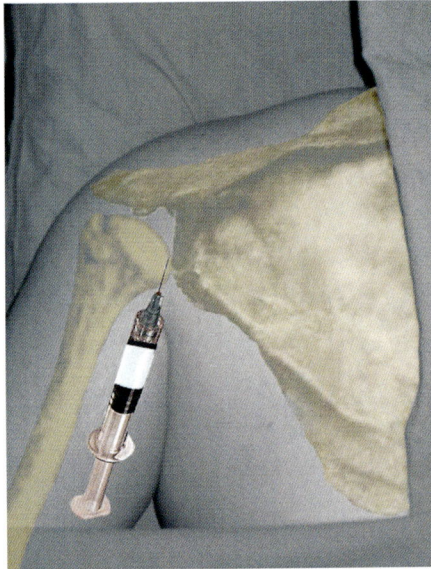

FIGURE 7A.4. Injection technique for shoulder, glenohumeral, posterior approach. The needle should be inserted 2 to 3 cm inferior to the poster lateral corner of the acromion. Palpate the coracoid as you insert the needle. Direct the needle anteriorly toward the coracoid process.

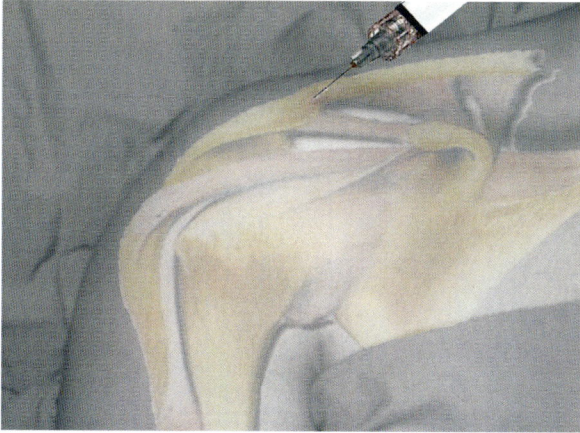

FIGURE 7A.5. Injection technique for shoulder, acromioclavicular. Patients are placed in the supine or seated position with the affected arm resting comfortably at their side. The AC joint is identified by palpating the clavicle from medial to lateral. At its most lateral point a slight depression will be felt at the joint articulation. The needle is inserted from a superior and anterior position into the AC joint.

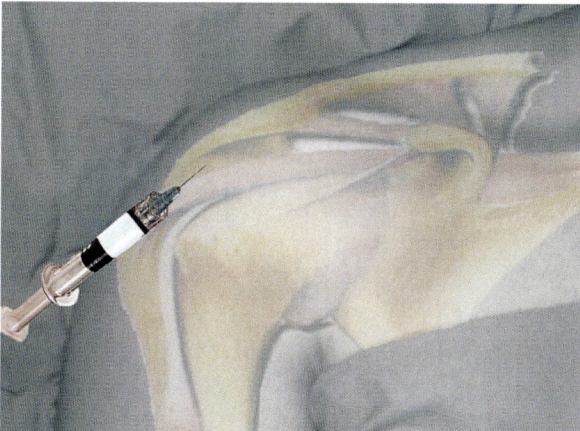

FIGURE 7A.6. Injection technique for shoulder, subachromial injection. This injection is best performed in a seated position so as to allow gravity to pull the arm and humeral head away from the acromion. The distal, lateral, and posterior edges of the acromion are palpated. It is sometimes helpful to mark these with a skin marker. The needle is inserted just inferior to the posterolateral edge of the acromion.

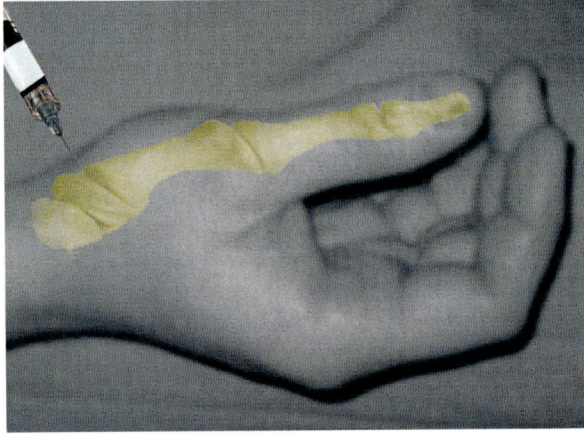

FIGURE 7A.7. Injection technique for first carpometacarpal joint. Move the thumb up and down while palpating the base of the metacarpal. The needle is placed just proximal to the first metacarpal on the extensor surface. Be sure to avoid the radial artery and the extensor pollicis tendons.

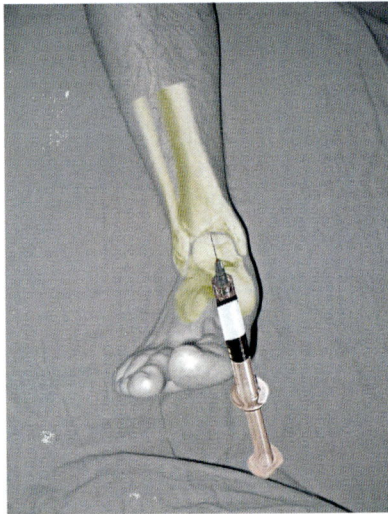

FIGURE 7A.8. Injection technique for ankle. Palpate between the dorsum of the foot between the medial border of the tibialis anterior tendon and the anterior border of the medial malleolus. Feel for the distal edge of the tibia and insert the needle within these landmarks. Advance the needle in a posterolateral direction.

Chapter 7B

Nerve Blocks

Elizabeth Demers
William Lavelle
Lori Lavelle

INTRODUCTION

Peripheral nerve blocks have been utilized in various pain management modalities. These include the diagnosis and treatment of chronic pain, intraoperative anesthesia, and postoperative pain control. Techniques of peripheral nerve blockade were described as early as the 1884, when Halsted and Hall described cocaine injections into peripheral nerves.[1,2] In the early 1900s, Heinrich F. W. Braun utilized epinephrine as an additive to local anesthetics to prolong the action of drugs.[3] The French surgeon Gaston Labat published the first definitive text on regional anesthesia while teaching his techniques in the 1920s at the Mayo Clinic.[4] Since that time, regional anesthesia continues to advance with new localization techniques and increased choices in anesthetic agents. Peripheral nerve blockade is an established element of comprehensive anesthetic care.[5]

UPPER EXTREMITY BLOCKS

Upper extremity regional anesthesia requires knowledge of the brachial plexus anatomy in order to optimize needle placement and determine the appropriate block required for pain control of a specific region.[6] (See Figures 7B.1 and 7B.2.)

Clinical Management of Bone and Joint Pain
© 2007 by The Haworth Press, Inc. All rights reserved.
doi:10.1300/5771_09

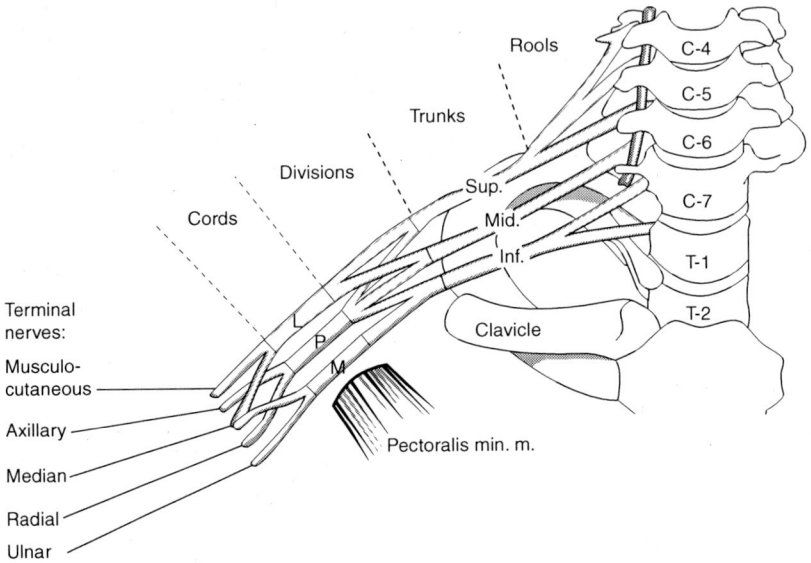

FIGURE 7B.1. Brachial plexus anatomy.

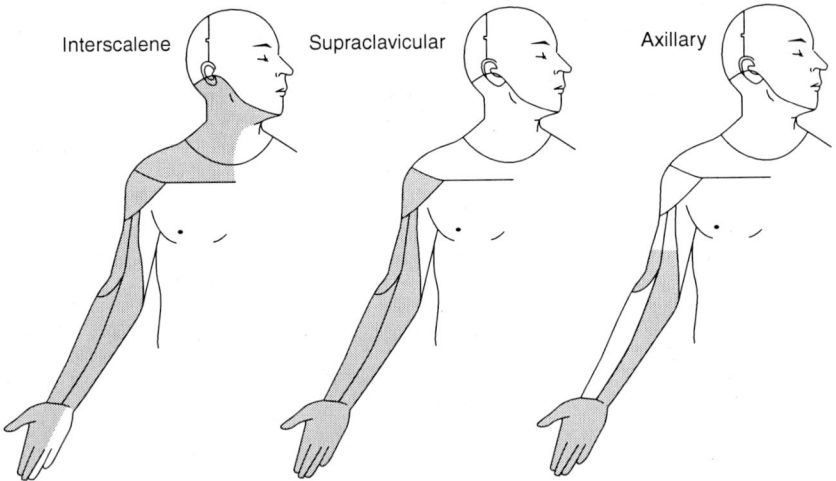

FIGURE 7B.2. Three upper extremity blocks (interscalene, supraclavicular, and axillary) and the regions affected by each.

Brachial Plexus Anatomy

The brachial plexus is a complex network of nerves which arise from the ventral rami of the fifth, sixth, seventh, and eighth cervical nerves (C5 to C8), as well as the first thoracic nerve (T1), with variable contributors including the fourth cervical (C4) and second thoracic nerve (T2).[7] There are seven major described configurations of the brachial plexus, with none having more than 57 percent representation.[8]

The classic schematic description of the brachial plexus provides useful anatomical knowledge for block insertion, keeping in mind that the anatomy may vary. The C5 and T1 rami unite to form three trunks in the space between the anterior and middle scalene muscles. The C5 and C6 rami unite to form the superior trunk, the C7 ramus becomes the middle trunk, and the C8 and T1 rami unite forming the inferior trunk. The roots and trunks of the brachial plexus can be accessed via the interscalene groove, a palpable depression between the anterior and middle scalene muscles. At the border of the first rib, the tree trunks separate into the anterior and posterior divisions. Three cords are formed as the divisions reorganize. The lateral cord is formed as the anterior divisions of the superior and middle trunks unite, the posterior cord is formed from all the posterior divisions of all three trunks, and the medial cord is formed from the anterior division of the inferior trunk. At the lateral border of the pectoralis minor, the three cords divide to give rise to the terminal branches of the plexus.[9]

In addition to the anatomy of the nerves at this level, vascular structures have clinical importance as both landmarks and structure to avoid. The vertebral artery enters a bony canal formed by the transverse process of C6. The cervical nerve roots course immediately posterior to the vertebral artery, which poses a potential site for intravascular injection. The external jugular vein overlies the interscalene groove at approximately C6, which can serve as a basic anatomic landmark.[8] The subclavian artery lies in close proximity to the brachial plexus at the level of the first rib. Vascular positions may be altered by arm position or external pressure applied during the placement of a nerve block.

The nerves of the upper extremity have been approached at every anatomic division of the brachial plexus.[10] The sensory innervation of the arm is important to understand to determine which level or nerves need to be blocked for adequate pain control.[6]

Interscalene Block

Clinical Uses

The principal use of the interscalene block is for surgery of the shoulder. Local anesthetic spread includes the upper and middle trunks of the brachial plexus.[11] Interscalene nerve blocks may spare the C8-T1 nerve distribution.

Placement Technique

The interscalene block relies on the correct identification of the interscalene groove, between the anterior and middle scalene muscles. Surface landmarks to assist in correct identification of the groove include the clavicle, the posterior border of the clavicular hear of the sternocleidomastoid muscle (SCM), and the external jugular vein. This block is most easily performed with the patient in the supine position with the head turned away from the side of the intended block. At the level of the cricoid cartilage, the posterior border of the SCM should be palpated. This is facilitated by requesting the patient to lift his or her head. Then the palpating fingers should slowly be moved posteriolaterally until they fall into the interscalene groove. At this level, the external jugular vein may overlie the intersection although it is not always a reliable landmark. For needle placement, the use of a nerve stimulator with approximately 0.8 mA, or elicitation of a paresthesia is recommended. Also, an ultrasound probe may be useful in the identification of the brachial plexus. A 22- to 25-gauge 4 cm needle should be advanced in a slight caudal direction to prevent inadvertent insertion of the needle toward the spinal cord. The typical depth of insertion is 1 to 2 cm. Once the appropriate response is elicited, 35 to 40 ml of local anesthetic solution should be injected with intermittent aspirations. Because motor blockage precedes sensory blockade, after 2 to 3 min the patient should not be able to lift his or her shoulder from the table. Within 20 min, surgical anesthesia should be achieved.[12-14]

Side Effects/Complications

Diaphragmatic paralysis is caused by an ipsilateral nerve blockade and occurs in 100 percent of the patients undergoing this nerve block.[15]

The interscalene block should be avoided in patients with severe chronic respiratory disease or who use their accessory muscles of respiration while breathing at rest.

The risk of a pneumothorax exists as the dome of the pleura lies anteromedial to the inferior trunk of the brachial plexus. The risk of pneumothorax is low when the needle is correctly placed at the C5-C6 level.[16]

Severe hypotension or bradycardia have been reported and are presumed to be caused by stimulation of the intracardiac mechanoreceptors be decreased venous return.[17]

Total spinal anesthesia can occur with this block. Nerve stimulation should not be seen with current intensities of less than 0.2 mA to avoid injection into the dural sleeve. Also, the needle should not be directed in a cephalad direction.

As with all nerve blocks, the risk of hematoma, vascular puncture, local anesthetic toxicity, and nerve injury exist.

Supraclavicular Block

Clinical Uses

The supraclavicular block is indicated for surgeries of the elbow, forearm, and hand.[6] The blockade is performed at the level when the brachial plexus is in its most compact from, the level of the proximal divisions or the trunk level. Advantages of this technique including the rapid onset of the sensory blockade and complete and reliable anesthesia for surgery are explained by the compactness of the nerve bundle at this level.[18] This block is also useful because it can be performed with the patient's arm in any position.

Technique

The supraclavicular block is performed where the neurovascular bundle lies inferior to the clavicle approximately at its midpoint. The first rib acts as a medial barrier to prevent the needle from reaching the pleural dome. The patient should be positioned supine with his or her head facing the side away from the block. With the classic insertion technique, the interscalene groove should be identified, as mentioned earlier, and the location should be noted, approximately 1 to 2 cm posterior to the midpoint of the clavicle. This position can be confirmed with the palpation of the subclavian artery at this point. A 22-gauge 4 cm should be directed in a caudad, medial, and posterior direction. Elicitation of a nerve twitch or paresthesia should be encountered, or the position of the needle should be visualized with an ultrasound probe. If the first rib is contacted, the needle should be walked anteriorly and posteriorly along the plexus until the subclavian artery or plexus is identified. The typical depth of insertion is 3 to 4 cm. Once the appropriate response is elicited, 20 to 30 ml of local anesthetic solution should be injected with intermittent aspirations.[7]

Side Effects/Complications

The most common complication of a supraclavicular nerve blockade is a pneumothorax, with the incidence of 0.5 to 6 percent. The initial symptoms of this complication include cough, dyspnea, and pleuritic chest pain. Frequently the onset of symptoms may be delayed and may not present until 24 hours post procedure.

Phrenic nerve blockade occurs in 40 to 60 percent of cases, thus rendering the technique less valuable in patients with known respiratory compromise. Horner's syndrome may also occur with this blockade.[7]

The supraclavicular block carries a high risk of hematoma and vascular puncture, as the subclavian artery lies adjacent to the brachial plexus at this point.[19] Local anesthetic toxicity and nerve injury are possible complications.

Infraclavicular Block

Clinical Uses

The infraclavicular nerve block is indicated for surgery of the hand and arm. The infraclavicular block has been shown to provide more consistent anesthesia over the distribution of the musculocutaneous and axillay nerves than did the axillary block, albiet with a longer time to onset.[6] The blockade occurs at the level of the cords in the infraclavicular fossa, anatomically where the pectoralis minor and major muscles lie anteriorly, the ribs lie medially, the clavicle and the coracoid process lie superiorly, and the humerus lies laterally.[13]

Technique

The brachial plexus is blocked below the level of the clavicle in the proximity of the coracoid process. The patient should be positioned supine with the head turned to the opposite side and the ipsilateral arm abducted to a 90° angle. Landmarks should be identified and marked, including:

1. Medial head of the clavicle
2. Coracoid process
3. Acromioclavicular joint
4. Midpoint of the clavicle between the acromion and the sternal head of the clavicle

The needle insertion should be 3 cm caudal to the midpoint of a line connecting the medial clavicular head and the coracoid process. A 22-gauge 10 cm needle should be inserted at a 45° angle and advanced parallel to the line connecting the medial clavicular head and the coracoid. This technique should be performed with a nerve stimulator or ultrasound, as there are no vascular landmarks to guide the position of the needle. The nerve stimulator should initially be set at 1.5 mA and a pectoralis twitch will be elicited, then the nerve stimulator should be lowered to 1.0 mA. After the pectoralis stimulation fades the needle should be advanced slowly and twitches in the hand should be seen. A biceps or deltoid twitch should not be accepted as the musculocutaneous and axillary nerves may leave the brachial plexus before the coracoid process. A 20 to 30 ml injection of local anesthetic should be performed with intermittent aspirations during the injection after an appropriate nerve response is seen.[12,20,21]

Side Effects/Complications

The most common complication for the infraclavicular block is intravascular injection because of the blind approach to the plexus. An often feared but rare complication is a pneumothorax. This is avoided by ensuring that the needle is directed away from the chest cavity. Local anesthetic toxicity and nerve injury are also possible complications.

Axillary Block

Clinical Uses

The axillary nerve block is the most widely used, studied, and modified approach to the brachial plexus. It is used for hand and forearm surgeries, although it may require supplementation with a musculocutaneous nerve block, typically performed with a separate injection near the belly of the coracobrachialis.[12] This is the most popular approach due to its ease of performance, reliability, and low risk for complications.[22]

Technique

The axillary block anesthetizes the brachial plexus around the axillary artery. Notably, the neurovascular bundle is compartmental, and shorter onsets to block and improved reliability have been seen with multiple injections.[23] Anatomically, the median nerve is superior to the artery, the ulnar nerve is inferior, and the radial nerve is posterior and somewhat lateral to the axillary artery. The patient should be placed supine with the arm abducted 90° and the forearm with external rotation. The axillary artery is the main landmark and a line can be drawn along its course from the lower axilla as proximally as possible. The artery should be fixed against the humerus proximally. The nerves can be localized using several techniques for identification:

1. *Paresthesias:* A 25-gauge 2 cm needle is advanced slowly at a 45° angle cephalad toward the axillary pulse until a paresthesia is obtained, usually a depth of about 1 to 2 cm. A 35 to 50 ml dose of local anesthetic should be injected. This technique has an 85-90 percent success rate.
2. *Transarterial approach:* A 25-gauge 2 cm needle is advance toward the axillary artery until bright red blood is aspirated during continuous advancement. The needle should then be advanced through the wall of the artery until no blood is aspirated. The needle tip should lie about 1 mm posterior to the wall of the artery. A 40 to 50 ml local anesthetic injection should be given in 5 ml increments with aspirations in the interim. Alternatively, after 20 ml is injected, the needle can be repositioned a second

time at the posterior aspect of the artery and the remaining 20 ml can be injected. This technique allows confirmation of the needle tip in close proximity to the vessel wall. The transarterial technique has an approximately 100 percent success rate.

3. *Nerve stimulator for needle position identification:* This technique does not require the elicitation of paresthesias, which may reduce the risk of nerve damage.[26] With an insulated needle, the axillary pulse is felt and approached slowly with the nerve stimulator set to 0.5 to 1.0 mA. Upon confirmation of hand twitching, usually a depth of 1 to 2 cm, the injection should proceed. A 35 to 50 ml dose of local anesthetic should be injected. The biceps twitch should not be accepted as it represents musculocutaneous nerve stimulation.[24,25]

Side Effects/Complications

Nerve injury and local anesthetic toxicity are the most significant complications associated with the axillary approach. Hematomas and infection are rare complications. This block does not carry risk of central neural blockade or pneumothorax as do the other approaches to the brachial plexus.[6]

LOWER EXTREMITY NERVE BLOCKS

Similar to upper extremity regional anesthesia, lower extremity nerve blocks require knowledge of the anatomy of the lumbosacral plexus. Unlike the compact anatomy seen in the upper extremity, however, the lower extremity consists of a nerve supply that is widely separated as it enters the thigh. Anatomically, the lumbar plexus and sacral plexus represent two distinct entities.[26] With the exception of a small cutaneous portion of the buttock, the innervation of the entire lower extremity is derived entirely from the lumbosacral plexus.[27]

Lumbar Plexus Anatomy

The lumbar plexus supplies the nerves to the muscles of the anterior and medial thigh. It arises from the ventral rami of the twelfth thoracic nerve (T12), as well as the first, second, third, and fourth lumbar nerves

(L1-4). The plexus lies within the psoas compartment between the psoas major and the quadratus lumborum.[9] At the border of the psoas compartment, it branches into the iliohypogastric, ilioinguinal, genitofemoral, lateral femoral cutaneous, femoral, and obturator nerves as it emerges laterally, medially, and anteriorly.[27] L2-4 primarily innervate the anterior and medial thigh, with the anterior divisions forming the obturator nerve and the posterior divisions forming the femoral nerve. The posterior divisions of L2-3 also form the lateral femoral cutaneous nerve.

Sacral Plexus Anatomy

The muscles of the buttocks, posterior thigh, and the muscles below the knee are all supplied by the nerves of the sacral plexus. The sacral plexus is produced by the joining of the fourth and fifth lumbar nerves (L4-5) and the first and second sacral nerves (S1-2).[28] Five of the 12 branches of the sacral plexus innervate the pelvis, and the remaining 7 branches emerge from the pelvis to innervate the buttock and lower extremity. The most important branches of the sacral plexus are the sciatic nerve and the posterior cutaneous nerve.[7]

Psoas Compartment Block

Clinical Uses

The psoas compartment block offers a single-shot injection technique to anesthetize the entire lumber plexus, with consistent anesthesia in the distribution of the femoral, lateral femoral cutaneous, and obturator nerves. It is useful for postoperative pain control in patient undergoing hip and knee surgery. It is also used for anterior thigh surgery anesthesia and in the treatment of chronic hip pain.[29] When combined with a sciatic block, this can be used for nerve block to the entire lower extremity.

Technique

The patient should be placed in the lateral position, operative side up, with the hips flexed. A line is drawn across bilateral iliac crests, at the L4 level. The needle entry point should be 1 cm cephalad to the intercristal line at a point two-thirds the distance from the midline to the posterior superior iliac spine line.[27] At this point, the lumbar plexus lies at a depth of approximately 8 cm in men and 7 cm in women, with the depth correlating with the patient's gender and body mass index. The distance from the transverse process to the lumbar plexus remains consistent at a distance of less than 2 cm. Therefore, contacting the transverse process provides a consistent landmark for this block. A 21-gauge 10 cm needle should be directed perpendicularly through the entry point until the transverse process of L4 is contacted.[30] Then the needle should be carefully advance under the transverse process until quadriceps femoris twitches are obtained. Approximately 30 ml of anesthetic solution should be injected when the needle is in the proper position.

Complications

The deep needle placement in the psoas compartment block increases the risk of epidural, subarachnoid, or intravascular anesthetic injections. Epidural spread has been described in 9 to 16 percent of adults receiving this block[31,32] and in over 90 percent of children.[33] Renal hematoma, pneumocele, total spinal, intraabdominal injection, and intravertebral disc injections are associated with excessive needle depth.[34-36]

A side effect from the extravasation of the local anesthetic in the region is the development of a sympathetic block. This may decrease the desire to perform this block, as the benefit of this block over a spinal anesthetic is prevention of a sympathectomy.

Femoral Nerve Block

Clinical Uses

The femoral nerve supplies the anterior muscles of the thigh and the overlying skin from the inguinal ligament to the knee.[7] Indications for this technique include anesthesia for knee arthroscopy procedures, femoral shaft fracture repair, ACL reconstruction, quadriceps muscle biopsies, and TKA postoperative pain control. Chelly et al. found a 20 percent decrease in length of stay in patients with continuous femoral nerve blocks for major knee surgery versus IV PCA narcotics.[37]

It must be typically used in conjunction with an obturator and lateral femoral cutaneous nerve block for complete anesthesia during knee surgeries. This block has a very high success rate and is a low-risk technique that is simple to perform.

Technique

The femoral nerve enters the thigh posterior to the inguinal ligament and lateral and slightly deeper than the femoral artery. As the nerve passes into the thigh, it divides into an anterior and posterior division ,and then quickly divides into many branches. At the level of the inguinal ligament the femoral nerve lies beneath the dense fascial planes of the fascia lata and fascia iliaca.[27] With the patient supine, the ilioinguinal ligament should be identified with a line from the anterior superior iliac spine and the pubic tubercle. The femoral crease should be marked and the femoral arterial pulse should be identified and marked. A 22-gauge 4 cm needle should be inserted immediately lateral to the femoral artery. The correct position of the needle can be determined with the sensation of two "pops" as the fascia are traversed, the elicitation of paresthesias, or through nerve stimulation of the quadriceps muscle (the patellar twitch) with 0.2 to 0.5 mA. A sartorius muscle twitch should not be considered ideal position as the femoral nerve anterior branch may have left the femoral sheath at this point. The needle should be directed more laterally and slightly deeper.[38] When the needle is determined to be in ideal position, approximately 20 ml of local anesthetic should be injected with intermittent needle aspiration.[7]

Side Effects/Complications

Possible complications of a femoral nerve block include hematoma and intravascular injection because of the close proximity to the femoral artery. The femoral artery is anatomically separated from the femoral nerve and lies approximately 1 cm from the nerve. Care should be taken to avoid redirecting the needle medially in order to avoid this complication. This block should be avoided in patients with femoral vascular grafts. Nerve damage and infection are rare complications.

Obturator Nerve Block

Clinical Uses

The obturator nerve innervates the adductor compartment of the thigh, including the external obturator, the adductor magnus muscles, and the knee.[27] Blockade of the obturator nerve is clinically useful in treating or diagnosing adductor spasm in patients with cerebral palsy or other muscle or neurologic diseases. It can also assist in diagnosis of hip pain.[7] Typically, the obturator nerve block is used to supplement the sciatic, femoral, and lateral femoral cutaneous nerve blocks on operations above the knee.

Technique

It leaves the psoas compartment at its medial border and passes along the side wall of the pelvis, exiting into the thigh through the obturator foramen. The patient is positioned supine, and a 22-gauge 8 to 10 cm needle is introduced perpendicularly to the skin 1 to 2 cm below and lateral to the pubic tubercle. It is advanced in a slightly medial direction until the pubic ramus is contacted, at approximately 2 to 4 cm. The needle is then withdrawn and redirected cephalad until it passes through the obturator canal. A local anesthetic volume of 10 to 15 ml is injected after negative aspiration.

Side Effects/Complications

Complications are rare but include damage to neural and vascular structures within the obturator canal. Hematoma, intravascular injection, and nerve damage are possible complications.

Sciatic Nerve Block

Clinical Uses

The sciatic nerve is a combination of two trunks, the tibial and the common peroneal, initially bound together with connective tissue.[27] The tibial trunk comprises ventral branches of the anterior rami from L4-S3, and the common peroneal trunk is derived from the dorsal branches of the anterior rami from L4-S3. At or above the level of the popliteal fossa, these trunks separate with the tibial nerve passing medially and the common peroneal passing laterally.[7] Because of its large distribution, a sciatic nerve block can be used for any procedure below the knee not requiring a tourniquet. Frequently, it is used in conjunction with a saphenous or femoral nerve block in these procedures. This block should not cause a sympathectomy and is therefore useful if hemodynamic stability is required.

Technique

The sciatic nerve exits the pelvis through the greater sciatic notch below the piriformis muscle. As it descends the thigh it lies posterior to the greater trochanter of the femur, and then lies on the posterior surface of the adductor magnus in the posterior medial thigh compartment.[8] The classic technique of Labat for the sciatic nerve block is a posterior approach with the patient positioned laterally with a slight forward tilt. The needle insertion point is 4 cm distal perpendicularly to the midpoint of a line connecting the posterior superior iliac spine and the greater trochanter of the femur.[39,40] A 22-gauge 10 to 12 cm needle should be inserted perpendicularly until sciatic nerve stimulation is observed with twitching of the hamstrings, calf, foot, or toes with a current of 0.2 to 0.5 mA. This typically is at a depth of about 5 to 8 cm. Approximately 20 ml of local anesthetic should be injected with intermittent aspirations.

The sciatic nerve can also be approached from an anterior location medial to the lesser trochanter of the femur,[41] medial location at the level of the lesser trochanter,[42] or posteriorly or laterally at or above the popliteal fossa. A popliteal fossa approach to the sciatic nerve is chiefly used in foot and ankle surgeries.[43-45] In order to block the sciatic nerve before its division at this level, the needle entry point should be at least 7 to 10 cm above the popliteal crease.[43] A 22-gauge 5 cm needle should be inserted 7 to 10 cm above the popliteal crease at a point 1 cm lateral to the line bisecting the apex and base of a triangle formed by the biceps and semimembranosus. The needle is advanced at a 45° angle until a paresthesia or nerve stimulation is attained. Alternatively, ultrasound can be used to visualize correct needle placement. After correct needle position, 30 ml of local anesthetic can be injected with intermittent aspirations. The popliteal approach has a 95 percent success rate.[43,46]

Side Effects/Complications

The classic sciatic nerve block can be technically difficult and painful for the patient. Hematoma formation is possible as well as nerve damage. A popliteal block may cause nerve damage. Intravascular injection into any of the vascular structures in the popliteal fossa may occur.[7]

Ankle

Clinical Uses

The five nerves that innervate the foot can all be blocked at the level of the ankle. Four of these nerves are terminal branches of the sciatic nerve: the posterior tibial, sural, superficial peroneal, and deep peroneal. The saphenous nerve is a cutaneous branch of the femoral nerve. An ankle block is highly effective in providing anesthesia for all podiatric surgeries and foot and toe debridement and amputations.

Technique

An ankle block involves the block of two deep nerves, the posterior tibial and deep peroneal, as well as three superficial nerves, the saphenous, sural, and superficial peroneal.

1. Blockade of the posterior tibial nerve: A 25-gauge 3 cm needle is inserted posterolaterally to the posterior tibial artery pulse. If a paresthesia is elicited, 3 to 4 ml of local anesthetic should be injected. If no paresthesia is elicited, 7 to 10 ml of local anesthetic should be injected.
2. Blockade of the deep peroneal nerve: The deep peroneal nerve runs below the layers o the peroneus longus, extensor digitorum longus, and extensor hallicus longus toward the front of the leg. The deep peroneal is located lateral to the tendon of the extensor hallicus longus at the level of the ankle. A 25-gauge 3 cm needle is inserted at this point and advanced until bone is touched. The needle should be withdrawn 1 to 2 mm and 2 to 3 ml of local anesthetic should be injected.
3. Blockade of the superficial nerves (saphenous, sural, and superficial peroneal): Blockade of these nerves is accomplished with a circumferential injection of local anesthetic.

Side Effects/Complications

There are almost no systemic complications that can be caused in the performance of an ankle block. As with all nerve blocks, possible complications include hematoma, vascular puncture, and nerve injury.[46,47]

Sympathetic Nerve Blocks

Sympathetic nerve blocks are typically utilized in the chronic pain management setting in order to establish a diagnosis of sympathetically mediated pain, such as in complex regional pain syndrome (CRPS). The effects of the local anesthetic injections, in these cases, can last for an extended duration as the block resets the sympathetic nervous tone to a normal state. Sympathetic blocks are also useful in increasing regional blood flow for patients with Reynaud's disease and peripheral vascular disease. Visceral pain can be alleviated with a sympathetic blockade, as in the case of a celiac plexus block.

Stellate Ganglion Block

Clinical Uses

The sympathetic innervations of the face and upper extremity pass through the stellate ganglion. Indications for a stellate ganglion block are for relief of sympathetic dystrophies of the upper extremity and for improvement of vascular flow.[7] Pain syndromes that can be alleviated or improved with a stellate ganglion block include CRPS I and II, postherpetic neuralgia, and phantom limb pain. Blood flow is improved to the upper extremity with the block in patients with Reynaud's disease, scleroderma, vasospasm, and vascular trauma. Patients who have undergone limb reimplantations and vascular reconstructions also benefit from stellate ganglion blocks.[48,49]

Technique

The stellate ganglion is formed by the fusion of the inferior cervical and first thoracic ganglion at the level of the vertebral body of C7. The patient should be positioned supine with slight extension of the neck and the head slightly rotated to the side opposite the block. Chassaignac's tubercle, the prominent transverse process of C6, should be located, with the sternocleidomastoid muscle and carotid sheath laterally and the trachea medially. With slight retraction of the sternocleidomastoid and the carotid sheath laterally, a 22-gauge 4 cm needle should be inserted at the point directly over the Chaissaignac tubercle in a perpendicular direction. After contacting the transverse process of C6, the needle should be withdrawn 1 to 2 mm and fixed. Proper needle placement can be confirmed with image-guided techniques such as CT or fluroscopy. After aspiration, 10 to 12 ml of local anesthetic should be injected carefully with intermittent aspiration. The onset of Horner's syndrome, nasal stuffiness, increased skin temperature, and vasodilation are signs of a successful blockade.[49]

Side Effects/Complications

Complications include intravascular injection, particularly due to carotid or internal jugular vein trauma. Local anesthetic toxicity can also be seen with intravascular injection into these vessels and seizures are possible. The local anesthetic can also spread locally causing hoarseness, difficulty swallowing, weakness of the upper extremity, and epidural and intrathecal blocks.[50]

TECHNIQUES FOR LOCALIZATION OF A NERVE

Regional nerve blocks aim to deliver a precise dosage of medication at a target nerve without incurring any risk of damage to the nerve or its surrounding structures.[52] Many techniques for the identification of the anatomy and location of the local anesthetic injection have been utilized. Knowledge of the anatomy as described above places the needle in the general location and allows avoidance of nearby structures. Facial "pops," elicitation of paresthesias, transarterial approaches, electrical stimulation, ultrasound, fluoroscopy, MRI, and CT have been used for nerve localization.

Continuous Catheter

Catheter placement has been performed with nerve blocks and provides longer-term pain relief. Catheters in the brachial plexus are particularly useful for chronic upper extremity pain control, CRPS, digit or upper extremity reimplantation, and elbow arthroplasty.[53] There are limited studies on the benefits of brachial plexus catheters. Nerve catheters have been placed for continuous blockade of the psoas compartment, sciatic nerve, femoral nerve, and popliteal fossa.[30,54,55] Continuous lower extremity nerve blockade has been demonstrated to provide better pain relief and fewer side effects after joint replacement.[55,56]

Choice of Anesthetic

The choice of local anesthetic depends on the duration of the surgical procedure. Blockade can last up to 24 hours with agents like bupivacaine and ropivacaine. High concentrations of local anesthetics are not recommended. Also, low concentrations of local anesthetics may not provide complete motor blockade. A common additive to the local anesthetic solution is a vasoconstrictor, such as epinephrine.[7] Blocks in areas with terminal blood supply, such as the digits, should avoid the usage of epinephrine. Clonidine, opioids, and ketamine have also been reported to enhance peripheral nerve blockade.[6]

REFERENCES

1. Halstead WS. Practical comments on the use and abuse of cocaine: Suggested by its invariably successful employment in more than a thousand surgical operations. *N Y Med J* 1885;42:294.

2. Hall RJ. Hydrochlorate of cocaine. *N Y Med J* 1884;40:643-646.

3. Braun H. *Local Anesthesia: Its Scientific Basis and Practical Use*, 3rd ed. Philadelphia, Lea and Febiger, 1914.

4. Labat G. *Regional Anesthesia: Its Technical and Clinical Application*. Philadelphia, WB Saunders, 1922.

5. Wedel DJ. Regional anesthesia and pain management: Reviewing the past decade and predicting the future. *Anesth Analg* 2000;90:1244-1245.

6. Neal, JM, Hebl JR, Gerancher JC, Hogan QH. Brachial plexus anesthesia: Eessentials of our current understanding. *Reg Anesth Pain Med* 2002;27:402-428.

7. Wedel DJ. Nerve blocks. In: Miller RD, Ed. *Miller's Anesthesia*, 6th ed. Churchill Livingstone Inc, Philadelphia, 2005, pp. 1685-1717.

8. Kerr AT. The brachial plexus of nerves in man, the variations in its formation and branches. *Am J Anat* 1918;23:285-395.

9. Brown DL. *Atlas of Regional Anesthesia*. 2nd ed. Philadelphia: W. B. Saunders; 1999.

10. Thompson GE, Brown DL. The common nerve blocks. In: Nunn JF, Utting JE, Brown BR, Eds. *General Anaesthesia*. 5th ed. London: Butterworths; 1989, pp. 1068-1069.

11. Lanz E, Theiss D, Jankovic D. The extent of blockade following various techniques of brachial plexus block. *Anesth Analg* 1983;62:55-58.

12. Brown DL, Bridenbaugh LD. The upper extremity: Somatic block. In: Cousins MJ, Bridenbaugh PO, Eds., *Neuronal Blockade in Clinical Anesthesia and Management of Pain*. Philadelphia, J.B. Lippincott-Raven Publishers, 1988, pp. 345-371

13. Chelly JE. *Peripheral Nerve Blocks. A Color Atlas*. Philadelphia, Lippincott, 1999.

14. Long TR, Wass CT, Burkle CM. Perioperative interscalene blockade: An overview of its history and current clinical use. *J Clin Anesth* 2002;14:546-556.

15. Urmey WF, Talts KH, Sharrock NE. One hundred percent incidence of hemidiaphragmatic paresis associated with interscalene brachial plexus anesthesia as diagnosed by ultrasonography. *Anesth Analg* 1991;72:498-503.

16. White JL. Catastrophic complications of interscalene nerve block. *Anesthesiology* 2001;95:1301.

17. Liguori GA, Kahn RL, Gordon J, Gordon MA, Urban MK. The use of metoprolol and glycopyrrolate to prevent hypotension/bradycardic Events during shoulder arthroscopy in the sitting position under interscalene block. *Anesth Analg* 1998;87:1320-1325.

18. Brown DL, Cahill DR, Bridenbaugh LD. Supraclavicular nerve block: anatomic analysis of a method to prevent pneumothorax. *Anesth Analg* 1993;76: 530-534.

19. Hickey R, Hoffman J, Ramamurthy S. Transarterial techniques are not effective for subclavian perivascular block. *Reg Anesth* 1990;15:245-249.

20. Maurer K, Ekatodramis G, Rentsch K, Borgeat A. Interscalene and infraclavicular block for bilateral distal radius fracture. *Anesth Analg* 2002;94:450-452.

21. Raj PP. Infraclavicular approaches to brachial plexus anesthesia. *Techniques in Reg Anesth and Pain Management* 1997;1:169-177.

22. deJong RH. Axillary block of the brachial plexus. *Anesthesiology* 1961; 22:215.

23. Thompson GE, Rorie DK. Functional anatomy of the brachial plexus sheaths. *Anesthesiology* 1983;59:117-122.

24. Selander D. Axillary plexus block: Paresthetic or perivascular. *Anesthesiology* 1987;66:726.

25. Hepp M, King R. Transarterial technique is significantly slower than the peripheral nerve stimulator technique in achieving successful block. *Reg Anesth Pain Med* 2000; 25:660.

26. Gray H. *Anatomy of the Human Body*. Philadelphia, PA: Lea & Fibiger; 1918.

27. Enneking FK, Chan V, Greger J, Hadzic A, Lang S, Horlocker TT. Lower-extremity peripheral nerve blockade: Essentials of our current understanding. *Reg Anesth Pain Med* 2005;30:4-35.

28. Snell RS (Ed). *Clinical Anatomy for Medical Students*, 2nd ed. Boston: Little Brown and Company, 1981, pp. 272, 479, 492.

29. Goroszeniuk T, di Vadi PP. Repeated psoas compartment blocks for the management of long-standing hip pain. *Reg Anesth Pain Med* 2001;26:376-378.

30. Capdevila X, Macaire P, Dadure C, Choquet O, Biboulet P, Ryckwaert Y, D'Athis F. Continuous psoas compartment block for postoperative analgesia after total hip arthroplasty: New landmarks, technical guidelines and clinical evaluation. *Anesth Analg* 2002;94:1606-1613.

31. Farny J, Girard M, Drolet P. Posterior approach to the lumbar plexus combined with a sciatic nerve block using lidocaine. *Can J Anaesth* 1994;41:486-491.

32. Parkinson S, Mueller J, Little W, Bailey SL. Extent of blockade with various approaches to the lumbar plexus. *Anesth Analg* 1989;68:243-248.

33. Dalens B, Tanguy A, Vanneuville G. Lumbar plexus block in children: A comparison of two procedures in 50 patients. *Anesth Analg* 1988;67:750-758.

34. Aida S, Takahashi H, Shimoji K. Renal subcapsular hematoma after lumbar plexus block. *Anesthesiology* 1996;84:452-455.

35. Pousman RM, Mansoor Z, Sciard D. Total spinal anesthetic after continuous posterior lumbar plexus block. *Anesthesiology* 2003;98:1281-1282.

36. Reddy MB. Pneumocoele following psoas compartment block. *Anaesthesia* 2002;57:938-939.

37. Chelly JE, Greger J, Gebhard R, Coupe K, Clyburn TA, Buckle R, Criswell A. Continuous femoral blocks improve recovery and outcome of patients undergoing total knee arthroplasty. *J Arthroplasty* 2001;16:436-445.

38. Vloka JD, Hadzic A, Drobnik L, Ernest A, Reiss W, Thys DM. Anatomical landmarks for femoral nerve block: A comparison of four needle insertion sites. *Anesth Analg* 1999;89:1467-1470.

39. Labat G. *Regional Anesthesia: Its Technical and Clinical Application*. Philadelphia, PA: Saunders; 1922.

40. Bailey SL, Parkinson SK, Little WL, Simmerman SR. Sciatic nerve block: A comparison of single versus double injection technique. *Reg Anesth* 1994;19:9-13.

41. Kilpatrick AW, Coventry DM, Todd JG. A comparison of two approaches to sciatic nerve block. *Anaesthesia* 1992;47:155-157.

42. Chowdary K, Splinter W. Sciatic nerve block: A new approach. *Can J Anesth* 2003;50:A51(abstr).

43. Rorie DK, Byer DE, Nelson DO, Sittipong R, Johnson KA. Assessment of block of the sciatic nerve in the popliteal fossa. *Anesth Analg* 1980;59:371-376.

44. Hansen E, Eshelman MR, Cracchiolo A. Popliteal fossa neural blockade as the sole anesthetic technique for outpatient foot and ankle surgery. *Foot Ankle Int* 2000;21:38-44.

45. Rongstad K, Mann RA, Prieskorn D, Nichelson S, Horton G. Popliteal sciatic nerve block for postoperative analgesia. *Foot Ankle Int* 1996;17:378-382.

46. Myerson MS, Ruland CM, Allon SM. Regional anesthesia for foot and ankle surgery. *Foot Ankle* 1992;13:282-288.

47. Reilley TE, Gerhardt MA. Anesthesia for foot and ankle surgery. *Clin Podiatr Med Surg* 2002;19:125-147.

48. Lamer TJ. Sympathetic nerve blocks. In: Brown DL, Ed., *Regional Anesthesia and Analgesia*, WB Saunders Co., 1996, pp. 362-366.

49. Cousins MJ, Lofstrom JB. Sympathetic neural blockade of upper and lower extremity. In: Cousins MJ, Bridenbaugh PO, Eds., *Neural Blockade in Clinical Anesthesia and Management of Pain,* 2nd ed. Philadelphia, JB Lippincott, 1988, pp. 479-481.

50. Scott, DL, Ghia JN, Teeple E. Aphasia and hemiparesis following stellate ganglion block. *Anesth Analg* 1983;62:1038.

51. Kapacz DJ, Thompson GE. Celiac and hypogastric plexus, intercostal, interpleural, and peripheral blockade of the thorax and abdomen. In: Cousins MJ, Bridenbaugh PO, Eds., *Neural Blockade in Clinical Anesthesia and Management of Pain,* 2nd ed., Philadelphia, Lippincott-Raven, 1998, pp. 451-488.

52. Peterson MK, Millar FA, Sheppard DG. Ultrasound-guided nerve blocks. *Br J Anesth* 2002;88:621-624.

53. O'Driscoll SW, Giori NJ. Continuous passive motion (CPM): theory and principles of clinical application. *J Rehabil Res Dev* 2000;37179.

54. Ilfeld BM, Morey TE, Wang RD, Enneking FK. Continuous popliteal sciatic nerve block for postoperative pain control at home: A randomized, double blinded, placebo-controlled study. *Anesthesiology* 2002;97:959-965.

55. Singelyn FJ, Deyaert M, Joris D, Pendeville E, Gouverneur JM. Effects of intravenous patient-controlled analgesia with morphine, continuous epidural analgesia, and continuous "3-in-1" block on postoperative pain and knee rehabilitation after unilateral total knee arthroplasty. *Anesth Analg* 1998;87:88-92.

56. Capdevila X, Barthelet Y, Biboulet P, Ryckwaert Y, Rubenovitch J, d'Athis F. Effects of perioperative analgesic technique on the surgical outcome and duration of rehabilitation after major knee surgery. *Anesthesiology* 1999;91:8-15.

Chapter 8

Opioids

Gary McCleane

Historically the derivatives of the opium poppy, *Papaver somniferum,* have been the mainstay of pain management in patients of all ages. Since the isolation of morphine from opium in 1801 by Serturner and the synthesis of codeine by Robiquet in the 1850s, the range of available opioids has increased to the extent that the clinician is confronted by a bewildering array of agents active at the opioid receptors. Not only have the number of different opioids increased but so to have the available modes of administration: We now have oral and parenteral formulations, formulations that allow administration transdermally, intrathecally, rectally, via the oral mucous membrane and even by inhalation.

While the use of so called "weak opioids" such as codeine is extensive, the same is not true of the "strong" members of this class. It is universally accepted that strong opioids are useful in the management of acute pain and that related to terminal illness. However, their use in management of chronic pain not related to a terminal condition provokes much controversy. Consequently, any view expressed on their use reflects a personal opinion. In this chapter an outline of the use of opioids in the management of bone and joint pain will be given with a personal view given at the end.

The pharmacological effects of the opioid analgesics are derived from their complex interaction with three opioid receptor types (mu, delta, and kappa). These receptors are found in the periphery, at presynaptic and postsynaptic sites in the spinal cord dorsal horn, and in the brain stem, thalamus, and cortex, in what constitutes the ascending

Clinical Management of Bone and Joint Pain
© 2007 by The Haworth Press, Inc. All rights reserved.
doi:10.1300/5771_10

pain transmission system, as well as structures that comprise a descending inhibitory system that modulates pain at the level of the spinal cord. The cellular effects of opioids include a decrease in presynaptic transmitter release, hyperpolarization of postsynaptic elements, and disinhibition. The antagonistic and partial agonistic effect at the opioid receptors of individual opioids varies, and this at least partially explains differing analgesics efficacy and side-effect profiles of these individual members of this class. Combined with differing receptor affinities are ranges of serum half-life, lipid solubility, and presence of active metabolites, among many other factors, which contribute to the individual identities of members of this class.

As with so many other therapeutic agents, it is now clear that the activity of opioids is not solely related to their activity at one identifiable receptor type. It appears that opioids have a range of effects which includes a non-competitive antagonistic effect at the N-methyl-D-aspartate (NMDA) receptor and an action on calcium channels on nociception-specific neurons.

PAIN AND ITS RESPONSIVENESS TO OPIOIDS

It is universally accepted that strong opioids are efficacious in reducing acute pain such as that occurring after surgery. Weaker opioids are commonly used for pain of a more chronic nature, including neuropathic pain. In the case of postoperative pain, McQuay and colleagues (1996) have shown that paracetamol alone is significantly more efficacious than codeine alone, while paracetamol given alone is almost as good as the combination of paracetamol and codeine. Presumably, however, side effects produced by the addition of codeine are significantly greater than those incurred by the use of paracetamol alone.

In the use of strong opioids much controversy exists. While in the past many doubted the efficacy of strong opioids in the treatment of chronic pain conditions, the balance of evidence now suggests that strong opioids, be it morphine, fentanyl, or oxycontin, can reduce the pain of multiple sclerosis, osteoarthritis, rheumatoid arthritis, and even neuropathic pain for example. However, if these agents are to be used successfully, then there must be a willingness to titrate the dose of the drug used to gain maximum effect and an appreciation that there may be a need to further increase dose to achieve the same degree of pain relief as time progresses (tolerance). Along with this may be an increase in side effects as the dose escalates.

So the balance of evidence is that strong opioids are efficaous in a wide range of pain conditions, although the issue still exists as to whether in individual cases they are the best choice, given that there are so many other proven options available. A few comparative studies have been carried out that show, for example, that opioids and tricyclic antidepressants are both effective in reducing the pain of postherpetic neuralgia, and because they have differing modes of action, both can legitably be used either alone or in combination.

EFFECT OF PERIPHERAL APPLICATION OF OPIOIDS FOR ACUTE PAIN

Two systematic reviews have examined the effect of peripheral application of opioids in acute pain. In that performed by Picard and colleagues (1997) they examined the studies that investigated the peripheral application of opioids when compared with placebo, local anesthetics, or systemic opioids. They found no evidence of a clinically relevant peripheral analgesic effect of opioids in acute pain.

In the systematic review of Gupta and colleagues (2001) examining the peripheral analgesic effect of intra-articular morphine when given after arthroscopy, they found that intra-articular morphine had a definite analgesic effect, but the extent to which a systemic effect contributed was impossible to define.

Why then is there a disparity between these reviews. We have seen from the animal literature that opioid receptors are present in uninjured tissue, but at relatively low concentrations. It is only after sciatic nerve ligation or paw inflammation that opioid receptors migrate to the site of injury. Could it therefore be that, in the case of patients with acute pain, the increases in density of peripheral opioid receptors have not yet occurred and, consequently, insignificant extra pain relief occurs when the opioid is administered peripherally? In the case of patients undergoing arthroscopy, pre-existing pain and inflammation are often present and an indication for arthroscopy, and hence the density of peripheral opioid receptors in the knee joint will have already have been increased by this inflammation and so pain relief is more evident.

CODEINE

Codeine is a weak opioid analgesic, so called because of its weak affinity for the mu opioid receptor. It has a half-life of around 2.5 to 3 hours. Despite the widespread use of codeine either on its own or in combination with other agents, it is likely that unaltered codeine has little intrinsic analgesic effect. It relies on *in vivo* O-demethylation to morphine to become active as an analgesic. This process is mediated by a cytochrome P450 enzyme, CYP2D6. Approximately 5 to 10 percent of Caucasians lack CYP2D6 activity and are termed poor metabolizers, while the remainder are termed extensive metabolizers. Poor metabolizers can expect little analgesia from the use of codeine alone.

Experimentally, codeine has been shown to reduce a number of pain-related parameters. It can increase pressure pain tolerance, pain threshold, and pain summation threshold, suggesting that it may be useful in clinical pain management.

Clinical studies have investigated the effect of codeine on its own and in combination with acetaminophen and nonsteroidal anti-inflammatory drugs. They suggest that codeine does have an analgesic effect in a range of pain conditions. Given that these studies must have included "poor metabolizers," it is likely that the extent of analgesia observed overall may have been greater in individuals who were "extensive metabolizers." The major drawback to these studies is the fact that they have investigated the analgesic effect of codeine administered over a short period of time. There are obviously clinical scenarios where pain is expected to be of short duration, but in many cases in the elderly patient the likelihood is that the pain will be of long duration. These studies fail to give reassurance that the analgesia apparent after short-term use is maintained with long-term use.

DIHYDROCODEINE

Like codeine, dihydrocodeine undergoes metabolism mediated by the CYP2D6 enzyme system. In contrast, dihydrocodeine does exhibit analgesic properties and its action does not depend on the presence of active metabolites. Therefore, the issue of "poor" and "extensive" metabolizers is of less relevance than in the case of codeine.

Dihydrocodeine is metabolized to dihydromorphine, dihydrocodeine-6-O-, dihydromorphine-3-O-, and dihydromorphine-6-O-glucuronide and nordihydrocodeine.

All of these metabolites have high the greatest affinity for the mu opioid receptor with dihydromorphine and dihydromorphine-6-O-glucuronide having affinities at least 70 times higher for the mu receptor as compared to the other metabolites.

They also have an affinity for the delta receptor and to a lesser extent the kappa receptor.

Both dihydrocodeine and dihydromorphine exhibit linear pharmacokinetics in extensive metabolizers.

TRAMADOL

Tramadol hydrochloride is a centrally active opioid analgesic with activity at the mu opioid receptor. It also causes inhibition of norepinephrine and serotonin reuptake, and can therefore augment the descending bulbospinal inhibitory pathways. Results from placebo-controlled studies show that tramadol can reduce the pain from diabetic neuropathy, polyneuropathy, postherpetic neuralgia, and osteoarthritis. Evidence from use in postoperative analgesia suggests that it is more effective than codeine alone or in combination with acetaminophen. There is a clinical impression that analgesic tolerance is less common, or less rapid in onset, when tramadol and codeine are compared. Tramadol is commonly used in combination with other analgesics and nonsteroidal anti-inflammatories, and the impression is of enhanced analgesic when these combinations are used. That said, confusion is possible when compound preparations are used and the risk of inadvertent overdose with particular components of the combination are possible.

The issue of coprescription of other mu opioid receptor active agents and of drugs such as the tricyclic antidepressants with documented effects on serotonin and norepinephrine has not yet been fully addressed.

Tramadol is available as normal-release and extended-release oral preparations. The analgesia from extended-release preparations is as good as normal-release tramadol with the advantage of a reduction in overall dose and a consequent reduction in the frequency and severity of side effects.

MEPERIDINE

A relatively weak mu opioid agonist with marked anticholinergic and local anesthetic properties. With a half-life of around 3 hours, it is most appropriately used for the treatment of acute pain of expected short duration. Its principle metabolite is normeperidine, which has epileptogenic properties, which again would suggest use in the short rather than the long term.

PROPOXYPHENE

This is a synthetic analgesic with a half-life of 6 to 12 hours. Only its D-sterioisomer, dextropropoxyphene, has analgesic effects. Its principle metabolite, norpropoxyphene has a half-life of 30 to 60 hours and may have a cardiotoxic effect. Propoxyphene has mu opioid agonist effects as well as some action on the NMDA receptor.

PENTAZOCINE

Pentazocine is a semisynthetic derivative of the benzomorphinanes with a delta and kappa opioid action. The effect on these receptors may contribute to its dysphoriant side effects. In addition to its delta and kappa agonist effects it also possesses mu antagonistic effects and is therefore classified as a mixed opioid agonist/antagonist.

MORPHINE

Despite its long history in medical practice, morphine still remains the gold standard in terms of strong opioids.

Morphine is metabolized chiefly through glucuronidation by uridine diphosphate glucuronosyl transferase enzymes in the liver.

The use of morphine in patients with postoperative pain and pain related to terminal illnesses is well accepted. Its use in those with chronic pain not related to terminal illness and in those with neuropathic pain is more controversial. Mounting evidence now suggests that morphine, when titrated to effect, is effective in a broad range of chronic pain conditions. Whether patients receiving this treatment continue to derive the same level of benefit when the morphine is administered over prolonged periods is more questionable. Often dose escalation is required to maintain effect. Some have suggested that rotation from one strong opioid to another will reduce the rapidity with which analgesic tolerance may develop. Others commend the use of other therapeutic agents that complement the analgesic effect of the morphine and minimize the dose required to achieve effect.

It is now suggested that single-dose administration of opioids can precipitate a reflex hyperalgesia and allodynia when the serum level of the opioid decreases. This would manifest itself to the patient as an increase in pain, which may prompt them to take additional opioids. Therefore, when short-acting opioids are used, analgesia rapidly followed by a reflex exaggeration of pain may complicate use. The logic is that sustained-release preparations should be used to avoid this type of on/off phenomenon with constant plasma levels being maintained, rather than the fluctuating levels found when immediate-release preparations are used.

It is suggested, therefore, that, when morphine is used in the management of chronic pain conditions, sustained-release preparations be used.

While the pharmacological mode of action of injected, oral immediate-release and oral sustained-release morphine are all the same, the clinical effect may be different. Patients often report that injected morphine and oral immediate release is more efficacious and helpful in a broader range of conditions than oral sustained-release morphine. Presumably, with the former modes of administration, peak serum levels are higher and all modes of action attributable to morphine use are operant. With use of sustained-release morphine, these peak levels are not achieved, and hence the difference in observable clinical effect.

Whether immediate-release morphine should be used in those with chronic painful conditions is therefore debatable.

Currently morphine is available in a broad range of formulations. Parenteral solutions are used for subcutaneous, intravenous, intramuscular, epidural, and intrathecal use. Immediate-release oral morphine in the form of tablet, suppository, and syrup preparations are available. In addition, sustained-release (12 and 24 hours) preparations are available for oral use. These include tablet and suspension forms. The sustained-release oral forms can be used rectally where the oral route is unavailable, although this use is outside the current product licence.

Case report evidence also suggests that morphine can be given in a nebulizer and can also be given through a urinary catheter for specific conditions. These aspects will be expanded upon when topical administration is considered.

DIAMORPHINE

This is a semisynthetic lipid-soluble opioid analgesic that is rapidly deacelyted to active metabolites 6-monoacetyl-morphine and morphine. Diamorphine has few advantages when compared with morphine. It is reputed to have a greater solubility than morphine, and therefore when high doses are required to be dissolved when used as a subcutaneous infusion, diamorphine may offer some advantage.

HYDROMORPHONE

Hydromorphone is a phenantrene derivative and a structural analog of morphine. It has strong affinity for the mu opioid receptor.

Quigley (2002) has analyzed all available studies investigating the analgesic effects of hydromorphone. While many of the studies analyzed were of poor quality or assessed small numbers of patients, the overall conclusions generated by his analysis were that in the context of both acute and chronic pain, hydromorphone appears to be a potent analgesic, but that there is little difference between it and morphine in analgesic effect or side-effect profile.

METHADONE

Methadone is a synthetic mu opioid receptor agonist and antagonist at the NMDA receptor. The pharmacokinetics and pharmacodynamics of methadone are highly variable and hence individualization of dose is necessary. Oral bioavailability varies from 40 to 90 percent, and intestinal metabolism varies to cause wide fluctuations in presystemic inactivation.

Methadone plasma levels follow a biexponential model of decline, and hence the variation between its analgesic action of 6 to 8 hours and its tendency to cumulate. Methadone does not have active metabolites and is excreted in feces and may therefore be a safer analgesic than the other strong opioids in those with renal impairment.

FENTANYL

Fentanyl has a long and established pedigree in postoperative pain management. More recently, the transdermal delivery of fentanyl has become popular in the treatment of chronic pain and that related to terminal illness.

Fentanyl possesses intense mu opioid related analgesic effects. When given intravenously, respiratory depression may complicate use. Fentanyl has a shorter duration of effect than morphine, with peak action diminishing after 20 min or so. Consequently immediate-release fentanyl has little place in the long-term management of chronic pain conditions, but may be useful in the acute management of pain of short duration such as may occur with change of wound or burns dressings or when a movement is anticipated in the presence of a movement-related pain condition, such as is seen with fractured ribs.

A number of preparations (apart from the transdermal delivery preparation) are currently available including a parenteral formulation, a sublingual tablet, and a lozenge-type formulation designed for rapid buccal absorption.

As well as parenteral and lozenge formulations, fentanyl is available in a transdermal fentanyl preparation. These are currently available in a 25, 50, and 75 µg/hour strengths, with larger doses requiring the use of a combination of these patches to achieve the required dosage. Each patch supplies drug for a 3-day period, and in opioid-naive patients' therapeutic levels of fentanyl and clinical effect is usually achieved within 12 to 18 hours.

The potential value of fentanyl patches include the known strong-opioid effect of fentanyl, the need to replace patches only once every

3 days (which may improve compliance), and the clinical impression of a slightly more favorable side-effect profile than other strong-opioid analgesics. In addition, their use continues to be appropriate even if the oral route of administration is unavailable because of, for example, intractable nausea or vomiting.

Menten and colleagues (2002) studied over 600 elderly patients using transdermal fentanyl for cancer-related pain. The fentanyl doses ranged from 25 to 950 μg/hour, and patient acceptance was found to be high. Constipation was recorded in 40 percent of patients, although this seemed to be related to the use of rescue doses of morphine. In those studies where transdermal fentanyl is compared with another strong opioid, pain relief is as good with fentanyl, and yet the incidence of opioid related side effects is less.

Ringe and colleagues (2002) have studied patients using transdermal fentanyl for back pain caused by vertebral osteoporosis. Their results give an indication of what might be expected from the use of transdermal fentanyl. The looked at 64 patients with at least one osteoporotic vertebral fracture that required the use of strong opioid analgesics. Pain and quality of life were recorded at baseline and after 4 weeks treatment. Of the 64 patients enrolled, 12 withdrew because of opioid-related side effects. In those who remained on treatment with fentanyl, pain at rest and on movement fell significantly (both by around 4 points on a 0 to 10 pain score) and quality of life also improved. Overall, 61 percent of patients were satisfied with their treatment.

Larsen and colleagues (2003) have examined dermal penetration of fentanyl in an *in vitro* model and found an intra-individual difference in absorption rates of around 18 percent. That said, when treatment is initiated, a process of gradual dose escalation to an effective dose is used, and this gradual process of dose increase will prevent an unexpectedly high dose being delivered in isolated individuals whose absorption characteristics are different to the majority. Larsen and colleagues also report that they found no difference in penetration of the drug when the patch was applied to either breast or abdominal skin.

Transdermal fentanyl, therefore, represents a useful method of administration of a strong opioid, and its use is probably associated with slightly fewer side effects than other strong opioids.

BUPRENORPHINE

This is a kappa agonist with a relatively long half-life and is available in oral, sub lingual, parenteral, and transdermal formulations. It is associated with dysphoriant side effects.

It is now presented (in the United Kingdom) in a transdermal delivery formulation with patches that deliver a measured dose over 3 or 7 days.

OXYCODONE

Oxycodone is now available in immediate- and sustained-release oral preparations as well as a parenteral form. Oxycodone undergoes extensive hepatic metabolism and conjugation to inactive metabolites.

Recent studies have shown that oxycodone can be effective in relieving osteoarthritis pain and that caused by diabetic neuropathy and postherpetic neuralgia.

Given that tricyclic antidepressants, antiepileptics, and capsaicin have all been shown to reduce the pain of diabetic neuropathy, the question arises as to which has most chance of being efficacious. Watson and colleagues (2003) have demonstrated in a randomized controlled trial that controlled-release oxycodone does have an analgesic effect when used in patients with painful diabetic neuropathy. They have calculated that the numbers needed to treat (NNT), that is the number of patients who need to be given the drug for one to obtain a 50 percent reduction in their pain, as being 2.6. With carbamazepine the NNT is 2.3, 2.1 for phenytoin, 3.8 for gabapentin, and 3.5 for tricyclic antidepressants. On this basis oxycodone is at least as good as other treatments conventionally used for painful diabetic neuropathy. Whether it should be used in preference to these other treatments is more debatable.

SIDE EFFECTS OF OPIOID ANALGESICS

It is clear that a substantial body of evidence supports the contention that opioid analgesics have a useful pain-relieving effect in a broad range of conditions. That is still not to say that they are necessarily the best agents for treating these pain conditions but merely that they can be logically considered.

A major influence on the decision to use an opioid is the risk of producing side effects. Some of these side effects are predictable and well know; others are less so. In treating acute pain immediate side effects are apparent: nausea and respiratory depression are the most obvious. With longer-term use others such as constipation often become apparent.

Cepeda and colleagues (2003) evaluated 8,855 patients given a variety of strong-opioid analgesics. Twenty-six percent had nausea and vomiting, while 1.5 percent had respiratory depression. They found that the risk of respiratory depression increased significantly in patients older than 60 years. Side effects were least frequent in the short term with meperidine.

Nausea and Vomiting

If the data supplied by Cepeda and colleagues (2003) are a true reflection of the incidence of nausea and vomiting after strong-opioid administration, then prophylactic administration of an antiemetic is warranted. When strong opioids are being initiated for chronic pain conditions, compliance may be reduced is nausea occurs. If it is prevented, then there is a greater chance that opioid treatment will be maintained by the patient. With the use of strong opioids on a chronic basis, antiemetic may only need to be given for the first 5 days of treatment. A variety of antiemetics are available: 5HT3 antagonists (ondansetron, granisetron, and tropisetron), dopamine receptor antagonist (metoclopramide and phenothiazines), muscarinic receptor antagonist (scopolamine), and H1 receptor antagonists (diphenhydramine).

In clinical practice, the following antiemetics may be useful. With acute parenteral use of strong opioids, cyclizine 50 mg or ondansetron 4 mg given with the opioid may be useful. When sustained-release preparations are used, then for the first 5 days ondansetron 4 mg twice daily or sustained-release metoclopramide 15 mg twice daily can be used.

Constipation

This is an almost inevitable consequence of long-term opioid use. As with nausea, prophylactic measures can avoid or minimize this side effect. Fecal softeners are a useful initial therapy with the use of stimulant laxatives if these prove inadequate.

Pruritis

This is most marked after intrathecal and epidural administration, but may also complicate oral and parenteral use. It usually responds to use of antihistamines such as chlorpheniramine given as 4 mg orally or 10 mg parenterally.

Tolerance

Analgesic tolerance, that is the need to increase the dose of opioid to derive the same level of pain relief, is common with opioids. A number of approaches to this issue can be made. First, opioids can be reserved for short-term use so that there is no risk of analgesic tolerance. Second, adjuvant agents can be given to either minimize the dose of opioid required to produce pain relief or to reduce the risk of tolerance developing. Third, a process of opioid rotation can be instituted where after a defined period of time the initial opioid is changed to another and then again to yet another after a similar period of time. Fourth, the dose of opioid can be substantially reduced by changing the route of administration: a fraction of the oral dose administered by the intrathecal route can achieve the same level of analgesia. Fifth, as tolerance occurs, the dose of opioid is increased to maintain the same level of analgesia, with the hope that analgesic tolerance is accompanied by tolerance to the principle side effects of that opioid.

Edwards and Salib (2002) found that 2.8 percent of elderly patients in a group of four practices were taking weak opioids for longer than 1 year. Using a "Diagnosis Criteria for Research" (DCR-10) criteria for dependence syndrome, they found that 40 percent of elderly patients taking weak opioids on a long-term basis fulfilled the DCR-10 criteria for dependence syndrome.

Effect on Cognitive and Motor Function

Clinical experience suggests that neuropsychological side effects due to opioid therapy usually decrease during the first weeks of therapy. A single dose of morphine has been shown to significantly reduce motor task reaction time. Other known adverse effects include mental clouding, sedation, and confusion. While these effects are well known and accepted in patients given a single dose of strong opioid since these patients are likely to be under supervision, these effects are less important than the issue of the effects of long-term administration of opioids in patients with pain of a more chronic nature. These patients may already experience cognitive impairment because of the severity of their pain or because of other medications taken for the pain. If medication is rationalized and pain reduced, then the burden of cognitive impairment induced by the opioid may be lessened or even removed because of the pain reduction consequent on its use.

An insight into the consequences of cognitive and motor impairment in elderly patients is given by the work of Eusrud and colleagues (2003). They found that the incidence of nonspine fracture in elderly community-dwelling females was significantly higher in those taking strong-opioid drugs.

When considering the effects of opioids on cognitive and motor function, it seems clear that stable use of sustained-release preparations such as controlled-release morphine and transdermal fentanyl are not associated with impairment of cognitive or motor performance. However, impairment of these functions may temporarily complicate the initiation phase of opioid treatment and probably at times when dose is increased. As cognitive and motor function impairment are such major issues in elderly patients, if they require the use of strong opioids, then controlled- or sustained-release preparations should be used to achieve a stable serum level of the drug, which will less adversely affect cognitive and motor function.

Effect on Endocrine Function

Acute administration of opioids increases prolactin, growth hormone, thyroid stimulating hormone (TSH), and ACTH while inhibiting leutenizing hormone (LH) release. When administered on a long-term basis, different endocrine results are observed. Abs and colleagues (2000) have extensively investigated 73 patients receiving intrathecal opioids for chronic nonmalignant pain. Their average duration of opioid treatment was 26 months. Decreased libido and impotence was present in 23 of the 24 men studied. Nine of the men had a significantly reduced testosterone level and most had a decreased LH level. All of the premenopausal females had either amenorrhea or an irregular cycle with ovulation in only one patient. All postmenopausal women had decreased LH and FSH levels when compared with control. The 24-hour urinary cortisol excretion was significantly lower than control in 14 of the 73 patients. Fifteen percent of all patients developed growth hormone deficiency. Therefore, in patients receiving intrathecal opioids on a long-term basis the majority of men and all women developed hypogonadotrophic hypogonadism, 15 percent developed central hypocorticism, and about 15 percent developed growth hormone deficiency.

Clearly, the results of this study are dramatic, but of course these patients were receiving intrathecal rather than oral opioids. It does, however, raise the question as to whether long-term, high-dose oral treatment may produce the same picture or at least upset the endocrine system to a lesser extent.

A single case report highlights a different possible side effect of fentanyl use. Kokko and colleagues (2002) report apparent inappropriate antidiuretic hormone (ADH) release in a patient with known lung tumor treated with fentanyl. Withdrawal of fentanyl terminated the ADH release, while reinstitution of fentanyl at a later date triggered of a further inappropriate ADH release.

Paradoxical Pain

While the primary aim of using opioid analgesics is pain relief, a strong body of evidence suggests that at times they can actually exacerbate, rather than relieve, pain.

In a study in rats, Yaksh and colleagues (1986) implanted intrathecally catheters and infused high concentrations of morphine. These rats exhibited features of pain behaviors that involved intermittent bouts of biting and scratching at the dermatomes innervated by levels of the spinal cord proximal to the catheter tip. In addition, during intervals between bouts of agitation, the animals displayed a clear, marked hyperesthesia where an otherwise innocuous stimulus (brush stroke) evoked significant signs of discomfort and consequent aggressive behavior. These effects were perfectly mimicked by a considerably lower dose of morphine-3-glucuronide.

Yaksh and Harty (1988), again using a rat model, have shown that morphine-3-glucuronide has a high chance of inducing this hyperesthesia, with dihydrocodeine and morphine having a lesser potential. They found that the opioids alfentanil, sufentanil, methadone, meperidine, oxycodone, levorphanol, and codeine, even when given at the highest does, did not induce pain behavior.

Vanderah and colleagues (2001) give an insight into the possible causes of this phenomenon. They found that rats implanted with pellets or osmotic minipumps delivering morphine displayed tactile allodynia and thermal hyperalgesia (i.e., "opioid-induced pain"); placebo pellets or saline minipumps did not change thresholds. Rostral ventromedial medulla (RVM) lidocaine, or bilateral lesions of the dorsolateral funiculus (DLF), did not change response thresholds in placebo-pelleted rats but blocked opioid-induced pain. These results suggest that opioids elicit pain through tonic activation of bulbospinal facilitation from the RVM.

In addition to this RVM effect, it is known that spinal dorsal horn dynorphin is increased after opioid administration. Although dynorphin was originally identified as an endogenous kappa-opioid agonist and may act as an endogenous antinociceptive agent under certain conditions, this peptide has significant nonopioid activity.

Considerable evidence now supports the conclusion that enhanced expression of spinal dynorphin is pronociceptive and promotes opioid tolerance.

A third possible mechanism that is implicated in opioid induced pain involves the peptide cholecystokinin (CCK). CCK, originally known as having effects solely on the gastrointestinal system, is now known to be represented in the central nervous system. CCK has an antiopioid effect and its levels are increased by chronic opioid administration (and by neural injury). Therefore, the long-term use of opioids may lead to an elevation of CCK levels that negates the analgesic effect of the opioid and endogenous enkephalins with an apparent magnification of pain. This latter mechanism is of importance because both animal and human studies shown that coadministration of a CCK antagonist may enhance the analgesic effect of the opioid and even reduce the rapidity and extent of analgesic tolerance.

It has been suggested that repeated opioids maintain their efficacy, but the concurrent expression of hyperalgesia counteracts antinociception, producing an impression of tolerance. Opioid-induced hyperalgesia has been hypothesized to result from unmasking of compensatory neuronal hyperactivity, which becomes evident after the opioid is removed or occurs intermittently between injections. Thus, opioid-induced hyperalgesia might result from repeated episodes of opioid withdrawal (mini withdrawals).

Hood and colleagues (2003) have shown that, in human volunteers with capsaicin induced hyperalgesia, the ultra-short-acting opioid remifentanil reduces the hyperalgesia and allodynia caused by the capsaicin while being administered. However, some time after the end of administration there is an increase in hyperalgesia and allodynia above what was apparent prior to remifentanil administration. The clinical implication of this study is that, while opioids may have an analgesic effect, as their plasma levels fall, there is a paradoxical increase in pain that may encourage further opioid consumption beyond the point where the original injury is inflicting pain.

Although the animal experiments investigating this phenomenon use intrathecally or systemically administered opioids at high doses, case reports from the human literature suggest that paradoxical opioid-induced pain may occur with intrathecally and intravenously administered morphine at less substantial doses. In a case report by Parisod and colleagues (2003), allodynia was apparent after a single intrathecal administration of 0.5 mg of morphine. If it appears that morphine, regardless of its mode of administration, is causing an increase in pain, then substitution of the morphine by another strong opioid may end the problem. We have seen that the work by Yaksh and Harty (1986) suggests that opioid-induced pain may occur with morphine and dihydrocodeine but, in animals, is less likely with meperidine, oxycodone and codeine.

The implication of the studies discussed is that strong opioids are not always the best option for the treatment of either acute or chronic pain. In some circumstances they may actually exacerbate rather than relieve pain. Because of the suggestion that this opioid-induced pain may be partially related to mini-withdrawal reactions, then, if opioids are to be used in the long term, controlled-release formulations that prevent rapid and frequent changes in plasma concentrations of the opioid, with associated mini-withdrawal reactions, are to be preferred.

Before using strong opioids in any patient, the following checklist may be used:

> Is a strong opioid the best form of treatment available for this pain?
> Will this opioid interact with any concomitantly administered medication?
> Can other therapeutic agents be added to minimize the dose of opioid required to achieve analgesia?
> Can other agents be added to minimize the risk of analgesic tolerance?
> Will other therapeutic agents be given to reduce the risk of side effects (e.g., laxatives, antiemetics)?
> Which route of administration is most appropriate?
> At what dose will the opioid be initiated?
> What is the expected duration of treatment?
> Will rules be imposed that limit the rate of dose escalation?
> Will there be a maximum dose of this opioid used?
> How will the effect of opioid treatment be measured?

CONCLUSIONS

Weak and strong opioids achieve their analgesic effect predominately by interacting with well-defined opioid receptors, and the strength of an opioid is related to its affinity for the receptor.

Codeine requires an enzyme-dependent metabolic step to become activated. A proportion of the population is deficient in this enzyme and will therefore gain little analgesia from codeine. Dihydrocodeine does not require this process.

Both weak and strong opioids have a proven analgesic effect in a broad range of pain conditions. They have well recognized side effects that include analgesic tolerance, nausea, constipation, mood disturbance, endocrine effects, and, at times, paradoxical pain associated with their use.

A careful process should be carried out before strong-opioid therapy is initiated in any patient.

BIBLIOGRAPHY

Mode of Action of Opioids

Bolton EA, Tallarida RJ, Pasternak GW. Synergy between mu opioid ligands: evidence for functional interactions among mu opioid receptor subtypes. *J Pharmacol Exp Ther* 2002; 303: 557-562.

Gharagozlou P, Demirci H, Clark JD, Lameh J. Activity of opioid ligands in cells expressing cloned mu opioid receptors. *BMC Pharmacology* 2003; 3: 1-8.

Inturrisi CE. Clinical pharmacology of opioids for pain. *Clin J Pain* 2002; 18: S3-S13.

McDowell TS. Fentanyl decreases Ca^{2+} currents in a population of capsaicin responsive sensory neurons. *Anesthesiology* 2003; 98: 223-231.

Narita M, Imai S, Itou Y, Yajima Y, Suzuki T. Possible involvement of mu1-opioid receptors in the fentanyl morphine-induced antinociception at supraspinal and spinal sites. *Life Sci* 2002; 70: 2341-2354.

Yamakura T, Sakimura K, Shimoji K. Direct inhibition of the *N*-methyl-D-aspartate receptor channel by high concentrations of opioids. *Anesthesiology* 1999; 91: 1053-1063.

Responsiveness of Pain to Opioids

Attal N, Guirimand F, Brasseur L, Gaude V, Chauvin M, Bouhassira D. Effects of IV morphine in central pain: A randomized, placebo controlled study. *Neurology* 2002; 58: 554-563.

Griessinger N, Sittl R, Jost R, Schaefer M, Likar R. The role of opioid analgesics in rheumatoid disease in the elderly population. *Drugs Aging* 2003; 20: 571-583.

Grilo RM, Bertin P, Scotto di Fazano C, Coyral D, Bonnet C, Vergne, Treves R. Opioid rotation in the treatment of joint pain. A review of 67 cases. *Joint Bone Spine* 2002; 69: 491-494.

Kalman S, Osterberg A, Sorensen J, Boivie J, Bertler A. Morphine responsiveness in a group of well defined multiple sclerosis patients: A study with IV morphine. *Eur J Pain* 2002; 6: 69-80.

Raja SN, Haythornwaite JA, Pappagallo M, Clark MR, Travison TG, Sabeen S, Max MB. Opioids versus antidepressants in postherpetic neuralgia: A randomised, placebo controlled trial. *Neurology* 2002; 59: 1015-1021.

Rowbotham MC, Twilling L, Davies PS, Reisner L, Taylor K, Mohr D. Oral opioid therapy for chronic peripheral and central neuropathic pain. *N Eng J Med* 2003; 348: 1223-1232.

Codeine

Arora S, Herbert ME. Myth: Codeine is a powerful and effective analgesic. *WJM* 2001; 174: 428.

Chew M, White JM, Somogyi AA, Bochner F, Irvine RJ. Precipitated withdrawal following codeine administration is dependent on CYP genotype. *Eur J Pharmacol* 2001; 425: 159-164.

Enggaard TP, Poulsen L, Arendt-Nielsen L, Honore-Hansen S, Bjornsdottir I, Gram LF, Sindrup SH. The analgesic effect of codeine as compared to imipramine in different human experimental pain models. *Pain* 2001; 92: 277-282.

Mullican WS, Lacy JR. Tramadol/acetaminophen combination tablets and codeine/acetaminophen combination capsules for the management of chronic pain: A comparative trial. *Clin Ther* 2001; 23: 1429-1445.

Pelso PM, Bellamy N, Bensen W, Thomson GT, Harsanyi Z, Babul, Darke AC. Double blind randomized placebo control trial of controlled release codeine in the treatment of osteoarthritis of the hip or knee. *J Rheumatol* 2000; 27: 764-771.

Wilder-Smith CH, Hill L, Spargo K, Kalla A. Treatment of severe pain from osteoarthritis with slow-release tramadol or dihydrocodeine in combination with NSAIDs: A randomised study comparing analgesia, antinociception and gastrointestinal effects. *Pain* 2001; 91: 23-31.

Williams DG, Patel A, Howard RF. Pharmacogenetics of codeine metabolism in an urban population of children and its implications for analgesic reliability. *Br J Anaes* 2002; 89: 839-845.

Yu A, Kneller BM, Rettie AE, Haining RL. Expression, purification, biochemical characterisation, and comparative function of human cytochrome P450 2D6.1, 2D6.2, 2D6.10 and 2D6.17 allelic isoforms. *J Pharmacol Exp Ther* 2002; 303: 1291-1300.

Dihydrocodeine

Ammon S, Hofmann U, Griese EU, Gugeler N, Mikus G. Pharmacokinetics of dihydrocodeine and its active metabolites after single and multiple oral dosing. *Br J Clin Pharmacol* 1999; 48: 317-322.

Schmidt H, Vormfelde S, Klinder K, Gundert-Remy U, Gleiter CH, Skopp G, Aderjan R, Fuhr U. Affinities of dihydrocodeine and its metabolites to opioid receptors. *Pharmacol Toxicol* 2002; 91: 57-63.

Schmidt H, Vormfelde SV, Walchner-Bonjean M, Klinder K, Freudenthaler S, Gleiter CH, Gundert-Remy U, Skopp G, Aderjan R, Fuhr U. The role of active metabolites in dihydrocodeine effects. *Int J Clin Pharmacol Ther* 2003; 41: 95-106.

Webb JA, Rostami-Hodjegan A, Abdul-Manap R, Hofmann U, Miku, Kamali F. Contribution of dihydrocodeine and dihydromorphine to analgesia following dihydrocodeine administration in man: A PK-PD modelling analysis. *Br J Clin Pharmacol* 2001; 52: 35-43.

Tramadol

Alder L, McDonald C, O'Brien C, Wilson M. A comparison of once daily tramadol with normal release tramadol in treatment of pain in osteoarthritis. *J Rheumatol* 2002; 29: 2196-2199.

Boureau F, Legallicier P, Kabir-Ahmadi M. Tramadol in post-herpetic neuralgia: A randomized, double-blind, placebo-controlled trial. *Pain* 2003; 104: 323-331.

Harati Y, Gooch C, Swenson M, Edelman S, Greene D, Raskin P, Donofrio P, Cornblath D, Sachdeo R, Siu CO, Kamin M. Double-blind randomized trial of tramadol for the treatment of pain of diabetic neuropathy. *Neurology* 1998; 50: 1842-1846.

Raffa RB, Friderichs E. The basic science aspect of tramadol hydrochloride. *Pain Rev* 1996; 3: 249-271.

Silverfield JC, Kamin M, Wu SC, Rosenthal N. Tramadol/acetaminophen combination tablets for the treatment of osteoarthritis flare pain: A multicenter, outpatient, randomized, double blind, placebo controlled, parallel group, add on study. *Clin Ther* 2002; 24: 282-297.

Sindrup SH, Andersen G, Madsen C, Smith T, Brosen K, Jensen TS. Tramadol relieves pain and allodynia in polyneuropathy: A randomised, double-blind, controlled trial. *Pain* 1999; 83: 85-90.

Morphine

Armstrong SC, Cozza KL. Pharmacokinetic drug interactions of morphine, codeine and their derivates: Theory and clinical reality. *Psychosomatics* 2003; 44: 167-171.

Caldwell JR, Rapoport RJ, Davis JC, Offenberg HL, Marker HW, Roth SH, Yuan W, Eliot L, Babul N, Lynch PM. Efficacy and safety of a once daily morphine formulation in chronic, moderate to severe osteoarthritis pain: Results from a randomized, placebo controlled, double blind trial and an open label extension trial. *J Pain Symptom Mang* 2002; 23: 278-291.

Gagnon B, Bruera E. Differences in the ratios of morphine to methadone in patients with neuropathic pain versus non-neuropathic pain. *J Pain Symptom Mang* 1999; 18: 120-125.

Maier C, Hildebrandt J, Klinger R, Henrich-Eberl C, Lindena G. Morphine responsiveness, efficacy and tolerability in patients with chronic non-tumor associated pain-results of a double blind placebo controlled trial. *Pain* 2002; 97: 223-233.

Rowbotham MC, Reisner-Keller LA, Fields HL. Both intravenous lidocaine and morphine reduce the pain of postherpetic neuralgia. *Neurology* 1991; 41: 1024-1028.

Walsh D, Tropiano PS. Long term rectal administration of high dose sustained release morphine tablets. *Support Care Cancer* 2002; 10: 653-655.

Wilkinson TJ, Robinson BA, Begg EJ, Duffull SB, Ravenscroft PJ, Schneider JJ. Pharmacokinetics and efficacy of rectal versus oral sustained release morphine in cancer patients. *Chemother Pharmacol* 1992; 31: 251-254.

Hydromorphone

Quigley C. Hydromorphone for acute and chronic pain. *Cochrane Database Syst Rev* 2002; 1: CD003447.

Fentanyl

Ackerman SJ, Mordin M, Reblando J, Xu X, Schein J, Vallow S, Brennan M. Patient reported utilization patterns of fentanyl transdermal system and oxycodone hydrochloride controlled release among patients with chronic non malignant pain. *J Manag Care Pharm* 2003; 9: 223-231.

Bredenberg S, Duberg M, Lennernas B, Lennernas H, Pettersson A, Westerberg M, Nystrom C. In vitro evaluation of a new sublingual tablet system for rapid oromucosal absorption using fentanyl citrate as the active substance. *Eur J Pharmac Sci* 2003; 20: 327-334.

Caplan RA, Ready LB, Oden RV, Matsen FA, Nessly ML, Olsson GL. Transdermal fentanyl for postoperative pain management. A double blind, placebo study. *JAMA* 1989; 261: 1036-1039.

Dellemijn PL, Vanneste JA. Randomised double blind active placebo controlled crossover trial of intravenous fentanyl in neuropathic pain. *Lancet* 1997; 349: 753-758.

Kornick CA, Santiago-Palma J, Moryl N, Payne R, Obbens EA. Benefit risk assessment of transdermal fentanyl for the treatment of chronic pain. *Drug Saf* 2003; 26: 951-973.

Larsen RH, Nieslen F, Sorensen JA, Nielsen JB. Dermal penetration of fentanyl: Inter and intraindividual variations. *Pharmacol Toxicol* 2003; 93: 244-248.

Menten J, Desmedt M, Lossignol D, Mullie A. Longitudinal follow up of TTS fentanyl use in patients with cancer related pain: Results of a compassionate use study with special focus on elderly patients. *Curr Med Res Opin* 2002; 18: 488-498.

Milligan K, Lanteri-Minet M, Borchert K, Helmers H, Donald R, Adriansen H, Moulin D, Haazen L. Evaluation of long term efficacy and safety of transdermal fentanyl in the treatment of chronic non cancer pain. *J Pain* 2001; 2: 197-204.

Mystakidou K, Parpa E, Tsilika E, Mavromati A, Smyrniotis V, Georgaki S, Vlahos L. Long term management of non cancer pain with transdermal therapeutic system fentanyl. *J pain* 2003; 4: 298-306.

Mystakidou K, Tsilika E, Parpa E, Kouloulias V, Kouvaris I, Georgaki S, Vlahos I. Long term cancer pain management in morphine pretreated and opioid naïve patients with transdermal fentanyl. *Int J Cancer* 2003; 107: 486-492.

Ringe JD, Faber H, Bock O, Valentine S, Felsenberg D, Pfeifer M, Schwallen S. Transdermal fentanyl for the treatment of back pain caused by vertebral osteoporosis. *Rheumatol Int* 2002; 22: 199-203.

Soares LG, Martins M, Uchoa R. Intravenous fentanyl for cancer pain: a "fast titration" protocol for the emergency room. *J Pain Symptom Manage* 2003; 26: 876-881.

Van Seventer R, Smit JM, Schipper RM, Wicks MA, Zuurmond WW. Comparison of TTS fentanyl with sustained release oral morphine in the treatment of patients not using opioids for mild to moderate pain. *Curr Med Res Opin* 2003; 19: 457-469.

Oxycontin

Oral oxycodone: New preparation. No better than oral morphine. *Prescrire Int* 2003; 12: 83-84.

Roth SH, Fleischmann RM, Burch FX, Dietz F, Bockow B, Rapaport, Rutstein J, Lacouture PG. Around the clock, controlled release oxycodone therapy for osteoarthritis related pain: Placebo controlled trial and long term evaluation. *Arch Int Med* 2000; 160: 853-860.

Watson CP, Babul N. Efficacy of oxycodone in neuropathic pain: A randomized trial in postherpetic neuralgia. *Neurology* 1998; 50: 1837-1841.

Watson CP, Moulin D, Watt-Watson J, Gordon A, Eisenhoffer J. Controlled release oxycodone relieves neuropathic pain: A randomized controlled trial in painful diabetic neuropathy. *Pain* 2003; 105: 71-78.

Side Effects of Opioid Analgesics

Adriaensen H, Vissers K, Noorduin H, Meert T. Opioid tolerance and dependence: An inevitable consequence of chronic treatment? *Acta Anaesthesiol Belg* 2003; 54: 37-47.

Cepeda MS, Farrar JT, Baumgarten M, Boston R, Carr DB, Strom I. Side effects of opioids during short term administration: Effect of age, gender and race. *Clin Pharmacol Ther* 2003; 74: 102-112.

Edwards I, Salib E. Analgesics in the elderly. *Aging Ment Health* 2002; 6: 88-92.

Cognitive Function

Allen GJ, Hartl TL, Duffany S, Smith SF, Van Heest JL, Anderson J, Hoffman JR, Kraemer WJ, Maresh CM. Cognitive and motor function after administration of hydrocodone bitartrate plus ibuprofen, ibuprofen alone, or placebo in healthy subjects with exercise-induced muscle damage: A randomized, repeated dose, placebo controlled study. *Psychopharmacology* 2003; 166: 228-233.

Ensrud KE, Blackwell T, Mangione CM, Bowman PJ, Bauer DC, Schwartz A, Nevitt MC, Whooley MA. Central nervous system active medications and risk for fractures in aged women. *Arch Intern Med* 2003; 163: 949-957.

Jamison RN, Schein JR, Vallow S, Ascher S, Vorsanger GJ, Katz NP. Neuropsychological effects of long term opioid use in chronic pain patients. *J Pain Symptom Manage* 2003; 26: 913-921.

Sabatowski R, Schwalen S, Rettig K, Herberg KW, Kasper SM, Radbruch L. Driving ability under long term fentanyl treatment with transdermal fentanyl. *J Pain Symptom Manage* 2003; 25: 38-47.

Tassain V, Attal N, Fletcher D, Brasseur L, Degieux P, Chauvin M, Bouhassira D. Long term effects of oral sustained release morphine on neuropsychological performance in patients with chronic non-cancer pain. *Pain* 2003; 104: 389-400.

Endocrine Effect

Abs R, Verhelst J, Maeyaert J, Van Buyten J-P, Opsomer F, Adriaensen H, Verlooy J, Van Havenbergh, Smet M, Van Acker K. Endocrine consequences of long term intrathecal administration of opioids. *J Clin Endocrinol Metab* 2000; 85: 2215-2222.

Grossman A. Brain opiates and neuroendocrine function. *Clin Endocrinol Metab* 1983; 12: 725-746.

Kokko H, Hall PD, Afrin LB. Fentanyl associated syndrome of inappropriate antidiuretic hormone secretion. *Pharmacotherapy* 2002; 22: 1188-1192.

Paice JA, Penn RD, Ryan WG. Altered sexual function and decreased testosterone in patients receiving intraspinal opioids. *J Pain Symptom Manage* 1994; 9: 126-131.

Su CF, Liu MY, Li MT. Intraventricular morphine produces pain relief, hypothermia, hyperglycaemia and increased prolactin and growth hormone levels in patients with cancer pain. *J Neurol* 1987; 235: 105-108.

Paradoxical Pain

Compton P, Athanasos P, Elashoff D. Withdrawal hyperalgesia after acute opioid physical dependency in non addicted humans: A preliminary study. *J Pain* 2003; 4: 511-519.

De Conno F, Caraceni A, Martini C, Spoldi E, Salvetti M, Ventafridda V. Hyperalgesia and myoclonus with intrathecal infusion of high-dose morphine. *Pain* 1991; 47: 337-339.

Heger S, Maier C, Otter K, Helwig U, Suttorp M. Morphine induced allodynia in a child with brain tumour. *BMJ* 319: 627-629.

Hood DD, Curry R, Eisenach JC. Intravenous remifentanil produces withdrawal hyperalgesia in volunteers with capsaicin-induced hyperalgesia. *Anesth Analg* 2003; 97: 810-815.

Ossipov MH, Lai J, Vanderah TW, Porreca F. Induction of pain facilitation by sustained opioid exposure: Relationship to opioid antinociceptive tolerance. *Life Sciences* 2003; 73: 783-800.

Parisod E, Siddall PJ, Viney M, McClelland JM, Cousins MJ. Allodynia after acute intrathecal morphine administration in a patient with neuropathic pain after spinal cord injury. *Anesth Analg* 2003; 97: 183-186.

Sjogren P, Jensen N-K, Jensen TS. Disappearance of morphine induced hyperalgesia after discontinuing or substituting morphine with other opioid analgesics. *Pain* 1994; 59: 313-316.

Sjogren P, Jonsson T, Jensen N-K, Drenck N-E, Jensen TS. Hyperalgesia and myoclonus in terminal cancer patients treated with continuous intravenous morphine. *Pain* 1993; 55: 93-97.

Vanderah TW, Gardell LR, Burgess SE, Ibrahim M, Dogrul A, Zhong C-M, Zhang E-T, Malan TP, Ossipov MH, Lai J, Porreca F. Dynorphin promotes abnormal pain and spinal opioid antinociceptive tolerance. *J Neurosci* 2000; 20: 7074-7079.

Vanderah TW, Ossipov MH, Lai J, Malan TP, Porreca F. Mechanisms of opioid induced pain and antinociceptive tolerance: Descending facilitation and spinal dynorphin. *Pain* 2001; 92: 5-9.

Vanderah TW, Suenaga NM, Ossipov MH, Malan TP, Lai J, Porreca F. Tonic descending facilitation from the rostral ventromedial medulla mediates opioid induced abnormal pain and antinociceptive tolerance. *J Neurosci* 2001; 21: 279-286.

Wolf CJ. Intrathecal high dose morphine produces hyperalgesia in the rat. *Brain Res* 1981; 209: 491-495.

Yaksh TL, Harty GJ. Pharmacology of the allodynia in rats evoked by high dose intrathecal morphine. *J Pharmacol Exp Ther* 1988; 244: 501-507.

Yaksh TL, Harty GJ, Onofrio BM. High dose of spinal morphine produce a non-opiate receptor mediated hyperaesthesia: Clinical and theoretical implications. *Anesthesiology* 1986; 64: 590-597.

Chapter 9

Acetaminophen

Nisar Soomro

Brodie and Axel Rod first described acetaminophen in 1956. Approximately 30 million people use acetaminophen each year safely and properly. As such it represents a tried-and-tested analgesic with which there is an extensive body of experience. This contrasts with some of the more recently introduced nonsteroidal drugs with which there has been a series of worrying revelations that have precipitated the issuing of safety notices and even the withdrawing of these drugs form the market.

Despite the familiarity of most patients and practitioners with acetaminophen, it remains a potent and useful analgesic option for patients with bone and joint pain.

STRUCTURE

Acetaminophen (4-acetamidophenol) is represented by the following formula:

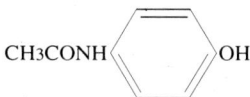

$C_8H_9NO_2$

M.W. 151.2

M.P. 169-172°C

pKa 9.5

MECHANISM OF ACTION

Among the substances involved in pain and inflammation are the prostaglandins. Inhibition of prostaglandin production by blocking the cyclo-oxygenase (COX) enzymes is known to be the mechanism of action of conventional nonsteroidal anti-inflammatory drugs (NSAIDs). Acetaminophen has no significant action on COX-1 or COX-2, and hence its lack of anti-inflammatory effects is of no surprise, as is its lack of significant gastrointestinal side effects so typical of the NSAIDs.

Recent research has, however, shown the presence of a new, previously unknown COX enzyme, COX-3, found in the brain and spinal cord, which is selectively inhibited by acetaminophen and is distinct from the two already known COX enzymes, COX-1 and COX-2. COX enzymes obtained from different tissues have different sensitivities to acetaminophen and NSAIDs. Acetaminophen is as effective as aspirin in inhibiting COX in brain tissue, but has less activity than aspirin against COX in the spleen. This may explain the effectiveness of acetaminophen against fever and pain but its lack of anti-inflammatory activity and its more acceptable gastrointestinal side effect profile.

ABSORPTION

Acetaminophen is rapidly absorbed, the soluble form being absorbed faster than the solid tablet form. Peak serum levels usually occur 30 min to 2 hours after ingestion. The peak blood level for both forms is similar and is usually less than 20 mg/l following a 1000 mg dose. Elimination from the body is rapid with a half-life of about 2 hours.

METABOLISM

In therapeutic doses, 90 percent of acetaminophen is metabolized in the liver by conjugation with glucuronide and sulphate. A small amount (5 percent) is metabolized by mixed function oxidase enzymes to form a highly reactive compound (*N*-acetyl-*p*-benzoquinoneimine, NAPQ), which is then immediately conjugated with glutathione and subsequently excreted as cysteine and mercaptopuric conjugates. Five percent of the ingested dose is excreted unchanged.

The effectiveness of acetaminophen depends on the type of pain being considered. One measure of effectiveness is the "numbers needed to treat" (NNT). The NNT of an analgesic is the number of patients who need to receive the drug for one to gain a 50 percent reduction in their pain. Acetaminophen 1000 mg has an NNT of between 3.5 and 4.6 compared with placebo. By comparison, codeine 30 mg with acetaminophen 500 mg when used for postoperative pain has an NNT of about 3.

TOXICITY

Acetaminophen and its two primary metabolites are relatively safe compounds. Hepatic toxicity arises through the 5 percent that is oxidized, that is, benzoquinoneimine, which is a highly reactive substance that normally combines with glutathione. As the dose of acetaminophen increases, the quantity of benzoquinoneimine produced increases too, and there comes a point at which the glutathione stores in the liver are completely exhausted. In this situation, the rate of production of new glutathione cannot keep up with the rate of production of the benzoquinoneimine. It is at this point that the benzoquinoneimine attaches to liver protein and causes liver injury. It takes approximately 3 to 4 days for this buildup and fatal liver damage to occur. It is estimated that liver injury may begin to occur at a single dose of acetaminophen of 15 g (30 standard tablets).

Acetaminophen-induced renal damage is mediated by a mechanism similar to hepatic toxicity.

In some countries acetaminophen can only be purchased in quantities of up to only 12 × 500 mg capsules or tablets to reduce the risk of accidental overdosage.

ANTIDOTE

N-acetylcysteine, administered intravenously, restores the liver's capacity to produce glutathione for combination with the benzoquinoneimine, and appears to have an additional protective effect on the liver.

Administration of the antidote within 12 hours of overdose is highly effective and is able to minimize the risk of liver injury. Antidote therapy is also very effective up to 24 hours, and there is evidence of benefit from antidote on occasions with administration up to 48 hours following overdose.

INDICATIONS

Relief for all kinds of mild to moderate pain, including headache, rheumatic pains, pains from minor injuries, and all the everyday aches and pains of normal life.

FORMULATIONS

Acetaminophen is available in the following formulations:

Oral (tablet, capsule)
Rectal
Parenteral

DOSE

Oral: 2 × 500 mg tablets or capsules every 4 to 6 hours. No more than eight tablets (each 500 mg) should be taken in 24 hours.
Rectal: 1 g 6-hourly.
Parenteral: 1 g in 100 ml by intravenous infusion over 20 min, repeated 12 hourly as required.

ARTHRITIC PAIN

Although articular cartilages lacks pain receptors, pain in osteoarthritis may arise from the fibrous capsule to subchondral bone, microfractures, or venous congestion caused by remodelling of subchondral trabeculae or from periarticular muscle or ligaments. Ligamentous sprains are common, especially in the unstable joint.

In patients with osteoarthritis with mild or intermittent pain without clinical evidence of inflammation, such as joint warmth or synovial effusion, an analgesic taken as needed and instruction of the patient in general measure of joint protection may be sufficient to relieve symptoms. Some individuals with osteoarthritis are unable to tolerate salicylates in any form because of dyspepsia or ototoxicity; for these patients acetaminophen (Tylenol) 650 mg every 4 to 6 hours provides comparable analgesia. Acetaminophen, however, can cause toxic hepatitis, and is thus contraindicated in those with prior liver disease.

Combined acetaminophen and NSAID treatment is more effective than treatment with NSAIDs alone.

There is also increasing evidence that using acetaminophen may help to protect against atherosclerosis by inhibiting the oxidation of certain low-density lipoproteins, which carry the "bad" form of cholesterol, hence preventing one of the main processes involved in the formation of arterial plaque, which contributes to many deaths per year from stroke and heart disease. Evidence suggests that acetaminophen may provide some protection from ovarian cancer.

INTERACTIONS

The severity of acetaminophen poisoning is dose related, but the following categories of patients are at high risk:

Preexisting liver disease
High alcohol intake
Poor nutrition anorexia nervosa and eating disorders
HIV infections

Enzyme-inducing drugs
Alcohol
Carbamazepine
Griseofulvin
Phenytoin
Prednisolone
Rifampicin

CONCLUSIONS

There are relatively few contraindications to the use of acetaminophen.
It is suitable for small children and the elderly.
At the recommended dosage there are few side effects.
Its analgesic (pain relief) and antipyretic (fever relief) effects are
  comparable to those of aspirin.
Interactions with other treatments are rarely problematical.
It can be taken by those sensitive to aspirin.
It is well tolerated by patients with peptic ulcers and asthma.

Chapter 10

Glucosamine

William Lavelle
Elizabeth Demers
Lori Lavelle

Glucosamine is an aminomonosaccharide and a normal component of the disaccharide units of glucosaminoglycans in cartilage and synovial fluid. Specifically, glucosamine is a precursor in proteoglycan synthesis.[5,13,16] Proteoglycans are ubiquitous in the natural lubrication and function of normal joints. Even though the use of supplemental glucosamine in therapeutic strategies for osteoarthritis has been investigated for over 30 years, their role and precise mechanism of action are yet to be defined. Still, many patients with joint pain have few nonsurgical alternatives and have turned to glucosamine as a method of mitigating joint pain and stemming the progression of their degenerative disease. Proponents of glucosamine feel that these possible effects, in addition to the favorable safety profile, constitute the rationale for the use of this agent.

HISTORY

Researchers in 1971 first found that exogenous glucosamine increased synthesis of glycosaminoglycans in cartilage cell cultures.[16] Radiolabeled exogenous glucosamine was later found to diffuse into articular cartilage after systemic administration.[16] That study spurred a plethora of laboratory trials in an attempt to better understand observations and elucidate an exact molecular mechanism that may

Clinical Management of Bone and Joint Pain
© 2007 by The Haworth Press, Inc. All rights reserved.
doi:10.1300/5771_12

be helpful in slowing the degenerative process. More recently, exogenous glucosamine has been found to stimulate the production of new proteoglycans in three-dimensional cellular cultures of human chondrocytes.[16]

Clinical investigations into the disease-modifying properties have led some to herald glucosamine as an effective symptom-modifying agent in itself.[26] Glucosamine along with chondroitin has been used in various forms in the treatment of osteoarthritis in Europe for more than 15 years.[16] It is only more recently that the use of glucosamine has become more popular in England and the United States. Despite its popularity, the medical community still holds a great deal of skepticism about the effectiveness of glucosamine.

MECHANISM OF ACTION

The basic premise for many of the proposed mechanisms of action of glucosamine is improved or augmented proteoglycan synthesis. Proteoglycans add to the compressive strength of articular cartilage. They are instrumental in helping cartilage capture water. By so doing, the hydrated proteoglycan component of the articular cartilage forms an elastic layer in the articular cartilage, thereby improving the mechanical characteristics of the articular cartilage.[13] Specifically, glucosamine, as an aminosaccharide, serves as a precursor to the synthesis of chondroitin sulfate, hyaluronic acid, and various other molecular constituents in the cartilage matrix.[8] The newly produced chondroitin sulfate is found in the extracellular cartilaginous matrix as a constituent of large aggregating-matrix proteoglycans, in particular aggrecan molecules. This is of particular interest to the elderly because, with aging, aggrecan molecules become much smaller and more variable in size, their keratan sulfate content increases, their chondroitin sulfate content decreases, and the proportion of these molecules that form large aggregates declines.[26] Some propose that, by supplementing the precursors to proteoglycan synthesis, the theoretical imbalance in osteoarthritis between the synthesis and degradation of proteoglycans will be ameliorated.[8] There is some laboratory evidence supporting this hypothesis to demonstrate a statistically significant increase in proteoglycan production by human chondrocytes cultured from osteoarthritic cartilage via three-dimensional culturing techniques.[16]

There is some debate on whether this observed increased proteoglycan synthesis occurs. One proposal involves regulatory mechanisms at the cellular level. In one study, cartilage samples were obtained from patients during knee replacement surgery. Cellular cultures were prepared and treated with a glucosamine solution. Assays for total matrix metalloproteinase activity were measured.[4] These are some of the enzymes proposed to be responsible for degradation of articular cartilage in the osteoarthritic patient. The assayed activity was found to be significantly decreased for the metalloproteinases. In particular, the genetic expression of aggrecanase-1 and aggrecanase-2 was found to be decreased in this study.[4] Previous laboratory studies in cartilage collected from animals support these findings.[6]

Another hypothesis involves pain relief through synthesis of hyaluronic acid. Glucosamine is a rate-limiting component in the synthesis of hyaluronic acid.[28] As outlined in Chapter 12, hyaluronic acids have been found to inhibit leukocyte migration, chemotaxis, and cellular adhesion in the destructive process of osteoarthritis leukocytes, mediate enzymatic and oxidative free radical reactions.[7] Theoretically, this would slow the degenerative process and thus abate pain. Hyaluronic acids have also been found to possess endogenous analgesic effects. In animal models, hyaluronic acid acted much like an anti-inflammatory agent. In early studies, hyaluronic acid was thought to directly bind pain peptides.[7] Later, in a model in which rats were administered intra-articular bradykinin to induce joint pain, the analgesic effect of the hyaluronic acid was not prevented by prior administration of a bradykinin antagonist.

CLINICAL TRIALS

The first clinical trials to show clinical efficacy were in the early 1980s. At that time, three large placebo-controlled studies were conducted.[7,8,24] The largest of these studies was conducted in Italy, where 80 patients with advanced osteoarthritis were enrolled in a placebo-controlled study. Subjects received either oral glucosamine at a standard dose of 500 mg three times daily or a placebo. The duration for treatment was 30 days. Patients receiving the treatment arm saw a symptom reduction of 73.3 percent as compared with the placebo group, who saw a 41.3 percent reduction. This difference was statistically significant.[8] Two smaller studies saw smaller enrollments. The study conducted by Crolle and D'Este saw symptomatic improvement increase from week 1 of treatment to week 2 of treatment by an additional 15 percent.[7] The second study by Pujalte et al. treated patients for 6 to 8 weeks. In addition to showing a significant difference between treatment and placebo, the study showed the treatment population showed a more complete resolution of symptoms as compared with the placebo group.[24]

A recent meta-analysis was completed in 2000. Thirty-seven studies were identified via a thorough literature search. Of the identified studies, the authors felt that only 15 appropriately met their inclusion criteria. The criteria set in this analysis was a double-blind, randomized, placebo-controlled trial of at least 4 weeks' duration. With these high standards, trials of glucosamine and chondroitin demonstrated moderate to large effects (Figure 10.1). As a meta-analysis, this paper is subject to all of the quality issues and bias of its constituent papers. The authors of this analysis concede to this fact and note that perhaps some of the included trials illustrated inflated estimates of benefit. This was as suggested by small effect sizes in their treated populations. In addition, most, if not all, of the trials received some form of manufacturer sponsorship.[16] It should also be noted that few adverse

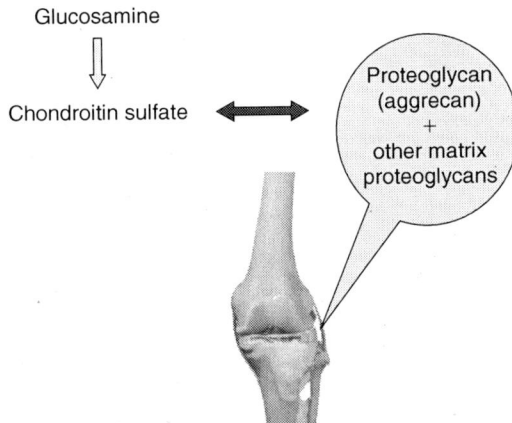

FIGURE 10.1. It has been proposed that extrinsic glucosamine and chondroitin influence the balance of proteoglycan synthesis and degradation.

side effects were reported in the analysis component studies, with the most common side effects being mild gastrointestinal upset.

In an additional analysis completed and published in 2005, a similar literature search was completed. Inclusion criteria was again limited to double-blind, randomized, placebo-controlled trials. However, the inclusion criteria also limited selection to studies of at least 1-year duration and also included outcomes measures such as symptom severity and disease progression as assessed by joint-space narrowing. Data was pooled from the remaining two studies that passed exclusion criteria. This analysis found that, with the pooled data, the risk of disease progression was reduced by 54 percent ($p = 0.0011$). The pooled effects for pain reduction and improvement in function were 0.41 ($p < 0.0001$) and 0.46 ($p < 0.0001$), respectively. Again, few side effects were reported.

As part of the previous meta-analysis, a randomized study on 212 patients with knee osteoarthritis was completed. Patients were randomly assigned to receive either 1500 mg oral glucosamine sulfate or placebo once daily for 3 years, with half of the population assigned to each group. Weight-bearing, anteroposterior radiographs were taken at enrolment and at 1- and 3-year follow-ups. Pain symptoms and function were scored by the Western Ontario and McMaster Universities (WOMAC) osteoarthritis index. Patients in the placebo group had progressive joint-space narrowing, while there was no significant joint-space loss in the 106 patients on glucosamine sulfate. WOMAC scores worsened in patients on the placebo compared with significant improvement observed in the patient population treated with glucosamine.[11]

A similar study—a 3-year, randomized, placebo-controlled, double-blind trial—was completed. Over 200 patients were enrolled to receive either once 1500 mg of oral glucosamine or a placebo. Changes in the radiographic joint space of the medial tibofemoral joint and symptoms were assessed using the Lequesne system described earlier and the WOMAC. Upon conclusion of the trial, there was no joint-space narrowing on an average in the glucosamine group, while the placebo saw a decreased joint space of 0.19 mm ($p = 0.001$). Symptoms improved modestly in the placebo group, while the glucosamine group saw approximately 25 percent improvement in WOMAC and Lequesne scores.[12]

Glucosamine has also been studied against the effectiveness of non-steroidal anti-inflammatory agent. Oral glucosamine was compared with ibuprofen (glucosamine sulfate 500 mg orally three times daily vs. ibuprophen 400 mg orally three times daily) for 4 weeks. The study was conducted on 200 hospitalized patients with osteoarthritis and active knee symptoms. Response was measured through the Lequesne severity index, which includes scores for pain, mobility, and limitations to activities of daily living. The study group found that the ibuprophen population improved 1 week sooner, but little difference was seen in the populations at 2 weeks. The success rates were 52 percent for the ibuprofen group and 48 percent for the glucosamine group ($p = 0.67$). Both groups saw a decrease in their average Lequesne index from 16 to 6; however, the ibuprophen group saw 35 percent of its population reporting adverse events with the most common event being gastric upset.[3]

SAFETY AND ADVERSE REACTIONS

The safety profile for glucosamine has been exceptional. Very few adverse reactions have been described and add support for the use of glucosamine despite questionable efficacy. Gastrointestinal upset is the most common of the rare adverse reactions and was reported as reversible upon discontinuation,[2,6] with one study reporting reversible gastrointestinal upset rate as high as 6 percent.[3] A multitude of other, rarer and perhaps anecdotal reactions have been observed including leg cramping, skin reactions, headache, and exhaustion.[8]

DISCUSSION

Oral glucosamine, although not an overwhelmingly strong pain reliever, has proven to be at least moderately effective in the treatment of osteoarthritis. Patients with this affliction have few nonsurgical alternatives. Nonsteroidal anti-inflammatory agents have the danger of causing gastric upset complicated by bleeding. Perhaps the greatest attraction of oral glucosamine is its safety profile. There are a few reports of complications, with the most common being mild gastric upset, which was relieved by discontinuing the drug. Glucosamine is often dosed at 500 mg orally three times daily, but may be dosed at 1500 mg orally once daily.[21] Glucosamine is available as an over-the-counter drug at a cost of approximately $30 for a month's supply at the time of publication of this text and is taken three times daily.

BIBLIOGRAPHY

1. Barclay TS, Tsourounis C, McCart GM. Glucosamine. *Ann Pharmacother* 1998;32:574-579.

2. Bassleer C, Rovati L, Franchimont P. Stimulation of proteoglycan production by glucosamine sulfate in chondrocytes isolated from human osteoarthritic articular cartilage in vitro. *Osteoarthritis Cartilage* 1998;6:427-434.

3. Bostrom M, Buckwalter J. The physiology of aging: Neuromuscular changes during aging and the effects on mobility. Koval, KJ (ed): *Orthopaedic Knowledge Update 7.* Rosemont, IL. American Academy of Orthopaedic Surgeons. 2002 Ch. 10, pp. 85-94.

4. Brief AA, Maurer SG, Di Cesare PE. Use of glucosamine and chondroitin sulfate in the management of osteoarthritis. *J Am Acad Orthop Surg* 2001;9:71.

5. Bruyere RF, Cucherat M, Henrotin Y, Reginster JY. Glucosamine and chondroitin effective for knee osteoarthritis. *J Fam Pract* 2003;52:919-920.

6. Cibere J, Thorne A, Kopec JA, Singer J, Canvin J, Robinson DB, Pope J, Hong P, Grant E, Lobanok T, Ionescu M, Poole AR, Esdaile JM. Glucosamine sulfate and cartilage type II collagen degradation in patients with knee osteoarthritis: Randomized discontinuation trial results employing biomarkers. *J Rheumatol* 2005; 32: 896-902.

7. Crolle G, D'Este E. Glucosamine sulphate for the management of arthrosis: A controlled clinical investigation. *Curr Med Res Opin* 1980;7:104-109.

8. da Camara CC, Dowless GV. Glucosamine sulfate for osteoarthritis. *Ann Pharmacother* 1998;32:580-587.

9. Drovanti A, Bignamini AA, Rovati AL. Therapeutic activity of oral Glucosamine sulfate in osteoarthrosis: A placebo-controlled double-blind investigation. *Clin Ther* 1980;3:260-272.

10. Fenton JI, Chlebek-Brown KA, Peters TL, Caron JP, Orth MW. Glucosamine HCl reduces equine articular cartilage degradation in explant culture. *Osteoarthritis Cartilage* 2000;8:258-265.

11. Forrester JV, Wilkinson PC. Inhibition of leukocyte locomotion by hyaluronic acid. *J Cell Sci* 1981;48:315-331.

12. Ghosh P, Guidolin D. Potential mechanism of action of intra-articular hyaluronan therapy in osteoarthritis: Are the effects molecular weight dependent? *Semin Arthritis Rheum* 2002;32:10-37.

13. Hungerford DS, Jones LC. Glucosamine and chondroitin sulfate are effective in the management of osteoarthritis. *J Arthroplasty* 2003;18:5-9.

14. Karzel K, Domenjoz R. Effects of hexosamine derivatives and uronic acid derivatives on glycosaminoglycan metabolism of fibroblast cultures. *Pharmacology* 1971;5:337-345.

15. Leeb BF, Schweitzer H, Montag K, Smolen JS. A metaanalysis of chondroitin sulfate in the treatment of osteoarthritis. *J Rheumatol* 2000;27:205-211.

16. McAlindon TE, LaValley MP, Gulin JP, Felson DT. Glucosamine and chondroitin for treatment of osteoarthritis: A systematic quality assessment and meta analysis. *JAMA* 2000;283:1469-1475.

17. McCarthy MF. Enhanced synovial production of hyaluronic acid may explain rapid clinical response to high-dose glucosamine in osteoarthritis. *Med Hypotheses* 1998;50:507-510.

18. Muller-Fassbender H, Bach GL, Haase W, Rovati LC, Setnikar I. Glucosamine sulfate compared to ibuprofen in osteoarthritis of the knee. *Osteoarthritis Cartilage* 1994;2:61-69.

19. Pavelka K Jr, Sedlackova M, Gatterova J, Becvar R, Pavelka K Sr. Glycosaminoglycan polysulfuric acid (GAGPS) in osteoarthritis of the knee. *Osteoarthritis Cartilage* 1995;3:15-23.

20. Pavelka K, Gatterova J, Olejarova M, Machacek S, Giacovelli G, Rovati LC. Glucosamine sulfate use and delay of progression of knee osteoarthritis: A 3-year, randomized, placebo-controlled, double-blind study. *Arch Intern Med* 2002;162: 2113-2123.

21. Persiani S, Roda E, Rovati LC, Locatelli M, Giacovelli G, Roda A. Glucosamine oral bioavailability and plasma pharmacokinetics after increasing doses of crystalline glucosamine sulfate in man. *Osteoarthritis Cartilage* 2005;13:1041-1049.

22. Poolsup N, Suthisisang C, Channark P, Kittikulsuth W. Glucosamine long-term treatment and the progression of knee osteoarthritis: Systematic review of randomized controlled trials. *Ann Pharmacother* 2005;39:1080-1087.

23. Presti D, Scott JE. Hyaluronan-mediated protective effect against cell damage caused by enzymatically produced hydroxyl (OH.) radicals is dependent on hyaluronan molecular mass. *Cell Biochem Funct* 1994;12:281-288.

24. Pujalte JM, Llavore EP, Ylescupidez FR. Double-blind clinical evaluation of oral glucosamine sulphate in the basic treatment of osteoarthrosis. *Curr Med Res Opin* 1980;7:110-114.

25. Reginster JY, Deroisy R, Rovati LC, Lee RL, Lejeune E, Bruyere O, Giacovelli G, Henrotin Y, Dacre JE, Gossett C. Long-term effects of glucosamine sulphate on osteoarthritis progression: A randomised, placebo-controlled clinical trial. *Lancet* 2001;357:251-256.

26. Richy F, Bruyere O, Ethgen O, Cucherat M, Henrotin Y, Reginster JY. Structural and symptomatic efficacy of glucosamine and chondroitin in knee osteoarthritis: A comprehensive meta-analysis. *Arch Intern Med* 2003;163:1514-1522.

27. Setnikar I, Giachetti C, Zanolo G. Absorption, distribution and excretion of radioactivity after a single intravenous or oral administration of [^{14}C] glucosamine to the rat. *Pharmatherapeutica* 1984;3:538-550.

28. Uitterlinden EJ, Jahr H, Koevoet JL, Jenniskens YM, Bierma-Zeinstra SM, Degroot J, Verhaar JA, Weinans H, van Osch GJ. Glucosamine decreases expression of anabolic and catabolic genes in human osteoarthritic cartilage explants. *Osteoarthritis Cartilage* 2005;1-8.

Chapter 11

Clinical Pharmacology
of Glucocorticoids

Muhammad A. Munir
Jun-Ming Zhang

INTRODUCTION

The natural adrenocortical hormones are steroid molecules produced and released by the adrenal cortex. The adrenal cortex synthesizes two classes of steroids: the *corticosteroids* and the *androgens*. The actions of corticosteroids are described as glucocorticoid (carbohydrate regulating) and mineralocorticoid (electrolyte regulating), reflecting their preferential activities. In humans, *cortisol (hydrocortisone)* is the main glucocorticoid and aldosterone is the main mineralocorticoid. Quantitatively, dehydroepiandrosterone (DHEA) in its sulfated form (DHEAS) is the major adrenal androgen.

Secretion of adrenocortical steroids is controlled by the pituitary release of corticotropin (ACTH). Secretion of the salt-retaining hormone aldosterone is primarily under the influence of angiotensin.

Adrenal cortex is an important source of both corticosteroids and androgens; however, patients with adrenal insufficiency can be restored to normal life expectancy by replacement therapy with corticosteroids alone. This points toward the role of corticosteroids in maintenance of life; however, addition of DHEA to the standard replacement regimen in patients with adrenal insufficiency may improve subjective well-being and sexuality.

Clinical Management of Bone and Joint Pain
© 2007 by The Haworth Press, Inc. All rights reserved.
doi:10.1300/5771_13

The effects of corticosteroids are numerous and widespread, and include alterations in carbohydrate, protein, and lipid metabolism; maintenance of fluid and electrolyte balance; and preservation of normal function of the cardiovascular system, immune system, kidney, skeletal muscle, endocrine system, and nervous system. In addition, corticosteroids endow the organism with the capacity to resist such stressful circumstances as noxious stimuli and environmental changes.

CORTICOSTEROIDS

Corticosteroids are grouped according to their relative potencies in Na^+ retention, effects on carbohydrate metabolism, and anti-inflammatory effects. In general, potencies of steroids as judged by their ability to sustain life in adrenalectomized animals closely parallel those determined for Na^+ retention, while potencies based on effects on glucose metabolism closely parallel those for anti-inflammatory effects. The effects on Na^+ retention and the carbohydrate/anti-inflammatory actions are not closely related and reflect selective actions at distinct receptors.

Based on these differential potencies, the corticosteroids are traditionally divided into mineralocorticoids and glucocorticoids. Estimates of potencies of representative steroids in these actions are listed in Table 11.1. Some steroids classified predominantly as glucocorticoids (e.g., cortisol) also possess modest but significant mineralocorticoid activity and thus may affect fluid and electrolyte handling in the clinical setting. In contrast, aldosterone is exceedingly potent with respect to Na^+ retention, but has only modest potency for effects on carbohydrate metabolism. At normal rates of secretion by the adrenal cortex or in doses that maximally affect electrolyte balance, aldosterone has no significant glucocorticoid activity and thus acts as a pure mineralocorticoid.

PHARMACODYNAMICS

Molecular Mechanism of Action

Glucocorticoids interact with specific receptor proteins in target tissues to regulate the expression of glucocorticoid-responsive genes,

TABLE 11.1. Some commonly used natural and synthetic corticosteroids.

Agent	Activity		
	Anti-inflammatory	Salt-retaining	Equivalent oral dose (mg)
Short- to medium-acting glucocorticoids			
Hydrocortisone (cortisol)	1	1	20
Cortisone	0.8	0.8	25
Prednisone	4	0.3	5
Prednisolone	5	0.3	5
Methylprednisolone	5	0	4
Intermediate-acting glucocorticoids			
Triamcinolone	5	0	4
Paramethasone	10	0	2
Fluprednisolone	15	0	1.5
Long-acting glucocorticoids			
Betamethasone	25-40	0	0.6
Dexamethasone	30	0	0.75
Mineralocorticoids			
Fludrocortisone	10	250	2
Desoxycorticosterone acetate	0	20	

thereby changing the levels and array of proteins synthesized by the various target tissues. As a consequence of the time required to modulate gene expression and protein synthesis, most effects of glucocorticoids are not immediate but become apparent after several hours. This fact is of clinical significance, because a delay generally is seen before beneficial effects of corticosteroid therapy become manifest.

The receptors for glucocorticoids are members of the nuclear receptor family of transcription factors that transduce the effects of a diverse array of small, hydrophobic ligands, including the steroid hormones, thyroid hormone, vitamin D, and retinoids. In the absence of the hormonal ligand, glucocorticoid receptors are primarily cytoplasmic, in oligomeric complexes with heat shock proteins (HSP). The most important of these are two molecules of Hsp90, though other proteins are certainly involved. Free hormone from the plasma and interstitial fluid enters the cell and binds to the receptor, inducing conformational changes that allow it to dissociate from the HSP.

After the glucocorticoid receptor (GR) dissociates from its associated proteins and translocates to the nucleus, it interacts with specific DNA sequences within the regulatory regions of affected genes. The short DNA sequences that are recognized by the activated GR are called *glucocorticoid responsive elements* (GREs) and provide specificity to the induction of gene transcription by glucocorticoids (see Figure 11.1).

In addition to binding to GREs, the ligand-bound receptor also forms complexes with and influences the function of other transcription factors, such as AP1 and NF-κB, which act on non-GRE-containing promoters, to contribute to the regulation of transcription of their responsive genes. These transcription factors have broad actions on the regulation of growth factors, proinflammatory cytokines, etc., and to a great extent mediate the antigrowth, anti-inflammatory, and immunosuppressive effects of glucocorticoids. The recognition that the

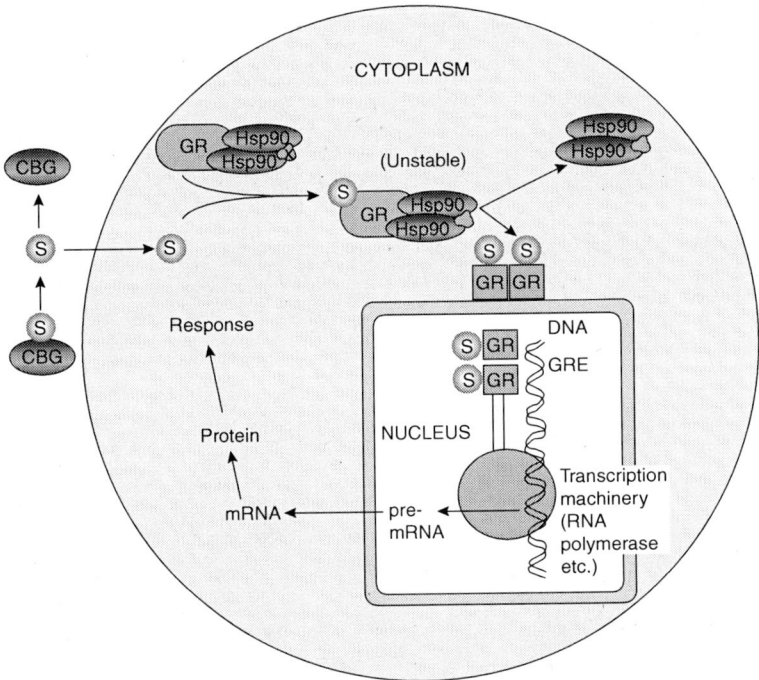

FIGURE 11.1. Mechanism of glucocorticoid action. GR: Glucocorticoid receptor; GRE: glucocorticoid-response element; HSP: heat shock proteins. S: steroid; CBG: corticosteroid-binding globulin or transcortin.

metabolic effects of glucocorticoids generally are mediated by transcriptional activation, while the anti-inflammatory effects are largely mediated by transrepression, suggesting that selective GR ligands may maintain the anti-inflammatory actions while lessening the metabolic side effects. Recent reports describe steroidal and nonsteroidal compounds that exhibit anti-inflammatory actions but have little effect on blood glucose, suggesting that such selective glucocorticoid agonists may emerge from ongoing research.

Some of the effects of glucocorticoids can be attributed to their binding to aldosterone receptors (AR). Indeed, ARs bind aldosterone and cortisol with similar affinity. A mineralocorticoid effect of cortisol is avoided in some tissues and results in corticosteroid specificity, particularly in the kidney, colon, and salivary glands by expression of 11β-hydroxysteroid dehydrogenase type 2, the enzyme responsible for biotransformation to its 11-keto derivative (cortisone), which has minimal affinity for aldosterone receptors (see Figure 11.2).

Physiologic Effects

The effects of corticosteroids are numerous and widespread, and include alterations in intermediary metabolism; maintenance of fluid and electrolyte balance; and preservation of normal function of the cardiovascular system, immune system, kidney, skeletal muscle, endocrine system, and nervous system.

The major metabolic consequences of glucocorticoid secretion or administration are due to direct actions of these hormones in the cell. However, some important effects are the result of homeostatic responses by insulin and glucagon. Many of the effects of glucocorticoids are dose related and become magnified when large amounts are administered for therapeutic purposes. However there are also certain other effects known as "permissive" effects, in the absence of which many normal functions become deficient. For example, the response of vascular and bronchial smooth muscle to catecholamines is diminished in the absence of cortisol and restored by physiologic amounts of this glucocorticoid. Furthermore, the lipolytic responses of fat cells to catecholamines, ACTH, and growth hormone are attenuated in the absence of glucocorticoids.

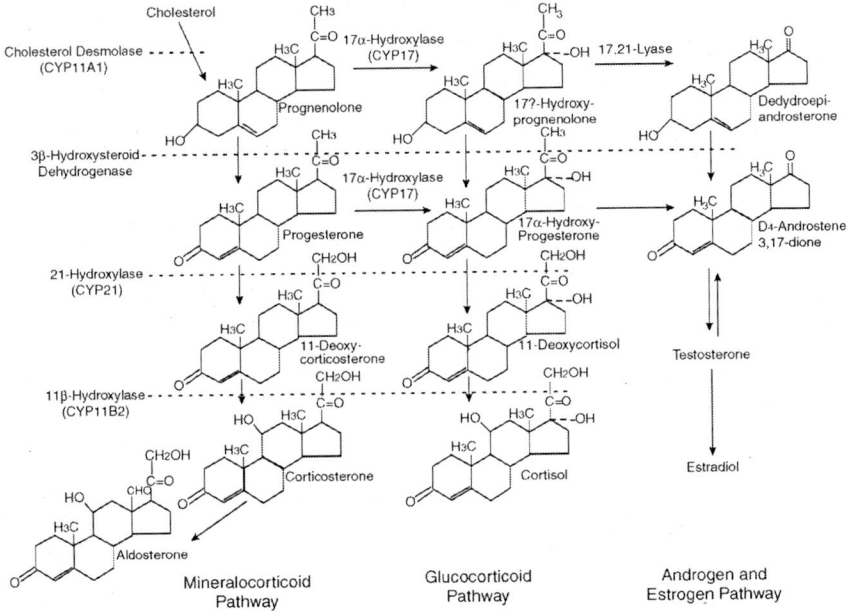

FIGURE 11.2. Synthesis of the various adrenal steroid hormones from cholesterol.

Carbohydrate and Protein Metabolism

Corticosteroids profoundly affect carbohydrate and protein metabolism. They stimulate the liver to form glucose from amino acids and glycerol and to store glucose as liver glycogen. In the periphery, glucocorticoids diminish glucose utilization, increase protein breakdown and the synthesis of glutamine, and activate lipolysis, thereby providing amino acids and glycerol for gluconeogenesis. The net result is to increase blood glucose levels. Because of their effects on glucose metabolism, glucocorticoids can worsen glycemic control in patients with overt diabetes and can precipitate the onset of hyperglycemia in patients who are otherwise predisposed.

Although glucocorticoids stimulate protein and RNA synthesis in the liver, they have catabolic and antianabolic effects in lymphoid and connective tissue, muscle, fat, and skin. Supraphysiologic amounts of glucocorticoids lead to decreased muscle mass and weakness and thinning of the skin. Catabolic and antianabolic effects on bone are the cause of osteoporosis in Cushing's syndrome and impose a major limitation in the long-term therapeutic use of glucocorticoids. In children, glucocorticoids reduce growth. This effect may be partially prevented by administration of growth hormone in high doses.

Lipid Metabolism

The effects of corticosteroids include the dramatic redistribution of body fat that occurs in settings of endogenous or pharmacologically induced hypercorticism, such as Cushing's syndrome. The other is the permissive facilitation of the lipolytic effect of other agents, such as growth hormone and α-adrenoceptor agonists, resulting in an increase in free fatty acids after glucocorticoid administration. With respect to fat distribution, there is increased fat in the back of the neck ("buffalo hump"), face ("moon facies"), and supraclavicular area, coupled with a loss of fat in the extremities.

Anti-Inflammatory and Immunosuppressive Action

Glucocorticoids dramatically reduce the manifestations of inflammation. This is due to their profound effects on the concentration, distribution, and function of peripheral leukocytes and to their suppressive effects on the inflammatory cytokines and chemokines and on other lipid and glucolipid mediators of inflammation. In addition to their effects on lymphocyte number, corticosteroids profoundly alter the immune responses of lymphocytes. These effects are an important facet of the anti-inflammatory and immunosuppressive actions of the glucocorticoids. Glucocorticoids can prevent or suppress inflammation in response to multiple inciting events, including radiant, mechanical, chemical, infectious, and immunological stimuli.

In addition to their effects on leukocyte function, glucocorticoids influence the inflammatory response by reducing the prostaglandin, leukotriene, and platelet-activating factor synthesis that results from activation of phospholipase A_2. Finally, glucocorticoids reduce expression of cyclo-oxygenase II, the inducible form of this enzyme, in inflammatory cells, thus reducing the amount of enzyme available to produce prostaglandins.

The anti-inflammatory and immunosuppressive effects of these agents are widely useful therapeutically but are also responsible for some of their most serious adverse effects.

Other Effects

The major action of glucocorticoids on the cardiovascular system is to enhance vascular reactivity to other vasoactive substances. Hypoadrenalism is associated with reduced response to vasoconstrictors such as norepinephrine and angiotensin II, perhaps due to decreased expression of adrenergic receptors in the vascular wall. Conversely, hypertension is seen in patients with excessive glucocorticoid secretion, occurring in most patients with Cushing's syndrome and in a subset of patients treated with synthetic glucocorticoids (even those lacking any significant mineralocorticoid action). Unlike hypertension caused by high aldosterone levels, the hypertension secondary to excess glucocorticoids is generally resistant to Na^+ restriction.

Glucocorticoids have important effects on the nervous system. Adrenal insufficiency causes marked slowing of the alpha rhythm of the EEG and is associated with depression. Increased amounts of glucocorticoids often produce behavioral disturbances in humans: initially insomnia and euphoria and subsequently depression. Large doses of glucocorticoids may increase intracranial pressure (pseudotumor cerebri). Glucocorticoids given chronically suppress the pituitary release of ACTH, GH, TSH, and LH.

Permissive concentrations of glucocorticoids are required for the normal function of skeletal muscle, and diminished work capacity is a prominent sign of adrenocortical insufficiency. Glucocorticoid excess over prolonged periods, either secondary to glucocorticoid therapy or endogenous hypercorticism, causes skeletal muscle wasting.

Large doses of glucocorticoids have been associated with the development of peptic ulcer, possibly by suppressing the local immune response against *Helicobacter pylori*. They also promote fat redistribution in the body, with increase of visceral, facial, nuchal, and supraclavicular fat, and they appear to antagonize the effect of vitamin D on calcium absorption. The glucocorticoids also have important effects on the hematopoietic system. In addition to their effects on leukocytes, they increase the number of platelets and red blood cells.

In the absence of physiologic amounts of cortisol, renal function (particularly glomerular filtration) is impaired, vasopressin secretion is augmented, and there is an inability to excrete a water load normally.

Glucocorticoids have important effects on the development of the fetal lungs. Indeed, the structural and functional changes in the lungs near term, including the production of pulmonary surface-active material required for air breathing (surfactant), are stimulated by glucocorticoids.

PHARMACOKINETICS

Hydrocortisone exerts a wide range of physiologic effects, including regulation of intermediary metabolism, cardiovascular function, growth, and immunity. Its synthesis and secretion are tightly regulated by the central nervous system, which is very sensitive to negative feedback by the circulating cortisol and exogenous (synthetic) glucocorticoids. Cortisol is synthesized from cholesterol (see Figure 11.2).

The rate of secretion of cortisol is 10 to 20 mg/day, whereas that of aldosterone is 0.125 mg/day. The concentration of cortisol in peripheral plasma increases up to 16 µg/100 ml in the morning and drops down by a factor of four (4 µg/100 ml) early in the evening. The rate of secretion follows a circadian rhythm governed by pulses of ACTH that peak in the early morning hours and after meals. In contrast, concentration of aldosterone remains constant through out the day (0.01 µg/100 ml) under usual circumstances and varies with water and electrolyte balance.

In plasma, cortisol is bound to circulating proteins. Corticosteroid-binding globulin (CBG), an α_2-globulin synthesized by the liver, binds 90 percent of the circulating hormone under normal circumstances. The remainder is free (about 5 to 10 percent) or loosely bound to albumin (about 5 percent) and is available to exert its effect on target cells. CBG is increased in pregnancy and with estrogen administration and in hyperthyroidism. It is decreased by hypothyroidism, genetic defects in synthesis, and protein deficiency states. Albumin has a large capacity but low affinity for cortisol, and for practical purposes albumin-bound cortisol should be considered free. Synthetic corticosteroids such as dexamethasone are largely bound to albumin rather than CBG.

The half-life of cortisol in the circulation is normally about 60 to 90 min; this half-life may be increased when hydrocortisone (the pharmaceutical preparation of cortisol) is administered in large amounts or when stress, hypothyroidism, or liver disease is present. Only 1 percent of cortisol is excreted unchanged in the urine as free cortisol; about 20 percent of cortisol is converted to cortisone by 11-hydroxysteroid dehydrogenase in the kidney and other tissues with mineralocorticoid receptors before reaching the liver. Most cortisol is inactivated in the liver by reduction and subsequent conversion to tetrahydrocortisol and tetrahydrocortisone by 3-hydroxysteroid dehydrogenase. There are small amounts of other metabolites. About one-third of the cortisol produced daily is excreted in the urine as dihydroxy ketone metabolites and is measured as 17-hydroxysteroids. Many cortisol metabolites are conjugated with glucuronic acid or sulfate at the C_3 and C_{21} hydroxyls, respectively, in the liver; they then reenter the circulation and are excreted in the urine.

Synthetic steroids with an 11-keto substituent, such as cortisone and *prednisone*, must be enzymatically reduced to the corresponding 11β-hydroxy derivative before they are biologically active. The type 1 isozyme of 11β-hydroxysteroid dehydrogenase catalyzes this reduction, predominantly in the liver, but also in specialized sites such as adipocytes, bone, eye, and skin. In settings in which this enzymatic activity is impaired, it is prudent to use steroids that do not require enzymatic activation (e.g., hydrocortisone and *prednisolone* rather than cortisone or prednisone). Such settings include severe hepatic failure and patients with the rare condition of cortisone reductase deficiency, who are unable to activate the 11-keto steroids because of a partial loss of 11β-hydroxysteroid dehydrogenase type 1 (11βHSD1) activity and a relative deficiency in the enzyme hexose-6-phosphate dehydrogenase, which supplies reducing equivalents to the 11β-hydroxysteroid dehydrogenase.

CLINICAL PHARMACOLOGY

A. Therapeutic Uses

Replacement Therapy

1. *Chronic Adrenal Insufficiency (Addison's disease):* Chronic adrenocortical insufficiency may result in fatigue, weight loss, hypotension, hyperpigmentation, and inability to maintain the blood glucose level during fasting. In such individuals, minor noxious stimuli may produce acute adrenal insufficiency with circulatory shock and even death.

In primary adrenal insufficiency, about 20 to 30 mg of hydrocortisone must be given daily, with increased amounts during periods of stress. Although hydrocortisone has some mineralocorticoid activity, this must be supplemented by a suitable amount of a salt-retaining hormone such as fludrocortisone. Synthetic glucocorticoids that are long-acting and devoid of salt-retaining activity should not be administered to these patients.

2. *Acute Adrenal Insufficiency:* The treatment for acute adrenocortical insufficiency must be instituted immediately. Therapy consists of correction of fluid and electrolyte abnormalities and treatment of precipitating factors in addition to large amounts of parenteral hydrocortisone.

   Hydrocortisone sodium succinate or phosphate in doses of 100 mg intravenously is given every 8 hours until the patient is stable. The dose is then gradually reduced, achieving maintenance dosage within 5 days. The administration of salt-retaining hormone is resumed when the total hydrocortisone dosage has been reduced to 50 mg/day.

3. *Congenital Adrenal Hyperplasia (CAH):* Congenital adrenal hyperplasia is characterized by specific defects in the synthesis of cortisol. The most common defect is a decrease in or lack of 21β-hydroxylase activity (see Figure 11.2). A lack of 21β-hydroxylase would lead to a reduction in cortisol synthesis and produce a compensatory increase in ACTH release. The gland becomes hyperplastic and produces abnormally large amounts of precursors such as 17-hydroxyprogesterone that can be diverted to the androgen pathway, leading to virilization. Metabolism of this compound in the liver leads to pregnanetriol, which is characteristically excreted into the urine in large amounts in this disorder and can be used to make the diagnosis and to monitor efficacy of glucocorticoid substitution. Nevertheless, the most reliable method of detecting CAH is the increased response of plasma 17-hydroxyprogesterone to ACTH stimulation.

   If the defect is in 11-hydroxylation, large amounts of deoxycorticosterone are produced, and because this steroid has mineralocorticoid activity, hypertension with or without hypokalemic alkalosis ensues. When 17-hydroxylation is defective in the adrenals and gonads, hypogonadism is also present. However, increased amounts of 11-deoxycorticosterone are formed, and the signs and symptoms associated with mineralocorticoid excess such as hypertension and hypokalemia are also observed.

When first seen, the infant with congenital adrenal hyperplasia may be in acute adrenal crisis and should be treated as described earlier, using appropriate electrolyte solutions and an intravenous preparation of hydrocortisone in stress doses.

Once the patient is stabilized, oral hydrocortisone, 12 to 18 mg/m^2/day in two unequally divided doses (two-thirds in the morning and one-third in late afternoon) is begun. The dosage is adjusted to allow normal growth and bone maturation and to prevent androgen excess. Alternate-day therapy with prednisone has also been used to achieve greater ACTH suppression without increasing growth inhibition. Fludrocortisone, 0.05 to 0.2 mg/day, should also be administered by mouth, with added salt to maintain normal blood pressure, plasma renin activity, and electrolytes.

4. *Postsurgical Replacement:* Cushing's syndrome is usually the result of bilateral adrenal hyperplasia secondary to an ACTH-secreting pituitary adenoma (Cushing's disease) but occasionally is due to tumors or nodular hyperplasia of the adrenal gland or ectopic production of ACTH by other tumors. The manifestations are those associated with the chronic presence of excessive glucocorticoids. This disorder is treated by surgical removal of the tumor producing ACTH or cortisol, irradiation of the pituitary tumor, or resection of one or both adrenals. These patients must receive large doses of cortisol during and following the surgical procedure. Doses of up to 300 mg of soluble hydrocortisone may be given as a continuous intravenous infusion on the day of surgery. The dose must be reduced slowly to normal replacement levels, since rapid reduction in dose may produce withdrawal symptoms, including fever and joint pain. If adrenalectomy has been performed, long-term maintenance is similar to that outlined above for adrenal insufficiency.

Nonendocrine Disorders

The synthetic analogs of cortisol are useful in the treatment of a diverse group of diseases unrelated to any known disturbance of adrenal function. The usefulness of corticosteroids in these disorders is a function of their ability to suppress inflammatory and immune responses. In disorders in which host response is the cause of the major manifestations of the disease, these agents are useful. In instances where the inflammatory or immune response is important in controlling the pathologic process, therapy with corticosteroids may be dangerous but justified to prevent permanent damage from an inflammatory response if used in conjunction with specific therapy for the disease process.

Since the corticosteroids are not usually restorative, the pathologic process may progress while clinical manifestations are suppressed. Therefore, chronic therapy with these drugs should be undertaken with great concern and only when the consequence of the disorder warrants their use and less dangerous measures have been exhausted.

In general, attempts should be made to bring the disease process under control using medium- to intermediate-acting glucocorticoids, such as prednisone and prednisolone, as well as all supplementary measures possible to keep the dose low. Where possible, alternate-day therapy should be utilized. Therapy should not be decreased or stopped abruptly. When prolonged therapy is anticipated, it is helpful to obtain chest X-rays and a tuberculin test, since glucocorticoid therapy can reactivate dormant disease. The presence of diabetes, peptic ulcer, osteoporosis, and psychologic disturbances should be taken into consideration, and cardiovascular function should be assessed.

Rheumatic Disorders

Glucocorticoids are used widely in the treatment of a variety of rheumatic disorders and are a mainstay in the treatment of the more serious inflammatory rheumatic diseases, such as systemic lupus erythematosus, and a variety of vasculitic disorders, such as polyarteritis nodosa, Wegener's granulomatosis, Churg-Strauss syndrome, and giant cell arteritis.

Initially, prednisone (1 mg/kg per day in divided doses) often is used, generally followed by consolidation to a single daily dose, with subsequent tapering to a minimal effective dose as determined by clinical variables.

To facilitate drug tapering and/or conversion to alternate-day treatment regimens, the intermediate-acting glucocorticoids such as prednisone and methylprednisolone are generally preferred over longer-acting steroids such as dexamethasone.

Alternatively, patients with major symptomatology confined to one or a few joints may be treated with intra-articular steroid injections. Depending on joint size, typical doses are 5 to 20 mg of *triamcinolone acetonide* or its equivalent.

In noninflammatory degenerative joint diseases (e.g., osteoarthritis) or in a variety of regional pain syndromes (e.g., tendinitis or bursitis), glucocorticoids may be administered by local injection for the treatment of episodic disease flare-up. In the case of repeated intraarticular injection of steroids, there is a significant incidence of painless joint destruction, resembling Charcot's arthropathy. It is suggested that intra-articular injections be performed with intervals of at least 3 months to minimize complications.

Except in patients receiving replacement therapy for adrenal insufficiency, glucocorticoids are neither specific nor curative, but are palliative because of their anti-inflammatory and immunosuppressive actions. Therefore, its use should be considered very seriously after carefully viewing the risks of therapy and potential benefits.

B. Diagnostic Uses

It is sometimes necessary to suppress the production of ACTH in order to identify the source of a particular hormone or to establish whether its production is influenced by the secretion of ACTH. In these circumstances, it is advantageous to employ a very potent substance such as dexamethasone because the use of small quantities reduces the possibility of confusion in the interpretation of hormone assays in blood or urine.

The dexamethasone suppression test is used for the diagnosis of Cushing's syndrome and has also been used in the differential diagnosis of depressive psychiatric states. As a screening test, dexamethasone, 1 mg, is given orally at 11 PM, and a plasma sample is obtained in the morning. In normal individuals, the morning cortisol concentration is usually less than 3 µg/dl, whereas in Cushing's syndrome the level is usually greater than 5 µg/dl. The results are not reliable in the presence of depression, anxiety, concurrent illness, and other stressful conditions or if the patient receives a medication that enhances the catabolism of dexamethasone in the liver. To distinguish between hypercortisolism due to anxiety, depression, and alcoholism (pseudo-Cushing's syndrome) and true Cushing's syndrome, a combined test is carried out, consisting of dexamethasone (0.5 mg orally every 6 hours for 2 days) followed by a standard corticotropin-releasing hormone (CRH) test (1 mg/kg given as a bolus intravenous infusion 2 hours after the last dose of dexamethasone).

In patients in whom the diagnosis of Cushing's syndrome has been established clinically and confirmed by a finding of elevated free cortisol in the urine, suppression with large doses of dexamethasone will help to distinguish patients with Cushing's disease from those with steroid-producing tumors of the adrenal cortex or with the ectopic ACTH syndrome. Dexamethasone is given in a dosage of 0.5 mg orally every 6 hours for 2 days, followed by 2 mg orally every 6 hours for 2 days, and the urine is then assayed for cortisol or its metabolites (Liddle's test); or dexamethasone is given as a single dose of 8 mg at 11 PM and the plasma cortisol is measured at 8 AM the following day. In patients with Cushing's disease, the suppressant effect of dexamethasone will usually produce a 50 percent reduction in hormone levels. In patients in whom suppression does not occur, the ACTH level will be low in the presence of a cortisol-producing adrenal tumor and elevated in patients with an ectopic ACTH-producing tumor.

Toxicity

The benefits obtained from use of the glucocorticoids vary considerably. Use of these drugs must be carefully weighed in each patient against their widespread effects on every part of the organism. Two categories of toxic effects result from the therapeutic use of corticosteroids: those resulting from withdrawal of steroid therapy and those resulting from continued use at supraphysiological doses. The side effects from both categories are potentially life threatening and mandate a careful assessment of the risks and benefits in each patient.

When the glucocorticoids are used for short periods (less than 2 weeks), it is unusual to see serious adverse effects even with moderately large doses. However, insomnia, behavioral changes (primarily hypomania), and acute peptic ulcers are occasionally observed even after only a few days of treatment. Acute pancreatitis is a rare but serious acute adverse effect of high-dose glucocorticoids.

Steroid Withdrawal

The most frequent problem in steroid withdrawal is flare-up of the underlying disease for which steroids were prescribed. There are several other complications associated with steroid withdrawal. The most severe complication of steroid cessation, acute adrenal insufficiency, results from overly rapid withdrawal of corticosteroids after prolonged therapy has suppressed the hypothalamic-pituitary-adrenal (HPA) axis. The therapeutic approach to acute adrenal insufficiency is already discussed. Many patients recover from glucocorticoid-induced HPA suppression within several weeks to months; however, in some individuals the time to recovery can be 1 year or longer. Patients who have received supraphysiological doses of glucocorticoids for a period of 2 to 4 weeks within the preceding year should be considered to have some degree of HPA impairment in settings of acute stress and should be treated accordingly.

In addition to this most severe form of withdrawal, a characteristic glucocorticoid withdrawal syndrome consists of fever, myalgias, arthralgias, and malaise, which may be difficult to differentiate from some of the underlying diseases for which steroid therapy was instituted. Finally, *pseudotumor cerebri*, a clinical syndrome that includes increased intracranial pressure with papilledema, is a rare condition that sometimes is associated with reduction or withdrawal of corticosteroid therapy.

Prolonged Glucocorticoids Use

Besides the consequences that result from the suppression of the HPA axis, there are a number of other complications that result from prolonged therapy with corticosteroids. These include fluid and electrolyte abnormalities, hypertension, hyperglycemia, increased susceptibility to infection, osteoporosis, myopathy, behavioral disturbances, cataracts, growth arrest, and the characteristic habitus of steroid overdose, including fat redistribution, striae, and ecchymoses.

Most patients who are given daily doses of 100 mg or more of hydrocortisone or the equivalent amount of synthetic steroid for longer than 2 weeks undergo a series of changes that have been termed iatrogenic Cushing's syndrome. The rate of development is a function of the dose and the genetic background of the patient. Fat tends to be redistributed from the extremities to the trunk, the back of the neck, and the supraclavicular fossae. In the face, rounding, puffiness, and plethora usually appear (moon facies). There is an increased growth of fine hair over the face, thighs, and trunk. Steroid-induced punctate acne may appear, and insomnia and increased appetite are noted. The underlying metabolic changes accompanying them can be very serious by the time they become obvious. The continuing breakdown of protein and diversion of amino acids to glucose production increase the need for insulin and over a period of time result in weight gain; visceral fat deposition; myopathy and muscle wasting; thinning of the skin, with striae and bruising; hyperglycemia; and eventually the development of osteoporosis, diabetes, and aseptic necrosis of the hip. Wound healing is also impaired under these circumstances.

Other serious side effects include peptic ulcers and their consequences. The clinical findings associated with certain disorders, particularly bacterial and mycotic infections, may be masked by the corticosteroids, and patients must be carefully watched to avoid serious mishap when large doses are used. The frequency of severe myopathy is greater in patients treated with long-acting glucocorticoids. The administration of such compounds has been associated with nausea, dizziness, and weight loss in some patients. It is treated by changing drugs, reducing dosage, and increasing potassium and protein intake.

Hypomania or acute psychosis may occur, particularly in patients receiving very large doses of corticosteroids. Long-term therapy with intermediate- and long-acting steroids is associated with depression and the development of posterior subcapsular cataracts. Psychiatric follow-up and periodic slit lamp examination are indicated in such patients. Increased intraocular pressure is common, and glaucoma may be induced. Benign intracranial hypertension also occurs. High dose of corticosteroids and prolonged treatment may result in growth retardation in children.

Steroids such as cortisone and hydrocortisone, which have mineralocorticoid effects in addition to glucocorticoid effects, cause some sodium and fluid retention and loss of potassium when given in amounts greater than physiologic ones. In patients with normal cardiovascular and renal function, this leads to a hypokalemic, hypochloremic alkalosis and eventually a rise in blood pressure. In patients with hypoproteinemia, renal disease, or liver disease, edema may also occur. In patients with heart disease, even small degrees of sodium retention may lead to heart failure. These effects can be minimized by using synthetic non-salt-retaining steroids, sodium restriction, and judicious amounts of potassium supplements.

Patients receiving these drugs must be monitored carefully for the development of hyperglycemia, glycosuria, sodium retention with edema or hypertension, hypokalemia, peptic ulcer, osteoporosis, and hidden infections.

The dosage should be kept as low as possible, and intermittent administration (e.g., alternate-day) should be employed when satisfactory therapeutic results can be obtained on this schedule. Even patients maintained on relatively low doses of corticosteroids may require supplementary therapy at times of stress, such as when surgical procedures are performed or intercurrent illness or accidents occur.

These agents must be used with great caution in patients with peptic ulcer, heart disease, or hypertension with heart failure, certain infectious illnesses such as varicella and tuberculosis, psychoses, diabetes, osteoporosis, or glaucoma.

CLINICAL SUMMARY

Glucocorticoids are administered in multiple formulations for a variety of disorders that share an inflammatory or immunological basis. However, glucocorticoids are not curative and rather provide palliative care for most nonendocrine and nonreplacement uses. The decision to start any particular patient with glucocorticoid therapy must be considered very carefully, considering the number and severity of side effects. In determining the dosage regimen to be used, the physician must consider the seriousness of the disease, the amount of drug likely to be required to obtain the desired effect, and the duration of therapy. However, a single dose of glucocorticoid, even a large one, is virtually without harmful effects, and a short course of therapy (less than 2 weeks) is unlikely to cause harm in the absence of specific contraindications. As the duration of glucocorticoid therapy increases beyond couple of weeks, adverse effects increase in a time- and dose-related manner.

BIBLIOGRAPHY

Axelrod L. Perioperative management of patients treated with glucocorticoids. *Endocrinol Meta Clin North Am* 2003; 32:367-383.

Bamberger CM, Bamberger AM, de Castro M, Chrousos GP. Glucocorticoid receptor-beta, a potential endogenous inhibitor of glucocorticoid action in humans. *J Clin Invest* 1995;95:2435.

Barnes PJ, Adcock I. Anti-inflammatory actions of steroids: Molecular mechanisms. *Trends Pharmacology Sci* 1993;14:436.

Bray PJ, Cotton RG. Variations of the human glucocorticoid receptor gene (NR3C1): pathological and in vitro mutations and polymorphisms. *Hum Mutat* 2003; 21:557-568.

Chin R. Adrenal crisis. *Crit Care Clin* 1991;7:23.

Chrousos GP. The hypothalamic-pituitary-adrenal axis and immune-mediated inflammation. *N Engl J Med* 1995;332:1351.

Coursin DB, Wood KE. Corticosteroid supplementation for adrenal insufficiency. *JAMA* 2002;287:236-240.

Coghlan, MJ, Elmore SW, Kym PR, Kort ME. The pursuit of differentiated ligands for the glucocorticoid receptor. *Curr Top Med Chem* 2003;3:1617-1635.

Dorr HG, Sippell WG. Prenatal dexamethasone treatment in pregnancies at risk for congenital adrenal hyperplasia due to 21-hydroxylase deficiency: Effect on mid-gestational amniotic fluid steroid levels. *J Clin Endocrinol Metab* 1993; 76:117.

Franchimont D, Kino T, Galon J, Meduri GU, Chrousos G. Glucocorticoids and inflammation revisited: The state of the art. *Neuroimmunomodulation* 2002; 10:247.

Hahn BH, Mazzaferri EL. Glucocorticoid-induced osteoporosis. *Hosp Pract (Off Ed)* 1995;30:45.

Hochberg Z, Pacak K, Chrousos GP. Endocrine withdrawal syndromes. *Endocrine Rev* 2003;24:523.

Norman AW, Mizwicki MT, Norman DP. Steroid-hormone rapid actions, membrane receptors, and a conformational ensemble model. *Nat Rev Drug Discov* 2004;3:27-41.

Saag KG. Glucocorticoid-induced osteoporosis. *Endocrinol Metab Clin North Am* 2003;32:135-157.

Tappy L, Randin D, Vollenweider P, Vollenweider L, Paquet N, Schrerrer U, Schneiter P, Nocod P, Jequier E. Mechanisms of dexamethasone-induced insulin resistance in healthy humans. *J Clin Endocrinol Metab* 1994;79:1063.

Chapter 12

Hyaluronic Acid

William Lavelle
Elizabeth Demers
Lori Lavelle

Hyaluronic acid is a gylcosaminoglycan occurring naturally in the human joints. It is principally responsible of the viscosity and normal lubrication of these joints. Fluid studies have revealed that the non-Newtonian properties of hyaluronic acid reduce shear rates and wear of articular cartilage.[1-5] The concentration and quality of hyaluronic acid has been found to decrease as degenerative arthritis progresses, but the exact mechanism by which joint degeneration causes pain is unclear.[2,6,7] Despite its known properties, it is difficult to determine how introducing extrinsic hyaluronic acid will either mitigate joint degeneration or, more importantly, relieve pain. A large segment of the medical community utilizes intra-articular injection of hyaluronic acid for the treatment of joint pain. Clinical data regarding the efficacy of hyaluronic acid in the treatment of joint pain has truly been mixed; however, patients with degenerative joint disease have few nonsurgical alternatives after failing nonsteroidal anti-inflammatory drugs (NSAIDs) and steroid injections.

HISTORY

Electron microscopy studies by Balazs, Bloom, and Swan found a thickened layer on the articular surface of older animals. This thickened layer was later found to contain hyaluronic acid.[8] In the late

Clinical Management of Bone and Joint Pain
© 2007 by The Haworth Press, Inc. All rights reserved.
doi:10.1300/5771_14

1960s the viscoelastic properties of hyaluronic acid were explored. It was at this time that Rydell and Balazs first proposed viscosupplementation. Hyaluronic acid was first prepared from rooster combs and umbilical cords and tested in dogs, monkeys, and horses with positive results.[8,9]

Since that time, commercial efforts have seen the development of injectable hyaluronic acid. Three forms are currently approved for use in the United States: sodium hyaluronate (Hyalgan), sodium hyaluronate (Supartz), and hylan G-F20 (Synvisc).

MECHANISM OF ACTION

The first proposed action of the injectable hyaluronic acid was the reconstitution of hyaluronic acid in synovial fluid.[6] Despite this seemingly logical contention, it was later determined that intra-articular hyaluronic acid is turned over quickly via local metabolism and the lymphatic system within 3 days.[10,11] Furthermore, hyaluronic acid turnover is doubled in inflamed joints.[12] It would seem clear that, for hyaluronic acid to provide true efficacy, as many physicians feel it has, another pathophysiology must exist.

Numerous cells involved in the degenerative process of osteoarthritis possess cellular adhesion molecules that bind hyaluronic acid.[1,13-25] Specifically, hyaluronic acid binds to CD44.[1,17] Other cellular receptors that also bind hyaluronic acid have been identified and include ICAM-1 and RHAMM;[1] however, the great majority of the described interactions involve CD44. The binding of hyaluronic acid to CD44 and RHAMM has been found to cause intracellular phosphorylation cascades, which lead to cell migration, proliferation, and endocytosis (see Figure 12.1).[1]

The effects of hyaluronic acid may be dependent on the molecular weight (Table 12.1). Lower molecular weight hyaluronic acid (1,000,000 d) may penetrate into arthritic and inflamed tissue more than that with higher molecular weight (2,000,000 d).[26,27] Low molecular weight hyaluronic acid may also differ in activity at the cellular level as well. Smaller hyaluronic acids (280,000 to 470,000 d) promoted chemokine expression by macrophages, while a preparation (6,100,000 d) closer to that of commercial preparations did not.[28] The varying activity we see may be explained by a need for formation

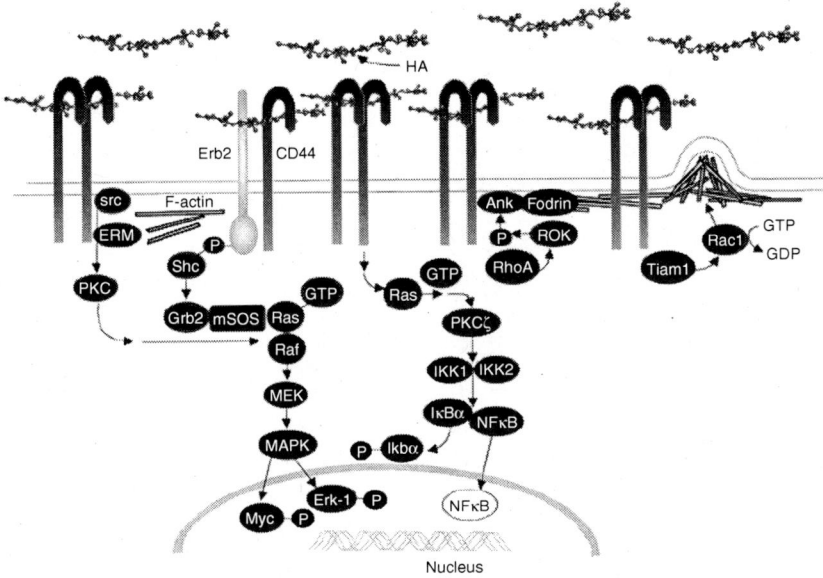

FIGURE 12.1. Diagrammatic representation of the CD44 cell surface receptors showing their possible intracellular signaling pathways, which can be activated by hyaluronic acid (HA). The four signaling cascades involving CD44 have been identified. Pathway (A) requires activation of the Src-related tyrosine kinases, (B) heterodimerization of CD44–Erb B2 may activate a MAP kinase (MAPK) cascade, (C) the nuclear transcription factor (NF-κB) may be activated through HA interaction with CD44 and a protein kinase C (PKC) dependent cascade, and (D) activation of GTPases by HA–CD44 interaction can lead to reorganization of the actin cytoskeleton. *Source:* Reprinted from *Seminars in Arthritis and Rheumatism, 32,* P Ghosh and D Guidolin, Potential mechanism of action of intra-articular hyaluronan therapy in osteoarthritis: are the effects molecular weight dependent? 10-37, (2002), with permission from Elsevier.

TABLE 12.1. Molecular weights of commercial hyaluronic acid.

Forms of hyaluronic acid	Molecular weight
Sodium hyaluronate (Hyalgan)	500,000-730,000
Sodium hyaluronate (Supartz)	620,000-1,170,00
Hylan G-F 20 (Synvisc)	80 percent Hylan A, 6,000,000 20 percent Hylan B, indeterminant molecular weight

of a specific and stable receptor complex. Interactions of multiple CD44 molecules by a single hyaluronic acid molecule may be required with this only occurring with hyaluronic acids of a particular size.[1]

In sharp contrast, higher molecular weight preparations (1,200,000 d) were more effective than lower molecular weight ones (176,000 and 668,000 d). The proposed mechanism for this finding was that a mesh-work developed, which allowed for protection from free radicals.[1,29]

It would appear that the exact mechanism of action by which hyaluronic acids relieve pain is unclear. Hyaluronic acids have been found to inhibit leukocyte migration, chemotaxis, and cellular adhesion.[30] In the destructive process of osteoarthritis leukocytes, they mediate enzymatic and oxidative free radical reactions.[1,29] Theoretically, this would slow the degenerative process and thus abate pain.

Hyaluronic acids have also been found to affect the synthesis of endogenous hyaluronic acid. The molecular weight of the hyaluronic acid affected this process as well. Endogenous hyaluronic acid synthesis by human synovial fibroblasts derived from arthritic joints was upregulated by extrinsic hyaluronic acid of molecular weight greater than 500,000 d.[1,31] Again, the proposed explanation for this difference was the need for formation of a specific and stable receptor complex, though perhaps with a different architecture than that described here.

Molecular weight is also important in the ability of hyaluronic acid to inhibit phagocytosis. High molecular weight hyaluronic acid interferes with the phagocytotic ability of macrophages.[10,32] Low molecular weight hyaluronic acid did not inhibit phagocytosis.

Hyaluronic acids have also been found to prevent the destruction of articular cartilage. In osteoarthritis, fibronectin fragments induce catabolic cytokines in human cartilage, which, in turn, suppress proteoglycan synthesis and induce matrix metalloproteinases to decrease the proteoglycan content. Hyaluronic acid has been reported to prevent proteoglycan depletion induced by fibronectin fragments. This effect was associated with coating of the articular surface, suppression of fibronectin-fragment-enhanced stromelysin-1 release, increased proteoglycan synthesis, and restoration of proteoglycans in damaged cartilage.[10,33]

Cartilage destruction may also occur via a neutrophil-mediated process. Hyaluronic acid has been found *in vitro* to interfere with the ability of neutrophils to adhere to the surface of articular cartilage. Molecular weight also played a role with this inhibition as well.[10,34]

In the forefront of treatment of osteochondral injuries, animal studies have been completed whereupon osteochondral injuries were created in 12 sheep. These animals subsequently underwent mosaic arthroplasty and were randomized to either receive intra-articular hyaluronic acid of a saline placebo. Better cartilage growth was seen in the experimental arm.[35]

Hyaluronic acids have been found to possess with their own endogenous analgesic effects. In animal models, hyaluronic acid acted much like an anti-inflammatory agent. In early studies, hyaluronic acid was thought to directly bind pain peptides.[1] Later, in a model where rats were administered intra-articular bradykinin to induce joint pain, the analgesic effect of the hyaluronic acid was not prevented by prior administration of a bradykinin antagonist. It was proposed that hyaluronic acid must be altering the pain pathway, either through the CD44 receptor or an alternative mechanism yet to be described.

CLINICAL TRIALS

With the multitude of proposed mechanism of actions, one must question the true efficacy of hyaluronic acid preparations. This question has been examined in the literature through a series of different types of studies, some more statistically valid than others. As would be expected, the more clinically relevant studies involved controlled trials with the best of these including arthrocentesis followed by saline injection.[26] Many patients demonstrated clinical benefit from this placebo. In addition, as cited earlier, molecular weight and dose are possible confounding factors as studies have found that the molecular weight and the concentration of the intra-articular hyaluronic acid may affect the result.

Ten placebo-controlled studies on Hyalgan that involved the use of arthrocentesis followed by saline injection were recently reviewed.[26,36-41] In nine of these studies, patients reported symptomatic relief for up to 6 months, with statistically significant differences in visual analog scores. There was only one study that failed to illustrate a statistically significant difference compared with arthrocentesis followed by saline injection.[26,39]

In a similar manner, two placebo-controlled studies, again involving arthrocentesis followed by saline injection, found that three Synvisc injections provided statistically significant pain relief.[26]

Intra-articular hyaluronic acid has also been compared directly to NSAID therapy. Naproxen and intra-articular saline were utilized as controls in a multicenter trial of Hyalgan. This study found comparable results between naproxen and hyaluronic acid. Both performed significantly better than saline injection.[40]

Intra-articular hyaluronic acid therapy has also been compared to intra-articular glucocorticoid therapy. Hyalgan was found to provide statistically significant improvement in pain relief when compared with a saline control. No statistical difference was seen when compared with intra-articular glucocorticoid therapy with either methylprednisolone or triamcinolone.[26,36,42] Researchers have also compared the cartilage of patients treated with either Hyalgan or methylprednisolone. Twenty-four subjects were compared. The Hyalgan group demonstrated a significant reconstitution of the superficial articular cartilage, similar to the reports described earlier.[43]

Most recently, a large meta-analysis of randomized controlled trials looking at the efficacy of hyaluronic acid was completed and published in the *Journal of Bone and Joint Surgery.* Twenty studies were included in the analysis. Overall, the analysis found significant improvements in pain and functional outcomes with few adverse events. Lower methodological quality such as single-blind or single-center design resulted in higher estimates of hyaluronic acid efficacy. The analysis also found that patients with advanced osteoarthritis by X-ray were less likely to benefit from intra-articular hyaluronic acid.[44]

SAFETY AND ADVERSE REACTIONS

As with all intra-articular injections, the most obvious and worrisome reaction to injection of hyaluronic acid is joint infection. Administrators of this agent should take care to maintain meticulous sterile technique as an iatrogenic joint infection would be devastating. The hallmark of an acute joint infection includes erythema, joint pain, warmth, a large effusion, and stiffness. Definitive diagnosis is determined through arthrocentesis followed by microbiological analysis of the aspirate consisting of a gram stain, cell count, and cell culture.

Unfortunately, a pseudoseptic reaction has been described for intra-articular hyaluronic acid. This process is also heralded by erythema, joint pain, warmth, a large effusion, and stiffness; however, the joint fluid revealed no trace of infection. Instead, large numbers of mononuclear cells and eosinophils were seen.[45-51] The reaction is typically seen with repeat injections and may represent a sensitization to the product. The long-term effects of these hypersensitivity reactions have not been described.[26] This pseudoseptic reaction has been observed in 2 to 8 percent of patients treated with Synvisc.[52-55]

The symptoms of erythema, joint pain, warmth, a large effusion, and stiffness related to hyaluronic acid therapy may also be due to an acute pseudogout attack. Pseudogout has been reported as a complication of infections with Hyalgan and Synvisc. These patients were reported to have done well with joint aspiration and conservative measures.[56-59]

DISCUSSION

Intra-articular hyaluronic injection offers a possible method for the treatment of chronic joint pain associated with osteoarthritis. Other agents have been studied more extensively and are considered "tradtional" means of treatment for osteoarthritis. These include NSAIDs, weight loss, and lifestyle changes. However, when faced with the alternative of surgery, intra-articular hyaluronic acid therapy offers another means of conservative therapy. Although currently covered by Medicare and some insurance plans, pertinent supportive data as to the need for intra-articular hyaluronic acid therapy should be maintained. Cost may also be another consideration, with a single injection costing approximately $230.[60]

REFERENCES

1. Ghosh P, Guidolin D. Potential mechanism of action of intra-articular hyaluronan therapy in osteoarthritis: are the effects molecular weight dependent? *Sem Arthritis Rheum* 2002;32:10-37.

2. Balazs EA, Watson D, Duff IF, Roseman S. Hyaluronic acid in synovial fluid. I. Molecular parameters of hyaluronic acid in normal and arthritis human fluids. *Arthritis Rheum* 1967;10:357-376.

3. Bothner H, Wik O. Rheology of hyaluronate. *Acta Otolaryngol Suppl* 1987; 442:25-30.

4. Balazs EA, Denlinger JL. Sodium hyaluronate and joint function. *Equine Vet Sci* 1985;5:217-228.

5. Scott D, Coleman PJ, Mason RM, Levick JR. Concentration dependence of interstitial flow buffering by hyaluronan in synovial joints. *Microvasc Res* 2000; 59:345-353.

6. Balazs EA, Denlinger JL. Viscosupplementation: A new concept in the treatment of osteoarthritis. *J Rheumatol Suppl* 1993;39:3-9.

7. Peyron JG. Intraarticular hyaluronan injections in the treatment of osteoarthritis: State-of-the-art review. *J Rheumatol Suppl* 1993;39:10-15.

8. Rydell N, Balazs EA. Effect of intra-articular injection of hyaluronic acid on the clinical symptoms of osteoarthritis and on granulation tissue formation. *Clin Orthop Relat Res* 1971;80:25-32.

9. Butler J, Rydell NW, Balazs EA. Hyaluronic acid in synovial fluid. VI. Effect of intra-articular injection of hyaluronic acid on the clinical symptoms of arthritis in track horses. *Acta Vet Scand* 1970;11:139-155.

10. Moreland LW. Intra-articular hyaluronan (hyaluronic acid) and hylans for the treatment of osteoarthritis: Mechanisms of action. *Arthritis Res Ther* 2003;5:54-67.

11. Fraser JRE, Brown TJ, Cahill TNP, Laurent TC, Laurent UBG. The turnover of hyaluronan in synovial joints. *Immunol Cell Biol* 1996;74:A10.

12. Fraser JR, Kimpton WG, Pierscionek BK, Cahill RN. The kinetics of hyaluronan in normal and acutely inflamed synovial joints: Observations with experimental arthritis in sheep. *Semin Arthritis Rheum* 1993;22(Suppl 1):9-17.

13. Knudson CB. Hyaluronan receptor-directed assembly of chondrocyte pericellular matrix. *J Cell Biol* 1993;120:825-834.

14. Culty M, O'Mara TE, Underhill CB, Yeager H Jr, Swartz RP. Hyaluronan receptor (CD44) expression and function in human peripheral blood monocytes and alveolar macrophages. *J Leukoc Biol* 1994;56:605-611.

15. Parkar AA, Kahmann JD, Howat SL, Bayliss MT, Day AJ. TSG-6 interacts with hyaluronan and aggrecan in a pH-dependent manner via a common functional element: implications for its regulation in inflamed cartilage. *FEBS Lett* 1998; 428:171-176.

16. Underhill CB, Nguyen HA, Shizari M, Culty M. CD44 positive macrophages take up hyaluronan during lung development. *Dev Biol* 1993;155:324-336.

17. Culty M, Miyake K, Kincade PW, Sikorski E, Butcher EC, Underhill C. The hyaluronate receptor is a member of the CD44 (H-CAM) family of cell surface glycoproteins. *J Cell Biol* 1990;111:2765-2774.

18. Rafi A, Nagarkatti M, Nagarkatti PS. Hyaluronate-CD44 interactions can induce murine B-cell activation. *Blood* 1997;89:2901-2908.

19. Hodge-Dufour J, Noble PW, Horton MR, Bao C, Wysoka M, Burdick MD, Strieter RM, Trinchieri G, Pure E. Induction of IL-12 and chemokines by hyaluronan requires adhesion-dependent priming of resident but not elicited macrophages. *J Immunol* 1997;159:2492-2500.

20. Chiu RK, Droll A, Dougherty ST, Carpenito C, Cooper DL, Dougherty GJ. Alternatively spliced CD44 isoforms containing exon v10 promote cellular

adhesion through the recognition of chondroitin sulfate-modified CD44. *Exp Cell Res* 1999;248:314-321.

21. Lesley J, Howes N, Perschl A, Hyman R. Hyaluronan binding function of CD44 is transiently activated on T cells during an in vivo immune response. *J Exp Med* 1994;180:383-387.

22. Siegelman MH, DeGrendele HC, Estess P. Activation and interaction of CD44 and hyaluronan in immunological systems. *J Leukoc Biol* 1999;66:315-321.

23. Fujii K, Tanaka Y, Hubscher S, Saito K, Ota T, Eto S. Cross-linking of CD44 on rheumatoid synovial cells up-regulates VCAM-1. *J Immunol* 1999;162: 2391-2398.

24. Ishida O, Tanaka Y, Morimoto I, Takigawa M, Eto S. Chondrocytes are regulated by cellular adhesion through CD44 and hyaluronic acid pathway. *J Bone Miner Res* 1997;12:1657-1663.

25. Aruffo A, Stamenko I, Melnick M, Underehill CB. Seed B. CD44 is the principal cell-surface receptor for hyaluronate. *Cell* 1990;61:1303-1313.

26. Kelly MA, Goldberg VM, Healy WL, Pagnano MW, Hamburger MI. Osteoarthritis and beyond: A consensus on the past, present, and future of hyaluronans in orthopedics. *Orthopedics* 2003;26:1064-1079.

27. Asari A, Miyauchi S, Matsuzaka S, Ito T, Kominami E, Uchiyama Y. Molecular weight-dependent effects of hyaluronate on the arthritic synovium. *Arch Histol Cytol* 1998;61:125-135.

28. Ohkawara Y, Tamura G, Iwasaki T, Tanaka A, Kikuchi T, Shirato K. Activation and transforming growth factor-beta production in eosinophils by hyaluronan. *Am J Respir Cell Mol Biol* 2000;23:444-451.

29. Presti D, Scott JE. Hyaluronan-mediated protective effect against cell damage caused by enzymatically produced hydroxyl (OH.) radicals is dependent on hyaluronan molecular mass. *Cell Biochem Funct* 1994;12:281-288.

30. Forrester JV, Wilkinson PC. Inhibition of leukocyte locomotion by hyaluronic acid. *J Cell Sci* 1981;48:315-331.

31. Smith MM, Ghosh P. The synthesis of hyaluronic acid by human synovial fibroblasts is influenced by the nature of the hyaluronate in the extracellular environment. *Rheumatol Int* 1987;7:113-122.

32. Forrester JV, Balazs EA. Inhibition of phagocytosis by high molecular weight hyaluronate. *Immunology* 1980;40:435-446.

33. Kang Y, Eger W, Koepp H, Williams JM, Kuettner KE, Homandberg GA. Hyaluronan suppresses fibronectin fragment-mediated damage to human cartilage explant cultures by enhancing proteoglycan synthesis. *J Orthop Res* 1999;17: 858-869.

34. Kawasaki K, Ochi M, Uchio Y, Adachi N, Matsusaki M. Hyaluronic acid enhances proliferation and chondroitin sulfate synthesis in cultured chondrocytes embedded in collagen gels. *J Cell Physiol* 1999;179:142-148.

35. Tytherleigh-Strong G, Hurtig M, Miniaci A. Intra-articular hyaluronan following autogenous osteochondral grafting of the knee. *Arthroscopy* 2005; 21:999-1005.

36. Bragantini A, Cassini M, De Bastiani G, Perbellini A. Controlled single-blinded trial of intra-articularly injected hyaluronic acid (hyalgan) in osteoarthritis of the knee. *Clin Trials J* 1987;24:333-340.

37. Dougados M, Nguyen M, Listrat V, Amor B. High molecular weight sodium hyaluronate (hyalectin) in osteoarthritis of the knee: A 1 year placebo-controlled trial. *Osteoarthritis Cartilage* 1993;1:97-103.

38. Huskisson EC, Donnelly S. Hyaluronic acid in the treatment of osteoarthritis of the knee. *Rheumatology (Oxford)* 1999;38:602-607.

39. Henderson EB, Smith EC, Pegley F, Blake DR. Intra-articular injections of 750 kD hyaluronan in the treatment of osteoarthritis: A randomised single centre double-blind placebo-controlled trial of 91 patients demonstrating lack of efficacy. *Ann Rheum Dis* 1994;53:529-534.

40. Altman RD, Moskowitz R. Intraarticular sodium hyaluronate (hyalgan) in the treatment of patients with osteoarthritis of the knee: A randomized clinical trial. Hyalgan Study Group. *J Rheumatol* 1998;25:2203-2212.

41. Dixon AS, Jacoby RK, Berry H, Hamilton EB. Clinical trial of intra-articular injection of sodium hyaluronate in patients with osteoarthritis of the knee. *Curr Med Res Opin* 1988;11:205-213.

42. Jones AC, Pattrick M, Doherty S, Doherty M. Intra-articular hyaluronic acid compared to intra-articular triamcinolone hexacetonide in inflammatory knee osteoarthritis. *Osteoarthritis Cartilage* 1995;3:269-273.

43. Guidolin DD, Ronchetti IP, Lini E, Guerra D, Frizziero L. Morphological analysis of articular cartilage biopsies from a randomized, clinical study comparing the effects of 500-730 kDa sodium hyaluronate (hyalgan) and methylprednisolone acetate on primary osteoarthritis of the knee. *Osteoarthritis Cartilage* 2001;9:371-381.

44. Wang CT, Lin J, Chang CJ, Lin YT, Hou SM. Therapeutic effects of hyaluronic acid on osteoarthritis of the knee. A meta-analysis of randomized controlled trials. *J Bone Joint Surg Am* 2004;86:538-545.

45. Adams ME, Lussier AJ, Peyron JG. A risk-benefit assessment of injections of hyaluronan and its derivatives in the treatment of osteoarthritis of the knee. *Drug Saf* 2000;23:115-130.

46. Pullman-Mooar S, Mooar P, Sieck M, Clayburne G, Schumacher HR. Are there distinctive inflammatory flares after hylan G-F 20 intraarticular injections? *J Rheumatol* 2002;29:2611-2614.

47. Puttick MP, Wade JP, Chalmers A, Connell DG, Rangno KK. Acute local reactions after intraarticular hylan for osteoarthritis of the knee. *J Rheumatol* 1995;22:1311-1314.

48. Allen E, Krohn K. Adverse reaction to hylan GF-20. *J Rheumatol* 2000;27:1572.

49. Martens PB. Bilateral symmetric inflammatory reaction to hylan G-F 20 injection. *Arthritis Rheum* 2001;44:978-979.

50. Rees JD, Wojtulewski JA. Systemic reaction to viscosupplementation for knee osteoarthritis. *Rheumatology (Oxford)* 2001;40:1425-1426.

51. Bernardeau C, Bucki B, Liote F. Acute arthritis after intra-articular hyaluronate injection: onset of effusions without crystal. *Ann Rheum Dis* 2001;60:518-520.

52. Neustadt DH. Long-term efficacy and safety of intra-articular sodium hyaluronate (Hyalgan) in patients with osteoarthritis of the knee. *Clin Exp Rheumatol* 2003;21:307-311.

53. Puttick MP, Wade JP, Chalmers A, Connell DG, Rangno KK. Acute local reactions after intraarticular hylan for osteoarthritis of the knee. *J Rheumatol* 1995; 22:1311-1314.

54. Chen AL, Desai P, Adler EM, Di Cesare PE. Granulomatous inflammation after Hylan G-F 20 viscosupplementation of the knee: a report of six cases. *J Bone Joint Surg Am* 2002;84:1142-1147.

55. Leopold SS, Warme WJ, Pettis PD, Shott S. Increased frequency of acute local reaction to intra-articular hylan GF-20 (synvisc) in patients receiving more than one course of treatment. *J Bone Joint Surg Am* 2002;84:1619-1623.

56. Luzar MJ, Altawil B. Pseudogout following intraarticular injection of sodium hyaluronate. *Arthritis Rheum* 1998;41:939-940.

57. Disla E, Infante R, Fahmy A, Karten I, Cuppari GG. Recurrent acute calcium pyrophosphate dihydrate arthritis following intraarticular hyaluronate injection. *Arthritis Rheum* 1999;42:1302-1303.

58. Ali Y, Weinstein M, Jokl P. Acute pseudogout following intra-articular injection of high molecular weight hyaluronic acid. *Am J Med* 1999;107:641-642.

59. Kroesen S, Schmid W, Theiler R. Induction of an acute attack of calcium pyrophosphate dihydrate arthritis by intra-articular injection of hylan G-F 20 (Synvisc). *Clin Rheumatol* 2000;19:147-149.

60. Modawal A, Ferrer M, Choi HK, Castle JA. Hyaluronic acid injections relieve knee pain. *J Fam Pract* 2005;54:758-767.

Chapter 13

Disease-Modifying Antirheumatic Drugs

Lori Lavelle
William Lavelle
Elizabeth Demers

INTRODUCTION

The immune system is an amazing and yet complicated part of the human body. It is composed of two portions: innate and acquired. The innate portion of the immune system includes primitive defense mechanisms such as the epithelial layers of skin, lungs, and intestines. Other components of the innate portion of the immune system include the complement system, as well as cytokines, or chemicals secreted into the cell environment, which stimulates the immune process.

The other half of the immune system, the acquired portion, is a strategy for the body to fight new viral, bacterial, and parasitic organisms it encounters. Acquired immunity also provides memory of organisms that have invaded the human body in the past, such that if the body encounters the same pathogen in the future, the immune system can mount a quicker and stronger defense.

Integrity of the acquired portion of the immune system relies on the interaction of three components: an antigen presenter cell (dendritic cell, macrophage, or monocyte), a T-cell, and a B-cell. Each of these three components signal to the other through an array of chemokines and cytokines released into the cell medium, in addition to a variety

Clinical Management of Bone and Joint Pain
© 2007 by The Haworth Press, Inc. All rights reserved.
doi:10.1300/5771_15

of ligands and proteins located on the cell surfaces. The exact mechanisms by which the antigen presenter cell, T-cell, and B-cell function are intricate and complex. The human body has pathways to ensure that the immune response is an appropriate action. However, the acquired immune system does occasionally mount an inappropriate response to an antigen that it should recognize as "self." When this occurs, an autoimmune disease originates. Also, as in the case of a transplanted organ, the immune system wants to mount a response to the foreign antigens it sees, but medication is required to halt this normally appropriate response. Medications such as disease-modifying antirheumatic drugs (DMARDs) are required to alter the immune system signaling mechanisms and provide a way for the human body to "reset" itself and maintain balance within the immune system.

ANTIMALARIALS

Antimalarial agents such as hydroxychloroquine (Plaquenil) have been used to treat autoimmune diseases such as rheumatoid arthritis and lupus for decades. The mechanism of action of Plaquenil is broad, and it is difficult to define its mechanism of action in a particular disease state. These medications act as weak bases raising the pH in cell environments, which interferes with chemical pathways that depend on a high-acid environment.[1] Antimalarials have been found to interfere with the binding of autoantigenic molecules called antigens to the surfaces of cells. This interferes with the body's inappropriate response to autoimmune diseases.[2] This class of medications also blocks the absorption of ultraviolet rays into the skin, which helps to heal skin lesions that occur in lupus.[3] Cholesterol values are affected by hydroxychloroquine, causing a decrease in total cholesterol, low-density lipoprotein (LDL), and very-low-density lipoprotein (VLDL).[4] Antimalarials also act as mild anticoagulants by interfering with platelet activity.[1] In patients with diseases such as rheumatoid arthritis or erosive osteoarthritis, they reduce swelling, stiffness, and pain. For patients with lupus, the addition of hydroxychloroquine improves fatigue and rashes, and decreases swelling and stiffness of joints.

Plaquenil is dosed as a 200 mg pill. A common dosage for patients with autoimmune diseases is one pill twice a day. It generally takes several months with this medication to notice a decrease in symptoms, as the half-life is 1 to 2 months.[5] The most common side effect is nausea or loss of appetite. If these side effects occur, patients are encouraged to take hydroxychloroquine with food or at bedtime. Antimalarial drugs have been shown to cause neuropathy, proximal muscle weakness from a myopathy, and cardiomyopathy. These symptoms have improved with discontinuation of hydroxychloroquine for several months.[6-8] This medication has, in rare cases, also been associated with deposition in the retina, causing altered vision. If this occurs, discontinuation of hydroxychloroquine most often alleviates the problem. It is recommended that patients who are taking Plaquenil have an eye exam every 6 months for the first year, then yearly thereafter.[9] If patients experience a change in vision, they are encouraged to see an ophthalmologist.

GLUCOCORTICOIDS

In any patient who suffers from a severe autoimmune disease, medication may be needed to reduce inflammation quickly. Glucocorticoids such as prednisone and methylprednisolone are medications that work quickly to reduce the immune system's activity. These medications are effective in controlling diseases such as lupus, vasculitis,[10] and rheumatoid arthritis.[11,12]

Steroids are very effective in controlling the inflammatory processes produced by the immune system, but it also can cause side effects, as listed here:[10]

Weight gain—stimulates the appetite and also causes water retention
Insomnia
Mood swings
Easy bruising of skin
Acne
Elevated high blood pressure
Elevated blood sugar
Risk of glaucoma or cataracts with prolonged use
Risk of osteopenia or osteoporosis, which could cause fractures
Muscle weakness
Avascular necrosis

For patients who are expected to be on a prolonged course of glucocorticoids, it is recommended that they take at least 1500 mg of calcium daily and 400 IU of vitamin D. Some patients whose bone mineral density is low before the introduction of steroids may need to take a bisphosphonate in addition to daily calcium and vitamin D.

METHOTREXATE

Another popular medication used as a steroid-sparing agent is Methotrexate (Rheumatrex). This medication is used to treat a variety of diseases including rheumatoid arthritis, polymyalgia rheumatica, vasculitis, and psoriatic arthritis.[13] It was originally used as part of chemotherapy regimens to treat cancer. Extensive research was done in the 1970s regarding the use of methotrexate in rheumatoid arthritis, and now this medication is often part of the standard regimen of treatment of many rheumatic diseases.

Methotrexate (MTX) is taken as a once a week dosing, either by mouth or as an injection. Traditionally once the amount of dose orally exceeds more than eight pills a week, the absorption of MTX is maximized by the intestines, and any additional amount of methotrexate will not be absorbed by the intestines. Patients who require more than 20 mg of methotrexate weekly are often switched to the weekly injectable form.

Common side effects of MTX include mouth sores, hair thinning, nausea, vomiting, loss of appetite, and diarrhea. Other rare side effects include pneumonitis, nodulosis, aplastic anemia, elevated liver enzymes, and cirrhosis.[13] Because of the risk of elevated liver enzymes, the consumption of alcoholic beverages should be severely limited or avoided. Antibiotics such as trimethoprim-sulfamethoxazole (Bactrim) should be avoided because it can deplete folic acid stores further. Blood work including complete blood count and hepatitis panel should be obtained every 2 to 3 months while on MTX. If patients experience shortness of breath or dry cough, a chest X-ray should be obtained and MTX discontinued because of the possibility of MTX-induced pneumonitis.

MTX interferes with the synthesis of purines by permanently binding to dihydrofolate reductase, thus inhibiting the production of a reduced state of folic acid and interfering with the way cells use folic acid. The etiology of most of the side effects listed in the previous paragraph is due to a depletion of folic acid. For this reason, patients should take a folic acid supplement of at least 1 mg/day.[14,15] If an increase in folic acid supplementation of up to 5 mg/day is unsuccessful in alleviating side effects, patients are then given folinic acid or leucovorin calcium. Folinic acid is reduced folate (the product that MTX does not allow to produce in cells), and thus is helpful in improving side effects caused by methotrexate.[16] This medication is provided in a 5 mg pill, which should be given 8 to12 hours after the weekly MTX dose.

MTX has been used as a gold standard in several studies. In the treatment of rheumatoid arthritis, MTX was used in combination with other medications, and "combination therapy" slowed the progression of arthritis compared with monotherapy.[17] With the addition of biologics in the treatment of diseases such as rheumatoid arthritis and psoriatic arthritis, MTX was used as a baseline treatment, with the biologics as "add-on" medications. In these studies, patients with rheumatoid and psoriatic arthritis had their diseases put into "remission," or had halt of radiologic progression of disease, owing to the combination of MTX and biologic agents.[18-22] This is a big advancement in the treatment of these diseases to date.

LEFLUNOMIDE

Leflunomide (Arava) is a medication that interferes with the production of pyridinamines, which is another foundation of DNA synthesis. Research has shown that leflunomide reduces joint swelling and radiographic progression in rheumatoid arthritis patients when used alone as well as in combination with MTX.[23-25] This medication is formulated in 10 mg, 20 mg, and 100 mg tablets. The 100 mg tablets are used as a loading dose, usually given daily for 3 days. The 10 mg and 20 mg pills are maintenance doses, and improvement in symptoms often takes 3 to 4 weeks.

While taking leflunomide, the most common side effects are diarrhea, nausea, and abdominal pain.[23] One other potential side effect is an elevation of liver enzymes,[26] and because of this, liver function tests are measured about every 4 to 8 weeks. Patients who are taking leflunomide should abstain from drinking alcoholic beverages because of its effects on the liver.

The half-life of leflunomide is about 2 weeks. If a patient taking leflunomide wishes to become pregnant or experiences hepatotoxicity, the patient must ingest a cholestyramine at a dose of 8 g three times daily for 10 days to 2 weeks to remove the medication from her body, since Arava has been found to be a teratogenic medication. If the patient refuses to take cholestyramine, the patient must discontinue the medication for at least 2 years before trying to conceive a child.[26]

SULFASALAZINE

Sulfasalazine (Azulfidine) is a medication that has been an effective treatment for rheumatoid arthritis, psoriatic arthritis, and inflammatory bowel disease. This medication is provided in 500 mg tablets, and patients are often asked to increase the dose gradually over several weeks. The typical maximum dose given is 1,000 mg twice a day. Symptom relief usually takes about 3 to 4 weeks, so this medication is often taken together with other DMARDs.

Sulfasalazine is absorbed by the small intestine and is then metabolized through the liver, forming a chemical called sulfapyridine. This form of the drug is thought to inhibit tumor necrosis factor[27] and an enzyme called nuclear factor κB,[28] which helps control the joint swelling in rheumatoid arthritis and psoriatic arthritis. The medication then enters back into the intestines by bile, where colonic bacteria changes sulfapyridine to a compound called 5-aminosalicylic acid (5-ASA). 5-ASA quiets the inflammation in inflammatory bowel disease as the metabolite works its way through the colon.[29] The side effects of sulfasalazine are listed as follows:

Abdominal pain
Nausea
Headache
Leukopenia (blood work should be checked 2 to 4 weeks after initiation)
Anemia
Skin rash

Kidney stones

Infertility in men (reverses about 3 months after stopping the
medication)

Because this medication contains sulfa, patients who have an allergy to sulfa products should not take Sulfasalazine. To this date,
there have been no official studies examining the effects of this medication on babies, so females who may be pregnant or are breast-feeding should not take Sulfasalazine.

Azulfidine has been found to work alone to treat rheumatoid arthritis,[30] but studies have found that combination therapy with DMARDs
works better than monotherapy. The most often used combination-
therapies with Sulfasalazine[17] are

- Methotrexate-Sulfasalazine and
- Methotrexate-hydroxychloroquine-Sulfasalazine.

While using Sulfasalazine, complete blood cell counts and liver
function tests should be obtained every 2 weeks during the first
3 months of treatment, monthly for the next 3 months, and then every
3 months. Women who continued Sulfasalazine throughout pregnancy
did not produce children with any birth defects, but no official studies
were done on pregnant women. Thus, Sulfasalazine is currently listed
as a "category B" medication.[31]

AZATHIPRINE

Azathioprine or Imuran was a medication first used in post-trans-
plant patients to prevent autorejection. Research was then performed
in patients with rheumatoid arthritis. Patients who used Imuran were
found to have less stiffness and synovitis of their joints. Generally,
this medication is used in patients who failed other DMARD therapies. Azathioprine is also used as a maintenance medication after
cyclophosphamide in the treatment of lupus nephritis, Wegener's
granulomatosis, and vasculitis.[32] This medication comes in 50 mg
tablets, and it is often dosed based on body weight at 1 to 1.5 mg/kg.
Once azathioprine enters into the bloodstream, it is converted to 6-mer-
captopurine (the active metabolite) by red blood cells.

This medication is metabolized through the cytochrome P-450 system, and thus it can counteract with many medications, including:

- Coumadin or warfarin
- Allopurinol (if combination needs to be used, decrease imuran dose by 50 percent)
- ACE inhibitors
- Methotrexate
- Alkylating agents, such as Cyclophosphamide, Melphalan, and Chlorambucil
- Trimethoprim

Possible side effects from taking azathioprine include nausea, vomiting, loss of appetite, oral ulcers, rash, and pancreatitis. Other more rare side effects include leukopenia and thrombocytopenia.[33] Malignancies such as squamous cell of the skin, lymphoma, and carcinomas of the vulva, cervix, and uterus have been seen in renal transplant patients who have taken azathioprine.[34] This medication has been found in studies to be teratogenic, so it is labeled as a category D medicine. Women who are pregnant or breast-feeding should not take azathioprine. Its reproductive effects have not been officially studied in men.[33]

CYCLOSPORINE

Cyclosporine, which was originally designed for prevention of rejection of a transplanted organ, has been approved as a DMARD for the treatment of rheumatoid arthritis. It has also been used in the treatment of other diseases such as psoriasis, lupus, and autoimmune ocular diseases such as keratoconjunctivitis sicca (in ophthalmic suspension).

The dosing of cyclosporine is based on weight, with usual dosing of 2.5 mg/kg, divided into twice daily dosing. If after about 8 weeks of treatment no response is seen, the dose can be increased by 0.5 to 0.75 mg/kg/day, and increased again if needed after 12 weeks. The maximum dose used is 4 mg/kg divided into two doses. If no response is seen after about 16 weeks, then discontinue the medicine.[35]

Cyclosporine works by inhibiting the production of a cytokine called IL-2, which in turn downregulates T-cells. It is dispensed as a 25 mg and 100 mg dose of capsules, oral solutions, and as an injection (50 mg/mL). Because the half-life of cyclosporine is 12 hours, this medicine must be taken at approximately the same times each day. If a dose of medication is missed, the patient should *not* double the dose. Physicians will often measure serum levels of cyclosporine weekly or biweekly when first initiating the medication, but once the levels are appropriate, serum levels are checked every few months.[36]

One of the most severe side effects of cyclosporine is elevated blood pressure. Therefore, blood pressure should be checked both at the office and by home monitoring. Another potentially severe side effect is elevated creatinine levels, and this is also checked frequently. Other less serious side effects include gum hyperplasia, headaches, nausea, tremor, hirsutism, and increase risk of infection.

Cyclosporine has been found to have multiple drug-drug interactions. Common medications that interact with cyclosporine are listed as follows:[37]

Allopurinol
Antibiotics such as erythromycin and clarithromycin
• Increase serum cyclosporine
Antibiotics such as rifampicin and nafcillin
• Decrease serum cyclosporine
Phenobarbital, phenytoin, and carbamazepine
• Lowers serum CyA
Ketoconazole
• Increases serum CyA
Calcium channel blockers
• Increases serum CyA
• Nifedipine increases the risk of gingival hyperplasia.

Cyclosporine should be avoided in pregnant patients if possible because it can cause miscarriages, IUGR, and premature delivery. However, in the medical literature there have been case reports of deliveries of healthy babies while moms have taken cyclosporine.

D-PENICILLAMINE

D-Penicillamine is a DMARD that is less commonly used today for the treatment of arthritic conditions because of the generation of newer medications. This medicine has been shown in the medical literature to help treat rheumatoid arthritis, juvenile rheumatoid arthritis, psoriatic arthritis, and scleroderma. It is dispensed in a 125 or 250 mg tablets, and is given either once or twice a day on an empty stomach. Because of drug interactions causing complexes with various minerals, patients should not ingest iron supplements while taking penicillamine.[38]

Side effects of penicillamine include neutropenia, thrombocytopenia, hematuria, and proteinuria. Because of this, a CBC and urinalysis are checked every 1 to 2 months. Other side effects include skin rashes, altered taste (due to binding with zinc, causing zinc deficiency), mouth sores, loss of appetite, heartburn, bleeding, and muscle weakness. There have been some reports of drug-induced lupus,[39] vasculitis affecting the kidney and lung,[40] and myasthenia gravis.[41] This medication should not be taken by women during pregnancy because of the risk of teratogenesis.

CYCLOPHOSPHAMIDE

Cyclophosphamide or Cytoxan is a potent medication used in the treatment of serious forms of diseases such as cancer, vasculitis from rheumatoid arthritis, renal and lung and central nervous system complications of lupus, Wegener's granulomatosis, and interstitial lung disease in scleroderma. This medication is offered in either an intravenous form or as a 50 mg pill. The intravenous form of cyclophosphamide is often administered in a monthly "pulse" dose simultaneously with solumedrol for at least 6 months, followed often by administration every 3 months for another 18 months. The dose of intravenous cyclophosphamide is calculated based on the patient's weight, height, total body surface area, and kidney function.

The oral preparation of cyclophosphamide is taken on a daily basis for between 6 months and 1 year, depending on the severity of the patient's symptoms. The dosage of the Cytoxan given is based on the patient's weight and creatinine value.

Patients who take oral cyclophosphamide must drink at least eight 8 oz glasses of water daily to avoid the side effect of hemorrhagic cystitis. Patients who receive intravenous Cytoxan can also take MESNA, which helps to protect the bladder from cyclophosphamide.

Other common side effects include hair loss, nausea, vomiting, blood abnormalities such as leukopenia, anemia, and thrombocytopenia, and risk of serious infections with opportunistic organisms. Because of its effects on lowering the immune system, patients are often given the antibiotic Bactrim 3 days a week, dapsone at a dose of 100 mg/day, or atovaquone at a dose of 1500 mg/day, to prevent *Pneumocystis cariini* pneumonia.

Blood work should be obtained between the 10th and 14th day after administration of IV cytoxan, or monthly while on oral cyclophosphamide to monitor for toxicity. Leukopenia, especially lymphopenia, is a concern during treatment, and the total white blood cell count should be more than 3500/mm^3 to avoid serious infections. If leukopenia occurs, the next cyclophosphamide dose may need to be lowered. Also, creatinine, liver enzymes, and a urinalysis should be checked monthly.

Cyclophosphamide is classified as a "category X" medication, as it has been linked to serious teratogenesis and miscarriages in pregnant women. Females of reproductive age who require Cytoxan are counseled about the fact that this medication given over a long period of time has been shown to cause ovarian failure in some patients. Because of the risk of infertility, women are encouraged to use birth control such as depomedrol or oral contraceptives. Intrauterine devices would prevent contraception, but will not offer protection to the ovaries.

Long-term effects of cyclophosphamide use include the increased risk of certain cancers such as lymphoma, leukemia, and bladder cancer. A urinalysis should be checked routinely after cyclophosphamide is given to a patient to monitor for hematuria, which could be an early sign for bladder cancer.[42]

MYCOPHENOLATE MOFETIL

Mycophenolate mofetil (Cellcept) (MMF) is an immune modulatory drug that has been used since the early 1990s in patients who have had organ transplantation to prevent rejection. Its primary use to date in autoimmune diseases is in the treatment of lupus,[43] especially to control lupus nephritis.[44] Once MMF enters into the bloodstream from the intestines, it is hydrolyzed to mycophenolic acid, which is active in the body for about 12 hours. Mycophenolic acid interferes with the purine synthesis of lymphocytes, which regulates the T-cells and B-cells in the immune system.

Cellcept is supplied as 500 mg tablets, and is often given as two pills twice daily. African-Americans have been found to metabolize MMF quicker than other races, so these patients are often given a higher dose of up to 3 g of medication daily. Common side effects include abdominal cramping, nausea, diarrhea, leukopenia, anemia, thrombocytopenia, and increased risk of infections. Blood work such as a complete blood count should be checked every 2 weeks when starting or increasing therapy, and then every 6 to 8 weeks thereafter to monitor for toxicity. Mycophenolate mofetil is labeled as a "category C" drug, so the medication should be avoided during pregnancy and lactation.[45]

GOLD

With the production of newer medications that have been proven to slow or halt the progression of rheumatoid arthritis, gold is not used often. Gold has been used in the treatment of juvenile rheumatoid arthritis, ankylosing spondylitis, and psoriatic arthritis. There are a few injectable forms of gold, and one oral form called auranofin (Ridaura). Studies have shown gold to be as effective as MTX in controlling rheumatoid and psoriatic arthritis symptoms in short term, but the long-term effectiveness of gold therapy in these diseases was controversial.

The usual dose for intramuscular gold shots is as follows:

- One test dose of 10 mg IM
- Another dose of 25 mg IM 1 week later
- Weekly doses of 50 mg IM until total dose of gold is 1 g, or until patients experience gastrointestinal side effects or lack of effect.

BIOLOGIC AGENTS

The introduction of biologic agents in the treatment of rheumatoid arthritis and other systemic rheumatologic diseases in 1998 has added a valuable new class of medications that have been shown in clinical studies to not only slow the progression of the disease, but actually place these diseases in a quiescent or "remissive" state. This class of medications prevents various chemokines from attaching to receptors on the surface of cells, thus stopping the inflammatory processes which drive these diseases. When studies were initially performed on patients with rheumatic diseases, they were tested in conjunction with the use of MTX, a medication that prior to the development of biologics was found to be the best DMARD to slow the progression of the disease state. Since the approval of combination therapy of MTX and biologic agents in treating different forms of arthritis, most of the biologic agents have also been found to be valuable in the treatment of both early and advanced forms of rheumatoid arthritis and psoriatic arthritis.

The biologics that will be discussed in this section are the following

- Tumor necrosis factor (TNF) inhibitors such as etanercept (Enbrel), infliximab (Remicade), and adalimumab (Humira)
- IL-1 inhibitors, such as Anakinra (Kineret)
- CD 20 inhibitors such as abatacept (Orencia)
- B-cell depletor, such as Rituximab (Rituxan)

Etanercept

Etanercept (Enbrel) was first introduced into the treatment regimen of rheumatoid arthritis in 1998. Since then, this medication has been found to be useful in various other diseases, including psoriasis, psoriatic arthritis, polyarticular juvenile rheumatoid arthritis, and ankylosing spondylitis. When Enbrel was first promoted, it was shipped in a powder form (at a dose of 25 mg of Etanercept) that when diluent was added, the powder transformed into a suspension that could be drawn up into a syringe and then injected subcutaneously. Because the half-life of the 25 mg strength of etanercept was found to be 102 ± 30 hours, the medication was administered twice a week. In 2003, etanercept became available as a prefilled syringe at a dose of 50 mg, which was injected subcutaneously once a week. Clinical trials did not show a difference in efficacy between the once a week and twice a week dosing.

Enbrel works by binding to TNF, a proinflammatory molecule in the serum and synovial fluid. During a normal immune response, TNF attaches to receptors on synovial cells. Once TNF binds to the cell surface, the synovial cells produce chemokines, which further drive the immune process. Etanercept is a dimeric fusion protein that looks similar to the receptors on the cell surface. When etanercept encounters TNF, the TNF binds to it. With TNF unable to bind to cell surface receptors, the autoimmune inflammatory process shuts down.

The research trials performed with etanercept have shown that both the 25 mg biweekly dose and 50 mg weekly dose can be used in the treatment of [46]

- Moderate to severe rheumatoid arthritis (both as monotherapy and additional therapy with other DMARDs),
- Polyarticular juvenile rheumatoid arthritis (dose is weight based),
- Psoriatic arthritis,
- Ankylosing spondylitis, and
- Chronic moderate to severe plaque psoriasis (at a dose of 50 mg subcutaneous biweekly for 3 months, followed by 50 mg subcutaneous [SQ] weekly).

The side effects of etanercept include these:[46]

- New onset or exacerbation of central nervous system demyelinating diseases, such as optic neuritis, multiple sclerosis, and new onset seizures
- Hematologic problems including pancytopenia and aplastic anemia
- Malignancies such as lymphoma and cancer of the colon, breast, lung, and prostate
- Serious infections, including sepsis with opportunistic infections and tuberculosis

Patients who have an allergy to latex should not use the 50 mg subcutaneous weekly dose. Enbrel should not be used in combination with Anakinra because the combination caused an increased rate of serious infections. Patients who have Class III or Class IV heart disease should not take etanercept because the drug could exacerbate congestive heart failure. Also, some patients with rheumatoid arthritis who took etanercept developed a positive antinuclear antibody and developed symptoms similar to a lupus-like reaction.[46]

Etanercept is listed as a "category B" medication, and although no official studies have been done on pregnant women, those who required etanercept delivered healthy babies.[46]

Infliximab

Infliximab (Remicade) is a chimeric monoclonal antibody composed of human and murine portions. It binds TNF-α and prevents its binding to cell receptors. It is shipped as a white powder containing 100 mg of infliximab, which is combined with 10 ml of sterile water and added into normal saline solution. The drug is then infused intravenously over about 2 hours.

The dose of infliximab infused into a patient varies depending on body weight (about 3 mg/kg when first starting the medication, up to 20 mg/kg). The medication is first infused on day 0, then day 14, and then every 4 to 8 weeks thereafter, depending on the patient's response. Evaluation for possible infections prior to infusing Remicade is recommended, since this medication has been found to cause serious infections due to altering the body's normal immune mechanisms.

Remicade is used for the treatment of the following diseases:[47]

- Early and advanced, moderate to severe rheumatoid arthritis (with the addition of methotrexate to prevent lupus-like syndrome)
- Active Crohn's disease (other immunosuppressants such as Azathioprine, Sulfasalazine, MTX, and steroids may be used to prevent infusion reactions)
- Fistulizing Crohn's disease (with other immunosuppressants)

Side effects are similar to Etanercept and include these:[47]

- Infusion reactions such as fever/chills, itching, hypotension, chest pain, dyspnea, hypertension, rash, and anaphylaxis
- Serious infections, including sepsis and tuberculosis
- Development of a positive antinuclear antibody/double-stranded DNA antibody causing lupus-like syndrome
- Hematologic disorders such as pancytopenia
- Elevated liver enzymes

- Nervous system disorders including multiple sclerosis and optic neuritis
- Malignancies such as lymphoma, breast, rectal, basal, and melanoma
- Congestive heart failure in patients with Classes III and IV heart disease

This medication should not be used in combination with Anakinra due to the possibility of severe infections with the combination. Infliximab is listed as a "category B" medication. A PPD should be placed before initiating treatment with infliximab to evaluate for tuberculosis.[47]

Adalimumab

Adalimumab (Humira) is a recombinant human monoclonal antibody that binds to TNF-α, which in turn does not allow TNF to bind to cell receptors. It is administered subcutaneously in a prefilled syringe at a dose of 40 mg every other week. It has been used effectively in the treatment of moderate to severe rheumatoid arthritis and psoriatic arthritis. Adalimumab may be used alone or in combination with other DMARDs such as methotrexate. Humira should not be used in combination with Anakinra, since the combination could cause serious infections.

A PPD should be placed prior to starting adalimumab to evaluate for the presence of tuberculosis. Like the other TNF inhibitors, Humira is labeled as a "category B" medication.

Side effects are similar to the other TNF inhibitors and include:[48]

- Risk of serious infections, including sepsis from opportunistic infections and tuberculosis
- Nervous system disorders including multiple sclerosis and optic neuritis
- Lupus-like syndrome
- Malignancies such as lymphoma, breast, colon, rectum, cervical, uterine, prostate, and melanoma
- Congestive heart failure in patients with Class III/IV heart disease

Anakinra

Anakinra (Kineret) regulates the immune system response through binding to IL-1. IL-1 is a cytokine involved in the immune process. In cases of autoimmune diseases, the overproduction of IL-1 causes destruction of cartilage and bone. Anakinra is a recombinant form of the human interleukin-1 receptor antagonist, which binds IL-1 before it can bind to the receptor on the cell surface.

This medication is supplied in a 100 mg prefilled syringe and is administered subcutaneously as a daily injection. Anakinra is indicated for the treatment of moderate to severe rheumatoid arthritis. With the introduction of TNF-inhibitors, Anakinra is now traditionally used after TNF inhibitors have failed to control rheumatoid arthritis.

Side effects of Anakinra include the risk of serious infections, especially in combination with etanercept and other TNF-inhibitors; thus, the combination is contraindicated. Caution should be taken when using Anakinra in patients with asthma and chronic obstructive pulmonary disease. Thus, a PPD is often placed on patients before starting Kineret.[49]

Also, neutropenia has been found in patients who use Anakinra. Thus, a complete blood count is checked monthly for 3 months, and then every 3 months thereafter. Malignancies such as lymphoma, breast, lung, and colon have been found in some patients taking Kineret. This medication is classified as "category B" in pregnant patients, so it should only be used if clinically indicated.[49]

Abatacept

Abatacept (Orencia) was approved by the Food and Drug Administration (FDA) in December 2005 for the treatment of moderate to severe rheumatoid arthritis. It downregulates the activity of the T-cell in the immune process. Usually for a T-cell to be activated, a cytokine attaches to a receptor on the cell surface. The T-cell then has another binding site adjacent to the "attached receptor," which must also be properly bound before the T-cell is officially activated. The "second receptor" on the surface of the T-cell is called CD 28. If CD 28 is not bound, and the receptor adjacent to CD 28 is bound, the T-cell will not be activated.

Abatacept takes advantage of this concept by blocking the "second receptor." This medication is effective in dow regulating T-cells by binding to CD 80 and CD 86, thereby blocking interaction with CD 28.[50] Research studies have shown abatacept to be effective as monotherapy and in combination with MTX. However, its current indication is for treatment of rheumatoid arthritis in patients who still have activity of disease with methotrexate treatment, or in patients who have failed TNF inhibitors. This medication should not be used in combination with TNF inhibitors or with Anakinra because of increased rates of serious infections.

Patients who start abatacept should be tested for tuberculosis first. Abatacept is administered as a vial containing 250 mg-strength powered solution. The powder is mixed with 10 ml of sterile water and placed into normal saline solution. It is then administered intravenously over a 30 min period. Patients receive the drug initially, 2 weeks later, 4 weeks after the initial infusion, and then every 4 weeks thereafter. The total dose administered depends on the patient's weight.[50]

Side effects of abatacept include the following:[50]

- Risk of serious infections and tuberculosis
- Infusion reactions
- Exacerbations of cough and dyspnea with patients who have chronic obstructive pulmonary disease (use with caution in this patient subtype)
- Malignancies including lymphoma and lung. Rare occurrences of cancer of skin, breast, bile duct, cervix, ovarian, uterine, renal, prostrate, and thyroid.

Abatacept is currently listed as a "category C" medication in pregnancy.[50]

Rituximab

Rituximab (Rituxan) was approved for the treatment of rheumatoid arthritis in early 2006. This medication is a monoclonal antibody which binds to and inhibits the CD 20 antigen on the surface of B-lymphocytes, thus down regulating the B-cell. CD 20 controls the life cycle of the B-cell. Once Rituximab attaches to CD 20 on the cell surface, it triggers the B-cell to self-destruct.

Rituxan is administered as a 1,000 mg intravenous injection initially and then 2 week later. The medication can be repeated every 6 months as needed. Common side effects of Rituximab include infusion reactions, skin rash, abdominal pain, anemia, dyspnea, hypotension, neutropenia, lymphopenia, and infections. A few cases of uveitis, optic neuritis, and vasculitis have been reported. The association of Rituximab with cancers is at the time of this publication unknown. Rituxan is classified as a "category C" medication, and females are encouraged to wait at least 1 year after treatment before conceiving.[51]

REFERENCES

1. Petri, M. Hydroxychloroquine use in the Baltimore Lupus Cohort: Effects on lipids, glucose, and thrombosis. *Lupus* 1996;5:S16.

2. Fox, R. Antimalarial drugs: possible mechanisms of action in autoimmune disease and prospects for drug development. *Lupus* 1996;5:S4.

3. Schaefer, B; Cahn, MM; Levy, EJ. Absorption of antimalarial drugs in human skin: Spectroscopic and chemical analysis in epidermis and corium. *J Invest Dermatol* 1958;30:341.

4. Tam, LS; Gladman, DD; Hallet, DC; et al. Effect of antimalarial agents on the fasting lipid profile in systemic lupus erythematosus. *J Rheumatol* 2000; 27:2142.

5. Furst, DE. Pharmacokinetics of hydroxychloroquine and chloroquine during treatment of rheumatic diseases. *Lupus* 1996;5:S11.

6. Estes, ML; Ewing-Wilson, D; Chou, SM. Chloroquine neuromyotoxicity: Clinical and pathologic perspective. *Am J Med* 1987;82:447.

7. Avina-Zubieta, JA; Johnson, ES; Suarez-Almazor, ME; et al. Incidence of myopathy in patients treated with antimalarials. A report of three cases and a review of the literature. *Br J Rheumatol* 1995;34:166.

8. Ratliff, NB; Estes, ML; Myles, JL; et al. Diagnosis of chloroquine cardiomyopathy by endomyocardial biopsy. *N Engl J Med* 1987;316:191.

9. Marmor, MF; Carr, RE; Easterbrook, M; et al. Recommendations on screening for chloroquine and hydroxychloroquine retinopathy: A report by the *American Academy of Ophthalmology* 2002;109:1377.

10. Saag, KG; Criswell, LA; Sems, KM; et al. Low dose corticosteroids in rheumatoid arthritis: A meta-analysis of their moderate-term effectiveness. *Arthritis Rheum* 1996;39(11):1818-1825.

11. Gotzsche, PC; Johansen, HK. Short-term low-dose corticosteroids vs. placebo and nonsteroidal anti-inflammatory drugs in rheumatoid arthritis. *Cochrane Database Syst Rev* 2003;1:CD000189.

12. Physician's Desk Reference 2005;59:1110-1112.

13. Physician's Desk Reference 2005;59:2966.

14. Morgan, SL; Baggot, JR; Vaughn, WH; et al. The effect of folic acid supplementation on the toxicity of low-dose methotrexate in patients with rheumatoid arthritis. *Arthritis Rheum* 1990;33:1.

15. Morgan, SL; Baggot, JE; Vaughn, WH; et al. Supplementation of folic acid during methotrexate therapy for rheumatoid arthritis: A double-blinded placebo-controlled trial. *Ann Intern Med* 1994;121:833.

16. Tishler, M; Caspi, D; Fishel, B; et al. The effects of leucovorin (folinic acid) on methotrexate therapy in rheumatoid arthritis patients. *Arthritis Rheum* 1988; 31:906.

17. O'Dell, JR; Leff, R; Paulsen, G; et al. Treatment of rheumatoid arthritis with methotrexate and hydroxychloroquine, methotrexate and sulfasalazine, or a combination of the three medications: Results of a two year, randomized, double-blind, placebo-controlled trial. *Arthritis Rheum* 2002;46:1164.

18. Weinblatt, ME; Kremer, JM; Bankhurst, AD; et al. A trial of etanercept, a recombinant tumor necrosis factor receptor: Fc fusion protein, in patients with rheumatoid arthritis receiving methotrexate. *N Engl J Med* 1999;340:253.

19. Klareskog, L; van der Heijde, D; de Jager, JP; et al. Therapeutic effect of the combination of etanercept and methotrexate compared with each treatment alone in patients with rheumatoid arthritis: Double-blinded, randomized controlled trial. *Lancet* 2004;363:675.

20. Keystone, EC; Kavanaugh, AF; Sharp, JT; et al. Radiographic, clinical, and functional outcomes of treatment with adalimumab (a human anti-tumor necrosis factor monoclonal antibody) in patients with active rheumatoid arthritis receiving concomitant methotrexate therapy: A randomized, placebo-controlled, 52 week trial. *Arthritis Rheum* 2004;50:140.

21. Maini, R; St Clair, EW; Breedveld, F; et al. Infliximab (chimeric anti-tumor necrosis factor alpha monoclonal antibody) versus placebo in rheumatoid arthritis patients receiving concomitant methotrexate: A randomized phase III trial. *Lancet* 1999;354:1932.

22. St Clair, EW; van der Heidje, DM; Smolen, JS; et al. Combination of infliximab and methotrexate therapy for early rheumatoid arthritis: A randomized, controlled trial. *Arthritis Rheum* 2004;50:3432.

23. Strand, V; Fox, R; Cohen, S; et al. Treatment of active rheumatoid arthritis with leflunomide compared with placebo and methotrexate. Leflunomide Rheumatoid Arthritis Investigators Group. *Archives Intern Med* 1999;159:2542.

24. Scott, DL; Smolen, JS; Kalden, JR; et al. Treatment of active rheumatoid arthritis with leflunomide: Two year follow up of a double blind, placebo controlled trial versus sulfasalazine. *Ann Rheum Dis* 2001;60:913.

25. Emery, P; Breedveld, FC; Lemmel, EM; et al. A comparison of the efficacy and safety of leflunomide and methotrexate for the treatment of rheumatoid arthritis. *Rheumatology* 2000;39:655.

26. Rozman, B. Clinical pharmacokinetics of leflunomide. *Clin Pharmacokinet* 2002;41:421.

27. Wahl, C; Lipty, S; Adler, G; et al. Sulfasalazine, a potent and specific inhibitor of nuclear factor kappa B. *J Clin Invest* 1998;101:1163.

28. Rodenburg, RJ; Ganga, A; van Lent, PL; et al. The anti-inflammatory drug sulfasalazine inhibits tumor necrosis factor alpha expression in macrophages by inducing apoptosis. *Arthritis Rheum* 2000;43:1941.

29. Craven, PA; Pfanstiel, J; Saito, R; et al. Actions of sulfasalazine and 5-amino-salicylic acid as reactive oxygen scavengers in the suppression of bile acid-increases in colonic epithelial cell loss and proliferative activity. *Gastroenterology* 1987; 92:1998.

30. Box, SA; Pullar, T. Sulphasalazine in the treatment of rheumatoid arthritis. *Br J Rheumatol* 1997;36:382.

31. Physician Desk Reference, Azulfidine, 59th edition, 2005.

32. Brandwein, S; Esdaille, J; Danhoff, B; et al. Wegener's granulomatosis. Clinical features and outcome in thirteen patients. *Arch Int Med* 1983;143:476

33. Physician's Desk Reference. Azathioprine, 59th Edition, 2005.

34. Penn, I. Cancers complicating organ transplantation. *N Engl J Med* 1990; 323:1767.

35. Holt, DW; Mueller, EA; Kovarik, JM; et al. Sandimmune Neoral Pharmacokinetics: impact of the new oral formulation. *Transplant Proc* 1995;27:1434.

36. Burckart, GJ; Canafax, DM; Yee, GC. Cyclosporine monitoring. *Drug Intell Clin Pharm* 1986;20:649.

37. Yee, GC; McGuire, TR. Pharmacokinetic drug interactions with cyclosporine. *Clin Pharmacokinet* 1990;19(4):319-332.

38. Chow, ST; McAuliffe, CA; Sayle, Bj. Metal Complexes of amino acids with derivatives-VIII. The reaction of D-Penicillamine with some transition and non-transition metal salts. *J Inorg Nucl Chem* 1973;35:4349.

39. Chalmers, A; Thompson, D; Stein, HE; et al. Systemic lupus erythematosus during penicillamine therapy for rheumatoid arthritis. *Ann Intern Med* 1982;97:659.

40. Nanke, Y; Akama, H; Terai, C; et al. Rapidly progressive glomerulonephritis with D-penicillamine. *Am J Med Sci* 2000;320:398.

41. Vincent, A; Newsome-Davis, J. Acetylcholine receptor antibody characteristic in myasthenia gravis. Patients with penicillamine-induced myasthenia or idiopathic myasthenia of recent onset. *Clin Exp Immunol* 1982;49:266.

42. Physician's desk reference. Cytoxan; 52nd edition, 2005.

43. Gaubitz, M; Schorat, A; Schotte, H; et al. Mycophenolate mofetil for the treatment of systemic lupus erythematosus: an open pilot trial. *Lupus* 1999;8:731.

44. Kingdon, EJ; McLean, AG; Psimenou, E; et al. The safety and efficacy of MMF in lupus nephritis: a pilot study. *Lupus* 2001;10:606.

45. Lipsky, JJ. Mycophenolate mofetil. *Lancet* 1996;348:1357.

46. Package insert for etanercept, Amgen and Wyeth pharmaceuticals, 2004.

47. Physician's Desk Reference, Remicade; 59th edition: 1117-1121.

48. Physician's Desk Reference, Humira; 59th edition: 473-475.

49. Physician's Desk Reference, Kineret; 59th edition: 588-590.

50. Package insert for Abatacept, Dec 2005.

51. Physician's Desk Reference, Rituxan, 59th edition: 958-960.

Chapter 14

Physical Therapy

Denis Martin

INTRODUCTION

Physiotherapists/physical therapists are rehabilitation profession-als. The titles physical therapist or physiotherapist denote expertise in functional maintenance and restoration across the range of health conditions (CSP 2002). This includes expertise in the management of neuromusculoskeletal-related pain, where, historically, physical thera-pists have used exercises and manual, thermal, and electrical/electro-magnetic techniques to relieve pain and heal damaged tissues.

Modern physical therapy, based on a biopsychosocial approach, has shifted from that position to place much more emphasis on help-ing people to understand their condition and develop practical strate-gies and tactics to minimize the effect of pain overall on their lives. This involves education and advice, promotion of general exercise and activity, and working with people as active participants in the management of their condition.

The aim of this chapter is to present physical therapy and, in paral-lel, neuromusculoskeletal-related pain within the context of func-tion. It is intended that this shared context of function will show the logic in the wider adoption of the biopsychosocial approach that still leaves room for targeted and more judicious use of more traditional approaches.

Clinical Management of Bone and Joint Pain
© 2007 by The Haworth Press, Inc. All rights reserved.
doi:10.1300/5771_16

FUNCTION

Function has become recognized as a fundamental concept of health and disability. With the support of the World Health Organisation, a working definition of health and disability has been developed that is both conceptually and practically useful—the International Classification of Functioning, Disability and Health (ICF) (WHO 2001). Within the ICF, positive health is framed as function and negative health is framed as dysfunction or disability. Functioning, in terms of the ICF, is positive health and negative health is dysfunctioning or disability. The ICF is a comprehensive and complex classification system intended to be relevant across the spectrum of health conditions. It has two parts: *Function* and *Context*. Function contains the two following components:

- Body structure and body functions
- Activity and participation

Anatomical structures like nerves, soft tissues, and bones are described as body structures. Sensory functions, mental functions, and movement-related functions are classed as body functions.

Two further important concepts within the ICF are activity and participation. Activity is concerned with what a person can do. It focuses on the person's capacity to execute a task or an action. Participation, on the other hand, is concerned with what a person does in practice. It focuses on the person's actual performance or involvement in social situations.

Disability is presented in similar terms to those used for function. The ICF describes three levels of disability—impairment, activity limitation, and participation restriction. Impairments relate to problems with body structures and body functions. Problems with the capacity to carry out tasks are activity limitations. Participation restrictions describe problems with performance in social situations.

Like function, context has two components. The first of these, personal factors, contains items such as age, sex, coping styles, and experience. The other component, environmental factors, contains items that include social support and attitudes, policies, and technology. In the ICF, a person's participation is considered in the context of a notional standard environment for that person.

The conceptual and practical usefulness of the ICF can be seen further by comparison with what it was designed to replace. The International Classification of Impairments, Disabilities and Handicaps (ICIDH) was the model of choice before the ICF. In the ICIDH, disability is kept distinct from health. Within that model health problems arise from an initial disease/disorder that develops into impairment, which in turn can lead to disability and, finally, handicap. The ICF links health and disability together under function, and the serial dependency between disease/disorder, impairment, disability, and handicap described are no longer relevant. The ICF describes dynamic relationships among body structures and body functions, and activity and participation that do not have to be serially dependent. Compared with the ICIDH, the importance of the environment is explicit and prominent in the ICF.

Rehabilitation is, in basic terms, the improvement of function (Stucki et al. 2002). So, the ICF, with its emphasis on function and the positive side of health, marks out a clear place for rehabilitation in health care. Also, the relevance of the ICF in the field of managing pain continues to be demonstrated (Soukup & Vollestad 2001; Chwastiak & Von Korff 2003; Steiner et al. 2002). This reinforces the value of rehabilitation professionals like physical therapists for people with neuromusculoskeletal-related pain.

ADDRESSING IMPAIRMENT: A BIOMEDICAL APPLICATION OF PHYSICAL THERAPY

An early edition of the International Association for the Study of Pain curriculum for pain defined one of the roles for physical therapy as the treatment of factors (such as inflammation) that are giving rise to the pain (Fields 1995). In terms of the ICF this can be interpreted as addressing impairment. The physical therapy techniques that are briefly described here are suited to addressing impairment.

Cold: Cryotherapy—the therapeutic use of cold—can be applied in a number of different ways ranging from ice packs held in contact with the skin to ethyl chloride sprays that quickly cool the skin surface. Cold is used as an immediate first aid measure following injury to decrease bleeding and swelling, and thus indirectly reduce pain. It can directly affect nerve activity and therefore it is also used with this aim of reducing pain.

Heat: Heat is another method that is commonly used by physical therapists. The aim of heating is to improve the extensibility of tissues, stimulate blood flow, and relieve pain through direct effect on nerve activity.

Heat is applied through heat packs that are placed in contact with the skin, water baths in which the body part is immersed, or infrared lamps that provide radiant heat without the need to be in contact with the skin. These methods supply heating to tissues that are mainly superficial.

Methods have been developed to heat deeper tissues. These include short-wave diathermy and ultrasound therapy, which deliver, respectively, radio frequency waves and ultrasonic waves into tissue to increase temperature.

Heat should not be applied during active inflammation or early repair because of the possibility of increasing bleeding and interfering with the restoration of the local circulatory system.

Athermal: Electromagnetic energy that does not produce heat—athermal energy—was developed to overcome the problems of heating tissue. The energy supplied by short-wave diathermy and ultrasound is pulsed rather than delivered in the continuous mode as used for heating. The time between each pulse allows the dissipation of energy so that there is no increase in temperature. The claimed therapeutic effects are by way of effects at cellular level. Low-level light/laser therapy is also used in this way. Again, the aim is to facilitate healing and relieve pain.

Electric current: Electric current is used to stimulate nerves with the aim of reducing pain, and there are also claims of optimizing the healing rate of tissue. The simplest method of electrical stimulation is transcutaneous electrical nerve stimulation (TENS). Another form of electrical stimulation is interferential current. Using the principles of wave interference, interferential current mixes two "medium frequency" currents with the aim of setting up an additional current at a low frequency similar to that used in TENS. It is used quite commonly with the aims of relieving pain and promoting healing. Whether it is sufficiently different from the much cheaper and more flexible TENS machines is arguable.

Acupuncture: Physical therapists are increasingly using acupuncture in its various forms.

Manual therapy: Physical manipulation and mobilization are commonly used to treat spinal and peripheral joint pain. The two methods are different in the force applied. In manipulation, the physical therapist applies high-velocity forceful thrusts to the structures. The aim is to make right a putitative biomechanical fault. In mobilization, the physical therapist moves the body parts in a more gentle fashion and there is no forceful thrust.

Massage, of which there are many different forms, is another manual technique used in physical therapy.

Exercise: Physical therapists can teach people specific exercises to improve the strength or extensibility of structures that have been identified as problematic. The issue of general exercise to improve overall fitness and wellbeing is dealt with further in the following text.

Claims of effectiveness for these methods have been made on the basis of mechanisms matching knowledge about their supposed biological or biophysical effects with knowledge about the structures and processes involved in pain and healing. While solid research evidence is developing, with various pictures emerging, there remains a consensus in systematic reviews that there is insufficient scientific evidence of clinical effectiveness and that the quality of trials is generally low. A further problem in evaluation of effectiveness is that in clinical practice the techniques are rarely used on their own. Rather, they tend to be used as part of a package of physical therapy that can vary considerably. Also, they can be delivered in a variety of doses and frequencies that need to be evaluated for relative effectiveness.

The development of physical therapy over the years has been dominated by thinking and practice that is consistent with a biomedical model of disease and cure. The methods detailed here have largely been developed within that context. This can be valid for acute pain following tissue trauma where it is possible to identify the impairment. However, the usefulness of the biomedical model tends to be limited when the person presents with persistent/chronic pain (Harding & Williams 1995; Martin & Palmer 2004). The problem here is that the impairment may not be identifiable or that any original impairment may have become dissociated with the pain-related disability that is the person's main problem. In such cases focusing on impairment may be at best palliative. This can be a problem in itself, however, if the treatment has been given in the context of an expectation of cure that subsequently does not transpire. The journey of people with chronic pain through health and social care is often one of raised expectations and dashed hopes, which serve to add to people's problems of negative thoughts and feelings, unhelpful behaviors, and misplaced beliefs, which are discussed in the following sections.

The next section will focus on the value of directly addressing activity and participation using methods to increase people's understanding of their condition and help them manage their lives despite pain.

ADDRESSING ACTIVITY AND PARTICIPATION: A BIOPSYCHOSOCIAL APPLICATION OF PHYSICAL THERAPY

From the perspective of a biomedical model, pain is a sensation that occurs as a result of tissue damage. As such, pain is seen as a symptom of an underlying injury or disease: treatment aims to primarily "cure" that injury or disease with the expectation that pain will then be relieved. This does not encompass the complexities involved when the pain is chronic. Chronic pain falls into the category of lived-in long-term conditions, which will remain with people for the rest of their lives and for which a cure is still unobtainable (Christianson et al. 1998). Recommendations to move health care systems for such conditions away from a biomedical model of disease and cure (Christianson et al. 1998; Von Korff et al. 2002) have begun to be adopted. These changes reflect a more biopsychosocial model of health that describes a dynamic interplay among physiological, psychological, and environmental factors (Hanson & Gerber 1989).

The biopsychosocial model allows for a more complex, more realistic view of pain than the biomedical model, and it has led to the development of a range of approaches to improve the management of pain (Keefe et al. 2004). From the perspective of a biopsychosocial model, pain has emotional and behavioral dimensions and is more than a sensation. Also, pain can be independent from tissue damage. This is consistent with the definition of pain as *an unpleasant sensory and emotional experience associated with actual or potential tissue damage, or described in terms of such damage* (Merskey & Bogduk 1994).

From a biopsychosocial perspective, the impact of pain can be physiological, psychological, and environmental. Also, physiological, psychological, and environmental factors can influence the impact of pain. Therefore, the biopsychosocial approach to pain sits comfortably with the ICF.

In accordance, physical therapy practice has developed within a biopsychosocial model to address the impact of pain on function rather than just focusing on the pain itself (Harding & Williams 1995; Jones & Martin 2003). In doing so, physical therapy has adopted the principles of cognitive-behavioral therapy into its approach to managing pain (Von Korff et al. 2005; Moseley 2002; Johnstone et al. 2002; Harding & Williams 1995).

Cognitive-Behavioral Therapy

Cognitive-behavioral therapy is an important part of the biopsychosocial approach to pain management (Vlaeyen & Morley 2005; Keefe et al. 2004; Morley 2004). Systematic reviews of the literature support the value of cognitive-behavioral approaches for chronic pain (Morley et al. 1999; van Tulder et al. 2000; Guzman et al. 2001).

The application of cognitive-behavioral therapy in pain management is based on an understanding that thoughts and emotions can have a large influence on the impact of pain (Stroud et al. 2000; Keefe et al. 2004).

People with chronic pain commonly talk about feelings of anger, frustration, anxiety, low mood, and depression. People also report having recurring negative thoughts such as:

- Why have I allowed this to happen to me?
- Will this pain never end?
- I can't handle this pain any more.

(It should be noted that these thoughts and feelings are perfectly normal given the presence of pain.) Negative feelings can develop further from such a pattern of negative thinking, which often becomes automatic, and the negative feelings can lead to more negative thoughts. This self-perpetuating cycle can also reinforce unhelpful behaviors such as inactivity, aggression, and social isolation from social contact, which in turn worsen the person's ability to cope with being in pain.

Cognitive-behavioral therapy aims to get people to recognize the pattern of negative thoughts and feelings and to understand how this causes them problems. People are encouraged and guided in ways of challenging and countering negative thinking and developing behaviors that are likely to help them to manage their condition and regain control of their lives.

Education: The biosychosocial approach emphasizes the importance of helping people to reach a practical understanding of their condition through education, advice, and experiential learning. Often people with pain have misplaced beliefs about their condition, which can exacerbate their problems. An example of this is seen in fear-avoidance behavior, when people with low back pain are afraid to move normally for fear of making things worse, despite the fact that such fear is unfounded (Vlaeyen & Linton 2000). Helping people with misplaced beliefs to understand more about pain and its impact aims to address these misplaced beliefs, and there is evidence that education can improve self-management and improve function (Moseley 2004; Burton et al. 1999). Misplaced beliefs are often reinforced within their environment in which there is likely to be a poor understanding about pain. Efforts can be made to address this through education of family members and carers (Ferrell & Ferrell 1991).

General exercise: Promotion of exercise is one of the main ways in which physical therapists can help people with chronic pain in terms of activity and participation. General exercise can improve fitness, increase activity levels, and improve mood—all areas that are affected by chronic pain.

There are any number of different methods of general exercise from simple walking to fashionably marketed, celebrity-endorsed regimes. The literature suggests that any type of general exercise aimed at increasing overall activity has potential benefits that can be long lasting (Liddle et al. 2004). For general exercise to be effective, it has to become a routine, but compliance with exercise is likely to be reduced with time. This may explain why supervision by the physical therapist can increase the effectiveness of general exercise (Liddle et al. 2004).

Pacing: Activity and participation can be hindered by an overactivity-underactivity cycle that is common in people who are struggling to cope with pain. The cycle is characterized by peaks of activity followed by spells of inactivity. These extremes of behavior are problematic because they lead to prolonged inactivity.

A typical scenario is that that the person is feeling particularly low and everyday tasks like housework, home maintenance, and self-care seem overwhelming. The person decides to rest rather than tackle these tasks. Then, when they feel more able, they attempt to make up for lost time and overdo things beyond their limits. This over activity results in fatigue and flare-up of pain and leads to another period of enforced inactivity. As with negative thoughts and feelings, this pattern can become self-perpetuating.

Physical therapists can help people to use techniques of pacing and goal setting to overcome this pattern of behavior and improve activity and participation (Harding & Williams 1995; Fey & Fordyce 1983). With pacing, people carry out tasks and activities as predetermined quota of activity rather than doing things on the basis that they feel motivated and/or capable of doing so.

Pacing requires some analysis to work out the levels of activity that bring on fatigue or flare-up—the *tolerance level*. Tolerance levels are specific to a particular activity and are defined in units of time or distance. Once determined, the tolerance level for a specific activity is then used to set a baseline for that activity. The baseline is set within the limits of the tolerance level. For example, the baseline may be 50 percent of the time taken to reach tolerance. (Others use baselines up to 80 percent of tolerance.) Pacing then entails the person carrying out the activity up to baseline level, taking a break from that activity, and then resuming up to baseline level again. Thus, a pattern of activity and rest is established that is more even than the peaks and troughs of the overactivity-underactivity cycle with less chance of triggering flare-up (Neilsen et al. 2001).

Sitting, standing, and walking are the usual activities that require initial attention, although pacing is adaptable to all activities.

In practice, setting tolerances and baselines is a matter of trial and error. For one thing, the effects of overactivity, fatigue or flare-up, may be delayed, and therefore, the physical therapist needs to spend time with the person to offer expert guidance and feedback on the calibration of levels.

Goal setting: Alongside pacing, goal setting complements pacing to help people improve activity and participation. In goal setting people are asked to define their aims and set specific targets. Often people will set goals that are too vague and targets that are unrealistic and very difficult to achieve. The inevitable failure leads to frustration and lack of compliance, which can further compound the problem that the person intended to resolve. As with pacing, physical therapists have a role to play in working with the person to help them set appropriate goals. This is best done by applying the SMART principles in which it is recommended that goals should be:

- *Specific:* The goal is very clearly defined. Wanting to dance is too vague. Wanting to dance for 10 min with the groom's father at your daughter's wedding is specific.
- *Measurable:* It is clear when the goal has been achieved.
- *Activity-related:* The goal involves actually doing something.
- *Realistic:* The goal is possible. There are many things other than chronic pain that can stop the achievement of a goal such as lack of finance.
- *Time-related:* A date is set by which time the goal should be achieved.

The physical therapist can discuss with the person and offer advice on dividing the main goal into a series of smaller, more realistic goals so that successful achievement of each minigoal gives reinforcement and motivation and takes the person closer to the main goal. The role of the physical therapist includes providing feedback on performance and giving guidance on techniques such as prioritization of tasks, delegation, and forward planning that help towards the achievement of the goals.

Flare-up management: Another role of the physical therapist in helping people to manage chronic pain is in flare-up management. As mentioned earlier, flare-up can occur after a period of overactivity. It can also come on unexpectedly and has been compared to breakthrough pain as seen in cases of cancer (Svendsen et al. 2005). Physical therapists can work with the person to identify triggers for flare-ups so that these can be avoided where possible.

It is recommended that people have a preordained plan of action that they follow during flare-up. (This is important because flare-up can be overwhelming and decision-making at the time can be difficult.) Here some of the methods, described earlier, as palliative for chronic pain, can be useful to make the situation more manageable. The physical therapist can offer advice on methods such as cold, heat, relaxation, pacing, TENS, positioning, and stretching that can be included in the plan.

CONCLUSION

Physical therapy has much to offer in the management of people with neuromusculoskeletal pain and can address function at each level of impairment (when appropriate), activity, and participation. The role is often best carried out in conjunction with other members of the rehabilitation team, for example, close working with vocational trainers in helping people return to work (Watson et al. 2004). Cognitive-behavioural therapy for people with pain is still developing and it should not be seen as a panacea for all (Vlaeyen & Morley 2005). However, the adoption of principles of cognitive-behavioral therapy into the practice of physical therapy has been a major development in expanding the role into one that places a strong emphasis on coaching and education rather than focusing on impairment. To misquote Homer J. Simpson, *less crackin', more yakkin'.**

REFERENCES

Burton A et al. Information and advice to patients with back pain can have a positive effect. A randomized controlled trial of a novel educational booklet in primary care. *Spine* 1999;24:2484-2491.

Christianson JB, Taylor R & Knutson D. *Restructuring Chronic Illness Management: Best Practices and Innovations in Team-Based Treatment.* San Francisco: Jossey-Bass 1998.

Chwastiak LA & Von Korff M. Disability in depression and back pain: Evaluation of the World Health Organization Disability Assessment Schedule (WHO DAS II) in a primary care setting. *J Clinical Epidemiology* 2003;56:507-514.

---

*In episode 258 of *The Simpsons,* Pokey Mom in 2001, Homer Simpson visited a chiropractor because of back pain. Homer admonished the chiropractor for talking too much with the phrase, "less yakkin', more crackin'."

CSP. *Curriculum Framework for Qualifying Programmes in Physiotherapy.* Chartered Society of Physiotherapy: London, UK, 2002.

Ferrell BA & Ferrell BR. Pain Management at home. *Clinics Geriatric Medicine* 1991;7:765-776.

Fey SG & Fordyce WE. Behavioral rehabilitation of the chronic pain patient. *Annual Review of Rehabilitation* 1983;3:32-63.

Fields HL. *Core Curriculum for Professional Education in Pain* (2nd ed.). IASP Press: Seattle WA, 1995.

Guzman J, Esmail R, Karjalainen K, Malmivaara A, Irvin E & Bombardier C. Multidisciplinary rehabilitation for chronic low back pain: Systematic review. *BMJ* 2001;322:1511-1516.

Hanson RW & Gerber KE. *Coping with Chronic Pain: A Guide to Patient Self-management.* New York: Guilford Publications, 1989.

Harding V & Williams AC de C. Extending physiotherapy skills using a psychological approach: Cognitive-behavioural management of chronic pain. *Physiotherapy* 1995;81:681-688.

Johnstone R, Donaghy M & Martin DJ. A pilot study of a cognitive-behavioural therapy approach to physiotherapy, for acute low back pain patients, who show signs of developing chronic pain. *Advances in Physiotherapy* 2003;2:182-188.

Jones D, Martin DJ. Chronic Pain. In Everett T, Donaghy M & Feaver S (Eds.) *Interventions for Mental Health: An Evidence Based Approach for Physiotherapists and Occupational Therapists.* Edinburgh: Butterworth-Heinemann 2003. Chapter 12:136-145.

Keefe FJ, Rumble ME, Scipio CD, Giordano LA & Perri LM. Psychological aspects of persistent pain: Current state of the science. *J Pain* 2004;5:195-211.

Liddle SD, Baxter GD & Gracey JH. Exercise and chronic low back pain: What works? *Pain* 2004;107:176-190.

Martin D J & Palmer S T. Soft tissue pain and Physical Therapy. Anaesthesia and intensive care medicine 2004.

Merskey H & Bogduk N. Classification of Chronic pain. Seattle: IASP Press, 1994.

Morley S. Process and change in cognitive behaviour therapy for chronic pain. *Pain* 2004;109:205-206.

Morley S, Eccleston C & Williams A. Systematic review and meta-analysis of randomized controlled trials of cognitive behaviour therapy and behaviours therapy for chronic pain in adults, excluding headache. *Pain* 1999;80:1-13.

Moseley GL. Physiotherapy is effective for chronic low back pain. A randomised controlled trial. *Australian J Physiotherapy* 2002;48:297-302.

Moseley GL. Evidence for a direct relationship between cognitive and physical change during an education intervention in people with chronic low back pain. *Eur J Pain* 2004;8:39-45.

Nielson WR, Jensen MP and Hill ML. An activity pacing scale for the chronic pain coping inventory: development in a sample of patients with fibromyalgia syndrome. *Pain* 2001;89:111-115.

Soukup MG & Vollestad NK. Classification of problems, clinical findings and treatment goals in patients with low back pain using the ICIDH-2 beta-2. *Disability Rehabilitation* 2001;23:462-473.

Steiner WA, Ryser L, Huber E, Uebelhart D, Aeschlimann A & Stucki G. Use of the ICF Model as a Clinical Problem-Solving Tool in Physical Therapy and Rehabilitation Medicine. *Physical Therapy* 2002;82:1098-1107.

Stroud MW, Thorn BE, Jensen MP & Boothby JL. The relation between pain beliefs, negative thoughts, and psychosocial functioning in chronic pain patients. *Pain* 2000;84:347-352.

Stucki G, Ewert T & Cieza A. Value and application of the ICF in rehabilitation medicine. *Disability Rehabilitation* 2002;24:932-938.

Svendsen KB, Andersen S, Arnason S, Arner S, Breivik H, Heiskanen T, Kalso E, Kongsgaard UE, Sjogren P, Strang P, Bach FW & Jensen TS. Breakthrough pain in malignant and non-malignant diseases: a review of prevalence, characteristics and mechanisms. *Eur J Pain* 2005;9:195-206.

van Tulder MW, Ostelo RWJG, Vlaeyen JWS, Linton SJ, Morley SJ, Assendelft WJJ. Behavioural treatment for chronic low back pain. (Cochrane Review). In: *The Cochrane Library Issue 2*. Oxford: Update Software, 2000.

Vlaeyen JWS & Linton SJ. Fear-avoidance and its consequences in chronic musculoskeletal pain: a state of the art. *Pain* 2000;85:317-332.

Vlaeyen JWS & Morley S. Active despite pain: the putative role of stop-rules and current mood. *Pain* 2004;110:512-516.

Vlaeyen JWS & Morley S. Cognitive-Behavioral Treatments for Chronic Pain: What Works for Whom? *Clinical Journal of Pain*. Special Topic Series: Cognitive-Behavioral Treatment for Chronic Pain 2005;21:1-8.

Von Korff M, Balderson BHK, Saunders K, Miglioretti DL, Lin EHB, Berry S, Moore JE & Turner JA. A trial of an activating intervention for chronic back pain in primary care and physical therapy settings. *Pain* 2005;13:323-330.

Von Korff M, Glasgow RE & Sharpe M. Organising care for chronic illness. *BMJ* 2002;352:92-94.

Watson PJ, Booker CK, Moores L & Main CJ. Returning the chronically unemployed with low back pain to employment. *Eur J Pain* 2004;8:359-369.

WHO. International Classification of Functioning, Disability and Health: ICF. Geneva: WHO, 2001.

Chapter 15

Acupuncture

Gira Patel

INTRODUCTION

The utilization of acupuncture in the United States has grown tremendously in the last decade. It is one of the most widely used forms of alternative or complementary procedures. Due to the clinical efficacy of this procedure, the National Institutes of Health (NIH) has drastically increased the budget to study acupuncture over the past 8 years. In 1997 the NIH had a Consensus Conference, which concluded acupuncture to be effective in the treatment of tennis elbow, fibromyalgia, low back pain, osteoarthritis, and headaches, to name a few.[1] This NIH Consensus Conference opened the door to hundreds of research grants for investigating the efficacy of acupuncture for different disorders and the proposed mechanisms of how acupuncture works. Although it is difficult to design randomized controlled trials (RCTs) for a dynamic and individual-based clinical procedure such as acupuncture, in recent years there is an increase of well-respected studies showing acupuncture as an effective method to treat various types of bone and joint pain. Clinical research investigating the mechanisms of acupuncture has been slow in the past, but increasing numbers of promising theories with preliminary evidence are being published each year. The effect of a local stimulation at an acupuncture point can now be observed with measures such as functional magnetic resonance imaging (fMRI) mappings of the brain, blood tests for specific hormones, or locally, such as the presence of endorphin, nor-epinephrine, cortisol, serotonin, substance P, etc., at

Clinical Management of Bone and Joint Pain
© 2007 by The Haworth Press, Inc. All rights reserved.
doi:10.1300/5771_17

the loci of stimulation[2] or at the target tissue. Outcome studies that examine the effectiveness of acupuncture demonstrate that, without any significant side effects, acupuncture does have a positive long-term effect on reducing acute and chronic pain.

HOW ACUPUNCTURE WORKS

The Gate theory is one of the earliest theories that attempts to explain how acupuncture is able to modulate pain, but it does not explain the long-lasting effects of acupuncture or its effect on the autonomic nervous system. Han and colleagues have demonstrated that electro-acupuncture can have analgesic effects at the spinal cord level and the central nervous system (CNS) level, promoting secretion of endorphin and dynorphin.[3] Acupuncture has been shown to influence pain perception by modulating the activity of key subcortical and brain stem sites along the descending pain modulating system pathway.[4] There are a number of nonopioid mechanisms of analgesia that may be involved as well. As an example, low-intensity and high-frequency electrical stimulation has a faster onset of action but does not have as prolonged of an effect as high-intensity and low-frequency stimulation. The former is thought to be serotonergic mediated and the latter opioid mediated.[5] One theory that may help better explain the long-term effect of acupuncture is that, by stimulating peripheral sensory afferents of the skin and muscle, sustained changes occur in the CNS via central neuromodulation. A fundamental concept that has emerged is that sustained nociceptive input can have profound effects on the CNS, causing pathological neuroplastic changes.[6] Acupuncture has been shown to suppress c-Fos expression in the spinal cord and the brain after noxious peripheral stimulation, suggesting a possible neuromodulatory mechanism that is independent of endogenous opioid release.[7] fMRI has made it possible to look into the effect acupuncture has on brain activation.[8] fMRI demonstrates some of the CNS pathways for acupuncture stimulation. Acupuncture at specific points has shown to activate structures of descending antinociceptive pathways and deactivate multiple limbic areas subserving pain association. "These findings may shed light on the CNS mechanism of acupuncture analgesia and endogenous pain modulation circuits in the brain."[9] Findings in the cortical and subcortical limbic/paralimbic structures in subjects who experienced deqi* demonstrate modulation of the cerebrocerebellar and limbic system activity that may constitute an important pathway of acupuncture action. "Acupuncture action involves the interplay between multiple neurotransmitters and modulators. Correlation of the distribution and the known function of these mediators in the cerebro-cerebellar and limbic systems with the hemodynamic response to acupuncture suggests that the down-regulation of dopaminergic and norepinephrinergic tone coupled with the up-regulation of serotonergic tone during the procedure may initiate a cascade of reactions that results in the more delayed effects of acupuncture."[10]

HISTORY AND PHILOSOPHY

Acupuncture is a medical procedure that entails the insertion of fine filliform needles into specific areas in the body to achieve clinical results either by modulating the course of a disease or by symptomatically reducing objective and subjective findings. Acupuncture is commonly practiced in conjunction with a technique called moxibustion. Moxibustion is a heat therapy in which a dried herb, *Artemisia vulgaris,* is burned to deliver a heat stimulus to an area or point on the surface of the skin.

Acupuncture is a medical practice that originated in China at least 3,000 years ago. Archeological findings of metallic acupuncture needles date back to the late Shang dynasty (1000 BC). Prior to that, bone chips and stone fragments were used to stimulate acupuncture points and meridians. With the development of the Chinese culture and civilization, from the time of the Spring-Autumn period (770 to 475 BC) onward, there appeared different schools of philosophical thought. It was during this period that the theories of Yin-Yang and Five Elements (Five Phases) were applied to medicine. The most important and influential work of this period is the Huangdi Neijing (Yellow Emperor's Internal Classic). Although it is said to have been written by the legendary Yellow Emperor, it was predominantly the work of a number of scholars and physicians living between the fifth and first centuries BC.[11] A large proportion of the Neijing deals with

---

*A sensation often described as heaviness, fullness, and dull ache at the site of acupuncture.

acupuncture and its related subjects, indicating that acupuncture had by this time developed into a special branch of Chinese medicine with its own sphere of learning. From the third century AD onward, acupuncture became a more specialized discipline in China, with many outstanding specialists and numerous valuable books devoted exclusively to it. Acupuncture as a medical discipline has spread to many countries throughout Asia, Europe, and America. As a result of this, many different forms of acupuncture have evolved. Though all disciplines of acupuncture are based on Chinese classic texts, one mayfind a great number of different styles including various Japanese styles, Korean hand acupuncture, and French energetics along with traditional Chinese acupuncture.

In order to understand the practice of acupuncture it is important to have a rudimentary understanding of the basis of traditional Chinese medicine (TCM) theory. One of the most important concepts in TCM is the idea of *"qi." Qi* (pronounced "chee") refers to an energy force in the body. There is no direct translation of this term into English. It is a force that allows for movement, growth, warmth, and development in the body. In good health, *qi* flows freely through the meridian system. An obstruction in the flow of *qi* can lead to a manifestation of disease or pain. According to TCM, acupuncture points are used to bring the body back into a state of equilibrium by balancing the flow of *qi* in the meridian system. There are 14 major meridians in the body; these meridians can be understood as virtual lines along which acupuncture points are found.* Eleven meridians in the body are associated with a major organ and three are not, as shown in the following list:

Upper extremity	Lower extremity
Lung meridian	Stomach meridian
Large intestine meridian	Bladder meridian
Small intestine meridian	Gall bladder meridian
Heart meridian	Liver meridian
Pericardium meridian	Spleen meridian
Triple warmer meridian	Kidney meridian
Conception vessel meridian	Governing vessel meridian

---

*Some acupuncture points can be found outside the meridian system and are called "extra points."

Utilizing the theory of TCM, acupuncture is able to treat a variety of diseases that impact the body even when the allopathic diagnosis is not conclusive. Diagnosis of disease using TCM includes taking a complete medical history and incorporating that with physical findings obtained through palpation of significant diagnostic zones on the body, as well as pulse and tongue diagnosis. Based on the findings, the practitioner is able to identify patterns that lead to a treatment protocol.[11] Regardless of the patients' complaint, it is imperative that the root of the medical problem be treated and not just from a symptomatic point of view. This ensures a long-lasting relief and not merely a temporary reduction in symptoms. The acupuncture practitioner has greater flexibility in treating a wide range of disorders using TCM, not being limited to a fixed diagnosis and able to view each patient on an individual basis. For example, a patient seeking acupuncture for pain resulting from a herniated disc who also suffers from hypertension should be evaluated by the acupuncturist for both problems as being one. In order for the patient to get the maximum relief from the herniated disc pain, it is imperative that the high blood pressure be addressed in the acupuncture treatment protocol first. The hypertension is seen as a constitutional problem and the pain syndrome as peripheral. The acupuncture treatment protocol for the constitutional or deeper lying problems already addresses the symptoms that the patient complains of. TCM is always looking for the underlying cause of a particular disease or symptom and the reason why it has not improved by the time the patient seeks help from the acupuncture practitioner.* This approach of combining a holistic medical investigation with palpation and meridian theory has proven to be a valuable tool in allowing the acupuncture practitioner to effectively treat a patients' complaint with the benefit of long-lasting effects. Often combining TCM with Conventional more symptomatic treatments such as steroid injections and/or nonsteroidal anti-inflammatory drugs (NSAIDs) can produce phenomenal results.[12] In this case, the constitutional (root) problems are addressed and the patients' body is now able to integrate and utilize a strong local, allopathic treatment with far less side effects and complications. It is important to understand that, in TCM, the treatment (points needled) will change as the clinical presentation

---

*A significant number of patients seeking help from acupuncture practitioners have undergone a variety of treatments ranging from medication therapies to surgery.

of the patient changes. This means that, in an acupuncture clinic, the patient will undergo a palpatory and verbal evaluation every time he or she comes for a repeat visit. The repeat differential diagnosis is usually much less time consuming but is necessary to the treatment outcome. Often, the treatment strategy will remain the same but the acupuncture points will change as a result of a change in palpatory findings and the patients' complaints. This ensures that the treatment is tailored for the individual patient in real time.

TREATMENT PRINCIPLES

Acupuncture can treat a very wide range of medical disorders, among them most bone and joint diseases.* Acupuncture used as the primary tool or used in conjunction with allopathic medicine (whether surgical or through medication) will address all subjective complaints of pain, discomfort, and unease. In addition it will also help many objective findings such as inflammation, swelling, contraction, and tightness of muscles and ligaments that accompany joint and bone disorders.

From a TCM perspective, there are three important parameters to evaluate when treating pain syndromes:

1. Bilateral structural evaluation of the musculoskeletal system
2. Meridians involved
3. Pre-existing internal diseases and other disorders in the patients' medical history

When a patient complaining of bone- or joint-related pain seeks acupuncture treatment, it is important to evaluate his or her entire structure so that structural imbalances leading to a disorder will not be ignored. This is a very useful approach for patients who have multiple-system problems and should not be treated based only on their symptomatic presentation. For example, a patient may come in with the main complaint of a right-sided knee pain. The structural assess-

---

*Acupuncture treatments will not cure genetic disorders, terminal disease, or fix advanced degenerative joint and bone problems, nor will acupuncture repair a broken or torn structure, which clearly demands surgery.

ment reveals that the patient also has a significant inversion of the foot, which must be included into the treatment protocol for the knee pain. According to Chinese medical theory, the foot inversion can be seen as an imbalance in the kidney and urinary bladder meridians. From an allopathic point of view it may simply be tightness in the IT band and inner thigh muscles or a local problem such as a degeneration of the medial meniscus. In TCM the problem is addressed by balancing these bladder and kidney meridians, not only correcting the structure of the foot but also balancing the IT band and the inner thigh, as well as influencing all other problems that the patient may present along the path of these meridians.*

Assessment of the meridians that cross the area of pain is another treatment strategy. Pain found along a meridian can be treated using distal points on the same or associated meridians. This type of meridian therapy is a quick and easy way for the practitioner to get a reduction in pain and inflammation without compromising the holistic approach. Often multiple meridians will pass through the painful area, and so it is important to determine which one has direct effect on the symptomatic presentation.

Pre-existing medical condition and family medical history are important in TCM when formulating a treatment strategy. In the majority of cases it is imperative to treat any type of pre-existing visceral problem the patient may present.[†] Problems in the organ systems may pose a major hindrance in the healing ability. It is also important to look at the family medical history for clues on how to approach the patients' complaints. Often patients have a hard time to heal due to a genetic predisposition to a disease. For example, some have a family history of diabetes and a difficult time healing from bone and joint problems. In this case, it is important to administer treatments that include the constitutional treatment for the diabetes as well as the more specific treatment addressing the bone or joint problem.

---

*The bladder meridian begins at the inner canthus of the eye and runs up crossing the vertex of the skull down the lateral aspect of the spine, posterior aspect of the leg crossing the lateral maleolus of the foot and ending at the lateral aspect of the fifth toe. The kidney meridian begins at the bottom of the foot runs up throught the medial maleolus up the inner thigh crossing the pelvis and the abdomen and ending at the throat.

†Anything from diabetes to asthma should be considered and added to the acupuncture treatment protocol.

Patients usually come for treatment once or twice a week depending on the severity of their main complaint. The total number of treatments varies from patient to patient depending on the chronicity and severity of the disorder. Patients usually see improvement in their condition within seven to ten acupuncture treatments. It is important to understand that the acupuncture treatments have a cumulative effect and that one treatment will not be sufficient to significantly change the clinical presentation of chronic pain problems.

CONDITIONS TREATED

Acupuncture can be very effective in treating painful bone and joint conditions associated with the neck, back, and the upper and lower extremities. Table 15.1 shows the most common bone and joint conditions treated with acupuncture. It is important to keep in mind that acupuncture can treat a wide variety of pain even if the diagnosis is unclear.

About 80 percent of adults in the United States suffer from osteoarthritis. Osteoarthritis commonly affects the hips, knees, and lower back, causing pain and decreased mobility. Acupuncture has been shown to produce long-term relief of symptoms due to osteoarthritis. A large study published in *Rheumatology* showed that acupuncture greatly improved pain in patients suffering from various types of osteoarthritis especially in the knees and hip.[13] This study took pain assessments prior to treatment, after treatment, and at 6 months post

TABLE 15.1. Common bone and joint conditions treated by acupuncture.

Location of pain	Condition
Low back and neck pain	Degenerative disc disease, osteoarthritis, herniated or bulging disc, spinal stenosis, postlaminectomy syndrome, sacro iliac
Shoulder	Rotator cuff problem—tendonitis/bursitis, adhesive capsulitis, arthritis, postoperative pain after breast surgery
Elbow	Lateral and medial epicondylitis, bursitis, repetitive strain, arthritis
Wrist/fingers	Arthritis, tendonitis, sprain, trigger finger, gout
Hip pain	Trochanteric bursitis, tendonitis, arthritis, postoperative pain
Knee pain	Arthritis, tendonitis, strain/sprains, Baker's cyst
Ankle/foot pain	Sprain/strain, fracture, arthritis, gout

treatment. Recently the NIH conducted one of the largest and most thorough clinical trials showing that "acupuncture reduces the pain and functional impairment of osteoarthritis of the knee" and that "these results also indicate that acupuncture can serve as an effective addition to a standard regimen of care and improve quality of life for knee osteoarthritis sufferers."[14]

Low back pain is the number-one cause of disability in people under the age of 45. In addition, it is one of the most common reasons patients visit their primary care physician. Despite advancements in surgical techniques and new medications, there is an abundance of patients who have little or no benefit from these procedures. This is in part because the diagnosis of low back pain is vague and in many instances is not precipitated by an injury. Acupuncture can be effective in the treatment of various types of acute and chronic back pain regardless of whether the etiology is known or defined in allopathic medicine. Often patients do not respond to allopathic approaches for low back pain because many of the treatments are too specific to the area of pain and do not take into consideration surrounding structures and muscles or the patients' medical history. This may explain why many patients do not get complete or long-term relief with conventional allopathic treatments. For example, a bulging or herniated disc may cause tightness and spasms in the muscles surrounding the affected area, leading to even more pain and discomfort. Therefore, a cortisone injection aimed at the disc may only have short-term pain relief. In this case, it is beneficial for the patient to receive acupuncture treatments before and after the injection in order to relax the musculature and enhance the effect of the local treatment. In a clinical setting, acupuncture has been effective in the treatment of low back pain associated with herniated discs, postlaminectomy syndrome, muscle spasms, piriformis syndrome, whiplash, degenerative disc disease, to name just a few. The diagnosis of low back pain can be quite variable and has proven to be a research challenge using any type of intervention including acupuncture. Despite the difficulties there have been a number of studies done in recent years with favorable outcomes. A meta-analysis, "Acupuncture for Low Back Pain," concluded that acupuncture "effectively relieves low back pain."[15] This study not only showed that acupuncture decreased pain but that it also increased functionality and decreased use of analgesic medications.

This data is very encouraging and should lead to a dramatic reduction in the use of opioid drugs to manage chronic pain. A study published by the Cochrane Review included 35 RCTs and concluded that acupuncture is an effective treatment for chronic low back pain.[16]

Pregnant women pose a great challenge in pain management as physicians lean toward nonpharmacological treatment options for them. Acupuncture has been used for thousands of years to treat pregnant women. This is safe and effective treatment modality for various types of bone and joint pain during pregnancy. Many women develop low back and pelvic pain during the second and third trimester. A recent study, "Acupuncture for Low Back Pain in Pregnancy," included two groups of women in the 15 to 30 weeks of pregnancy with low back and pelvic pain.[17] The study group received acupuncture with NSAIDs and the control group received only NSAIDs. After 8 weeks the study group reported a significant reduction in pain, decreased use of analgesics, and improved function compared with the control group. Another study done in Sweden with women in their third trimester presenting with girdle or low back pain showed that acupuncture provided a significant relief in pain and increased function compared with the control group that did not receive acupuncture treatments.[18]

Acupuncture is effective in treating various types of tendonitis in a clinical setting. Medial and lateral epicondylitis due to repetitive strain can be a very persistent disorder. Some of these patients benefit from cortisone injections and NSAIDs. There is a group of patients who have short-term or no relief from the allopathic treatment. In these patients, a more holistic approach should be implemented. Often, patients presenting with epicondylitis hold a posture that delays or inhibits healing or even causes the disorder. Structural alignment in these patients is often overlooked in the allopathic approach, but is integrated into the acupuncture treatment. A study published by the Cochrane Review in November 2001 provides promising preliminary results for the use of acupuncture in treating lateral elbow pain.[19] One RCT in the group clearly demonstrated patients that received real acupuncture verses sham acupuncture had a 55.8 percent reduction in pain compared with 15 percent in the sham group.[20]

Autoimmune disease such as rheumatoid arthritis and lupus contribute to bone and joint pain, which is often difficult to treat even with opioids. These patients benefit with acupuncture sessions especially if they are not responding and/or are having side effects to medications. In these cases, the acupuncture works to regulate the bodies' immune system and adrenal gland. To date there have been poorly designed studies, which have provided little evidence to support or refute the effectiveness of acupuncture in autoimmune diseases like rheumatoid arthritis. In a clinical setting it has been shown that acupuncture is effective in treating joint pain and inflammation associated with rheumatoid arthritis and lupus.

Patients who have been diagnosed as suffering from "fibromyalgia" constitute a growing population. Although fibromyalgia is not an orthopedic problem per se, many of them complain of joint pain such as bursitis, tendonitis, and reduced range of motion. Fibromyalgia is often quite difficult to treat because of the complex and ambiguous nature of this syndrome. These patients are perfect candidates for acupuncture since the treatment applied is based on a multisystem and holistic approach. There is a growing body of research that shows the benefit of acupuncture in this group of patients. A recent study showed that patients who received acupuncture had a 70 percent relief in pain and less stiffness than those in the control group.[21]

Acupuncture is a complex and effective procedure that can be a safe and cost-effective primary or complementary treatment for various types of orthopedic problems.

REFERENCES

1. Acupuncture, NIH Consensus Statement Online 1997 Nov 3-5; 15(5): 1-34.

2. Shah JP, Phillips TM, Danoff JV, Gerber LH. An in vivo microanalytical technique for measuring the local biochemical mileu of human skeletal muscle. *J Appl Physiol* 2005; 99: 1977-1984.

3. Chen XH, Han JS. Analgesia induced by electroacupuncture of different frequencies is mediated by different types of opioid receptors: Another cross-tolerance study. *Behav. Brain Res* 1992; 47: 143-149.

4. Mayer DJ. Biological mechanisms of acupuncture. *Prog Brain Res* 2000; 122: 457-477.

5. Debreceni L. Chemical releases associated with acupuncture and electric stimulation. *Crit Rev Phys Rehab Med* 1993; 53: 247-275.

6. Morgan JI, Curran T. Stimulus-transcription coupling in the nervous system: Involvement of the inducible proto-oncogenes fos and jun. *Ann Rev Neurosci* 1991; 14: 421-451.

7. Pan B, Castro-Lopes JM, Coimbra A. C-fos expression in the hypothalamo-pituitary system induced by electroacupuncture or noxious stimulation. *Neuro-Report* 1994; 5: 1649-1652.

8. Cho ZH, Chung SC, Jones JP, et al. New findings of the correlation between acupoints and corresponding brain cortices using functional MRI procedure. *National Acad Sci* 1998; 95: 2670-2673.

9. Wu M-T, et al. Central nervous pathway for acupuncture stimulation: localizing of processing with functional MR imaging of the brain—preliminary experience; *Neuroradiology* 1999; 212: 133-141.

10. Hui KKS, et al. The integrated response of the human cerebro-cerebellar and limbic systems to acupuncture stimulation at St36 as evidenced by fMRI. *Neuro Image* 2005; 27: 479-496.

11. Bensky OJD. *Acupuncture a Comprehensive Text*. Chicago, Illinois: Eastland Press 1981.

12. Albrecht F. Molsberger, Jochen Mau, Danuta B. Pawelec, Janos Winkler. Does Acupuncture improve the orthopedic management of chronic low back pain—A randomized, blinded, controlled trial with 3 months follow up. *Pain* 2002; 99: 579-857.

13. Linde K, Weidenhammer W, Streng A, Hoppe A, Melchart D. Acupuncture for osteoarthritic pain: An observational study in routine care. *Rheumatology* 2006; 45: 222-227.

14. Berman BM, Lao L, Langenberg P, Lee WL, Gilpin AM, Hochberg MC. Effectiveness of acupuncture as adjunctive therapy in osteoarthritis of the knee. *Ann Intern Med* 2005; 141: 901-910.

15. Manhelmer E, White A, Berman B, Forys K, Ernst E. Meta-analysis: Acupuncture for low back pain. *Ann Intern Med* 2005; 142: 651-663.

16. Furlan AD, van Tulder MW, Cherkin DC, Tsukayama H, Lao L, Koes BW, Berman BM. Acupuncture and dry needling for low back pain. *The Cochrane Database of Systematic Review* Issue 1.

17. Guerreiro da Silva JB, Nakamura MU, Cordeira JA, Kulay L. Acupuncture for low back pain in pregnancy. *Acupuncture in Medicine* 2004; 22: 60-67.

18. Kvorning N, Holmberg C, Greenert L, Aberg A, Akeson J. Acupuncture relieves pelvic and low back pain in late pregnancy. *Acta Ostet Gynecol Scand* 2004; 83: 246-250.

19. Green S, Buchbinder R, Barnsley L, Hall S, White M, Smidt N, Assendelft W. Acupuncture for lateral elbow pain. *The Cochrane Database of Systematic Review* 2002 Issue 1.

20. Molsberger A, Hille E. The analgesic effect of acupuncture in chronic tennis elbow pain. *Br J Rheumatol* 1994; 33: 1162-1165.

21. Berman BM, Ezzo J, Hadhazy V, Swyers JP. Is acupuncture effective in the treatment of fibromyalgia? *J Fam Pract* 1999; 48: 213-218.

Chapter 16

Botulinum Toxin

Charles Argoff

INTRODUCTION

Contrary to the way in which the medical literature has described this topic, botulinum toxin should not in fact be considered a single type of toxin but a group of botulinum toxins. Each of them is a product of the anaerobic bacterium, *Clostridum botulinum.* Of the seven known immunologically distinct serotypes of these extremely potent neurotoxins, types A, B, C1, D, E, F, and G, types A and B are the only ones available for routine clinical practice. Two type A preparations, Botox (Allergan, Inc., Irvine, CA) and Dysport (Ipsen Ltd., Berkshire, UK) have been developed for commercial use, and Dysport is currently being evaluated in the United States, while Botox is available. Type B toxin is currently commercially available as Myobloc in the United States and as Neurobloc in Europe. While each of these neurotoxins is similar in that they are proteins, they vary with respect to molecular weight, mechanism of action, duration of effect, and adverse effects. The bacteria synthesize each toxin initially as a single-chain polypeptide. Bacterial proteases then "nick" both type A as well as type B proteins, resulting in a dichain structure consisting of one heavy and one light chain. Type A is nicked more than type B, and there is less than a 50 percent homology between the two toxins.[1]

The mechanism of action of these toxins was initially linked to their ability to inhibit the release of acetylcholine from cholinergic nerve terminals; however, for many years it has been generally acknowledged that this effect does not appear to explain the apparent analgesic activity of some of these toxins.[2] In fact, much recent

Clinical Management of Bone and Joint Pain
© 2007 by The Haworth Press, Inc. All rights reserved.
doi:10.1300/5771_18

research has been directed toward examining other potential and actual mechanisms of action of these toxins that might better explain its analgesic effects. Inhibition of the release of glutamate, substance P, and calcitonin gene-related peptide reduced afferent input to the central nervous system through effects of the toxins on muscle spindles. Other possible effects on pain transmission independent of the effect on cholinergic transmission of these neurotoxins have been proposed based on the results of many laboratory experiments in which it has been proposed that, through a mechanism similar to that which inhibits the release of acetylcholine, these other neurotransmitters are inhibited as well.[3-5] In particular, Cui and colleagues have recently reported in a placebo-controlled study that subcutaneous injections of botulinum toxin type A (BTX-A) into the paws of rats before exposure to the formalin model of inflammatory pain experienced a significant dose-dependent inhibition of both the acute as well as secondary pain responses. In addition to the demonstration that glutamate release in the periphery was reduced in treated as opposed to control animals, inhibition of the expression of C-fos in the dorsal spinal cord in treated animals but not controls was observed. These findings have been summarized in two recent reviews, one by Aoki and the other by Borodic and colleagues, each suggesting that there are noncholinergic mechanisms of at least one of the botulinum toxins (BTX-A), which help to explain its analgesic effect.[6-9] Nevertheless, recent data from a randomized, placebo-controlled study designed to quantify the potential reduction in cutaneous nociception following subcutaneous injections of BTX-A in healthy human volunteers failed to show a difference in cutaneous nociception in treated and placebo groups 4 and 8 weeks following injection.[10] Whether or not the analgesic effect of BTX-A is maximized in a disturbed, abnormal state rather than normal state remains to be determined. In other words, perhaps only in certain abnormal states are the effects of botulinum toxin likely to be analgesic.

The mechanism by which acetylcholine is released by these neurotoxins is a multistep process. At present, it is clearly much better understood than the mechanism by which these neurotoxins may exert their analgesic effects, although much work has been recently completed regarding its potential analgesic effect. The toxin must be internalized into the synaptic terminal for it to exert its anticholinergic effect. The first step in this process is the binding of the toxin to a receptor on the axon terminals of the cholinergic terminals. Each botulinum toxin serotype binds specifically to its own receptor irreversibly, and each neither binds to nor inhibits the other serotypes' receptor.[11,12] After the toxin is bound, an endosome is formed that carries the toxin into the axon terminal. The final step involves cleavage of one of the known synaptic proteins, which are required for acetylcholine to be released by the axon. Botulinum toxins A, E, and C cleave synaptosome-associated protein-25 (SNAP-25). Botulinum toxins B, D, F, and G cleave synaptobrevin, also known as vesicle-associated membrane protein (VAMP). Botulinum toxin type C also cleaves syntaxin.[1] The specific manner in which each toxin type may cleave the synaptic protein and the specific differences in effect on inhibiting acetylcholine and other neurotransmitter release is under active investigation and quite fascinating but it is beyond the scope of this chapter. In addition, it is not known at present how these differences translate into various observed beneficial as well as adverse effects.

Following injection of the toxin into the muscle, weakness occurs within a few days to a week, peaks most often within 2 weeks, and then gradually resolves with a slow return to baseline. The recovery of strength is associated with sprouting of the affected axon and the return, for example, of cholinergic synaptic activity to the original nerve terminals. Regeneration of the cleaved synaptic protein is also required for recovery to occur. The duration of the clinical effect of the currently available neurotoxins appears to be approximately 3 months but may clearly vary from individual to individual.[4,13,14] In addition, the possible differences in duration of action of these toxins for different clinical conditions, for example, cervical dystonia versus migraine headache versus chronic low back pain has not been well studied to date. In my clinical experience, the analgesic effect of botulinum toxin depends on the serotype used (type A, Botox, typically longer than type B, Myobloc) but is almost always less than 12 weeks.

THE CURRENT USFDA-APPROVED USES OF THE BOTULINUM TOXINS

In 1989, BTX-A (Botox) became the first botulinum toxin to be approved by the USFDA for use in the United States. Although originally

U.S. Food and Drug Administration (USFDA) approved for the treatment of strabismus, blepharospasm, and hemifacial spasm, Botox was subsequently USFDA approved for the treatment of cervical dystonia and, most recently, for the treatment of glabellar wrinkles and axillary hyperhidrosis. The only other botulinum toxin to be currently USFDA approved, BTX-B, is currently approved only for cervical dystonia.[15] Despite the fact that neither currently USFDA-approved botulinum toxin is approved specifically as an analgesic, and of great interest is that, in initial published studies of the use of either BTX-A or BTX-B for cervical dystonia, the analgesic effects of these agents, e.g., the reduction in intensity of dystonia, appeared to be independent of the ability of these toxins to reduce the pain associated with cervical dystonia. In fact, the analgesic effect of the neurotoxins appeared to have a greater duration of action than other more direct neuromuscular effects.[16]

Therefore, the review of the use of any of the botulinum toxins in the management of painful states other than those noted above presently involves a discussion of these agents used in an "off-label" manner.

THE USE OF THE BOTULINUM TOXINS FOR THE TREATMENT OF CHRONIC HEADACHE

Migraine Headache

The botulinum toxins have been utilized for a number of different headache types with varying responses according to the individual study. Dr. William Binder, a plastic surgeon, serendipitously made the observation that many of his patients who had undergone BTX-A injections for the treatment of glabellar lines reported notable improvement in their headache control. Because of this observation, he coordinated a multicenter open-label trial of botulinum toxin type A in patients with migraine.[17] Of the patients, 36/77 (51 percent) with migraine as defined by the International Headache Society (IHS) noted complete relief of their headaches with a mean duration of effect of 4.1 months, and 27/77 (38 percent) reported a partial response. The site of injections varied from patient to patient but most often included the frontalis, temporalis, corrugator and procerus muscles, and, in a few patients, the suboccipital muscles. The dose of BTX-A also varied from patient to patient. Except for eyebrow ptosis, no significant adverse effects were experienced. Silberstein et al. reported the results of a multicenter, randomized, controlled study of BTX-A involving 123 patients with HIS-defined migraine who experienced between two and eight severe migraine headaches each month. Patients were randomized to one of three groups: placebo, 25 units of BTX-A, or 75 units of BTX-A. Eleven standard injection sites were utilized including the frontalis, temporalis, corrugator, and procerus muscles. Bilateral injections were performed. Compared with placebo, the patients receiving 25 units of BTX-A experienced significantly fewer and less severe migraine headaches each month, a reduction in the amount of acute headache medication used, and a lower incidence of emesis. There was no difference between the group receiving 75 units of BTX-A and those receiving placebo. No adverse effects were noted except for 2 cases of diplopia and 13 cases of ptosis.[18] Brin and his colleagues, in a separate study, presented the results of a randomized, placebo-controlled multicenter study of BTX-A in the migraine prophylaxis. Patients either received injections in the frontal and temporal regions, frontal only with placebo injections into the temporal region, temporal only with placebo injections into the frontal region, or placebo injections into both regions. Only patients who received BTX-A injections into both temporal and frontal regions experienced significantly greater pain relief than the placebo-only group.[19]

A variety of other studies have been reported more recently primarily as abstracts only. Regardless, some interesting observations have been made. In one study, 30 patients with HIS-defined migraine headache who were experiencing between two and eight attacks each month were randomized to receive either 50 units of BTX-A or placebo injections. Fifteen injection sites were utilized including the temporalis, frontalis, corrugator, procerus, trapezius, and splenius capitis muscles bilaterally. The patient's response was followed for up to 90 days. Compared with placebo-treated patients, who did not experience any significant change in their headache frequency or severity, those who received BTX-A injections had a significant reduction in headache frequency (at 90 days 2.5 versus 5.8; $p < 0.01$) as well as severity. No significant adverse effects were noted.[20]

In an open-label study evaluating the effects of BTX-A on disability in episodic and chronic migraine, treatment with 25 units of BTX-A (frontalis, temporalis, and corrugator muscles) resulted in decreased migraine-associated disability in 58 percent of the patients.[21] Two retrospective studies have emphasized the potential benefit of BTX-A as a "disease-modifying" treatment for patients with chronic migraine.[22,23] Each of these reports suggest (based on nonrandomized data) that there may be increasing benefit experienced with repeated treatments with BTX-A for patients with chronic migraine—these clinical observations, although not derived from randomized, controlled studies, are important as many injectors do, in fact, believe that, for maximal benefit to be realized from botulinum injections, a patient may indeed have to be treated with botulinum toxin on multiple occasions.

One open-label study involving the use of BTX-B for the treatment of chronic migraine headache has been reported. Forty-seven patients with at least four migraine headaches within a 4-week period were treated with a total of 5,000 units of BTX-B into at least three injection sites. On the basis of pain distribution, "trigger points," and glabellar lines, injection sites were chosen Thirty patients (64 percent) reported improvement in headache intensity and severity. One adverse effect experienced with BTX-B treatment in this study that was not experienced with BTX-A-treated patients was dry mouth.[24]

Tension-Type Headache

The use of botulinum toxin for the treatment of HIS-defined tension-type headache has been studied as well. Smuts et al. completed a randomized, controlled study of 37 patients with tension-type headache. Patients received either 100 units of BTX-A or placebo into six injection sites—two in the temporalis muscles and four in the cervical sites. By the third month post injection, a statistically significant reduction in headache severity was noted in the treatment group compared with the placebo-treated group.[25] Freund and Schwartz have published a retrospective study of 21 patients with chronic tension-type headache who experienced concurrent tenderness of the scalp or neck as well. Five injection sites were chosen and the patient received a total of 100 units of BTX-A. The injection sites were chosen based on the sites of maximal tenderness as reported by the patient. At least a 50 percent reduction in headache frequency was experienced by 18/21 patients, and 20/21 experienced at least a 50 percent reduction in scalp/neck tenderness to palpation.[26] There have been several other clinical reports of a small number of successfully treated patients; however, another small study reported by Zwart et al. of six patients with tension-type headache who were treated with BTX-A demonstrated no improvement in pain intensity following injection.[27-30] One reason for this study's negative outcome may have been that, in this study, patients received injections only into their temporalis muscle unilaterally. In a small randomized controlled study of ten patients with tension-type headache, BTX-A was no more effective than placebo.[31] Porta evaluated the difference in response between BTX-A injections and methylprednisolone injections in patients with tension-type headaches. Although both groups improved, patients who had undergone botulinum toxin injections experienced improvement for a greater duration of time (>60 days) compared with methylprednisolone-treated patients.[32]

Cluster Headache

There have been several reports of treatment of cluster headache with botulinum toxin. In 1996, Ginies and colleagues reported a single patient with cluster headache refractory to other treatment who was reported to respond to the injection of botulinum injection.[33] Two patients with intractable cluster headache were reported by Freund and Schwartz to respond to the unilateral injection of 50 units of BTX-A into five sites within the temporalis muscle on the affected side only. Within 9 days of treatment, the headaches abated for both patients.[34] In an open-label study, Robbins reported his observations that for seven patients with chronic cluster headache who were treated with BTX-A or BTX-B, treatment was at least moderately effective in four of the seven and not effective in three. He also treated three patients with episodic cluster headache with botulinum toxin, and two of the three patients had at least moderate improvement.[35]

Chronic Daily Headache

Multiple studies have been reported regarding the use of botulinum toxin in the management of one of the most difficult to treat types of headaches, chronic daily headache. Four of five treated patients in an open-label study of patients with chronic daily headache (CDH) by Klapper and Klapper benefited from injections.[36] The most recent report of a large randomized controlled study of patients with CDH who were treated with 150 to 225 units of BTX-A (Botox) or placebo did not meet its primary end points; however, analysis of the study did indicate that there was in fact a reduction of headache severity and intensity in patients who were treated with the toxin.[37] In a randomized trial of 56 patients with CDH, patients were divided into four groups involving both forehead and suboccipital injections. Only patients who received botulinum toxin injections into each region experienced significant benefit.[38] Argoff reported three patients with CDH who were successfully treated with a total of 5,000 units of BTX-B injected into the frontalis, temporalis, corrugator, splenius capitis, splenius cervicis, levator scapular, and trapezius muscles.[39]

A number of recent reviews regarding the use of botulinum toxin in the management of various headache disorders has in general been favorable toward the use of botulinum toxin, most notably BTX-A, although each of the reviews suggests the need for additional research to confirm the clinical observations.[40-43] In two reviews using an evidence-based analysis, the authors conclude that there is insufficient evidence for a treatment recommendation of migraine with botulinum toxin;[41,42] nevertheless, the same authors acknowledges that it is likely that there are subgroups of patients with headache who are likely to respond to treatment.[41,42]

THE USE OF BOTULINUM TOXIN IN THE MANAGEMENT OF MUSCULOSKELETAL PAIN

Among the painful musculoskeletal conditions that have been treated with botulinum toxin are chronic temporomandibular joint dysfunction (TMJ), chronic myofascial pain, chronic cervicothoracic pain, and chronic low back pain.

BTX-A has been utilized for a number of the temporomandibular disorders including myofascial dysfunction affecting this joint, bruxism, oromandibular dystonia, and masseter/temporalis hypertrophy.[44] The results of randomized, placebo-controlled study examining the effect of the use of BTX-A in the treatment of chronic facial pain associated with masticatory hyperactivity completed by von Lindern and colleagues have been recently reported.[45] There was a statistically significant difference in the reduction of pain in the treated group compared with the placebo group in this study.[45] In an open-label study of 46 patients with chronic temporomandibular pain, Freund and Schwartz injected BTX-A into both the masseter muscles (50 units each) and into the temporalis muscles (25 units each) under EMG guidance. Pain level as assessed by VAS scores, interincisal oral opening and tenderness to palpation were among the outcome measures that showed improvement. Approximately 60 percent of those treated experienced at least 50 percent improvement in these areas.[46] More recently, these same two investigators suggested that botulinum toxin injections could play an adjunctive role when performing an arthrocentesis of the temporomandibular joint.[47] In contrast, Nixdorf et al. completed a double-blind, placebo-controlled crossover trial evaluating the use of BTX-A in the management of chronic moderate to sever orofacial pain of myogenic origin. Just as in Freund and Schwartz's open-label study, 25 units of toxin were injected into each temporalis muscle and 50 units were injected into each masseter muscle. The crossover occurred at 16 weeks. The primary outcome variable utilized was pain intensity and unpleasantness. No significant difference was determined between placebo versus active treatment in this study; however, only 15 patients entered the study and only 10 patients completed it, suggesting that these small numbers may have made it difficult to see a statistical difference between the two groups.[48]

The doses of botulinum toxin used for treatment of the temporomandibular disorders depends on the sizes of the muscles involved as well as the type of toxin used. For the temporalis and medial pterygoid muscles, the recommended doses of BTX-A are between 5 and 25 units in multiple injection sites. For the masseter muscle, the recommended dose of BTX-A is 25 to 50 units also in multiple injection sites. For the lateral pterygoid muscle, the recommended dose of type-A toxin is between 5 and 10 units.[44] For each of these muscles, the recommended doses of type B toxin is between 1,000 and 3,000 units again with multiple injection sites within each muscle.[49]

A number of studies have examined the role of botulinum toxin in the treatment of chronic cervical or thoracic pain most often associated with myofascial dysfunction. One recently reported chart review compares type A and type B toxin for the treatment of myofascial pain syndrome and concludes that type-A-treated patients had a longer duration of benefit and fewer serious side effects.[50] Evidence against the use of a conventional trigger point injection technique in the use of botulinum toxin has been reported as well.[51] Two recently published randomized studies have concluded either that local anesthetic trigger point injections are equally effective as botulinum toxin injections for myofascial pain or that small doses of botulinum toxin injections fail to provide notable relief compared with placebo injections.[52,53] In their study of the use of BTX-A injections into cervical paraspinal, trapezius and, thoracic paraspinal muscles, Wheeler et al. were not able to detect any significant differences in pain reduction between treated and placebo patients.[54] In contrast and certainly noting a different treatment group and trial design, Freund and Schwartz in their randomized controlled study of 26 patients with chronic neck pain following "whiplash" injuries demonstrated a statistically significant reduction in pain for the patients who were treated with BTX-A compared with placebo. A hundred units of toxin were injected into five "tender" sites and these were compared with a similar number of saline injections. Improvement was noted after 4 weeks.[55] In another report of the use of BTX-A for whiplash, Juan reported benefit in treated patients.[56] Cheshire et al. injected myofascial trigger points in the cervical paraspinal or shoulder girdle area in six patients with either BTX-A (50 units spread out over two or three areas) or saline. Crossover occurred at 8 weeks in this randomized, controlled, crossover study. Four of the six patients experienced at least 30 percent pain reduction with toxin but not saline injections.[57] In a previous study by Wheeler et al., 33 patients with cervical myofascial pain were injected with either 50 or 100 units of BTX-A or placebo. No significant differences were seen between the two groups.[58]

Utilizing a novel injection technique, injecting the whole muscle in a grid-like pattern instead of the areas of tenderness only, and using doses of BTX-A ranging from 20 to 600 units, Lang, in an open-label study of the use of type A toxin in the treatment of myofascial pain, noted that 60 percent of the patients experienced good to excellent results 22 to 60 days following injection.[59] In a 12-week randomized, double-blind, placebo-controlled study, 132 patients with cervicothoracic myofascial pain were treated with BTX-A or saline by Ferrante et al. No significant differences in outcome were seen between each group. Patients receiving BTX-A were treated with 50 to 250 units of toxin total divided among five injection sites.[60]

Porta, in a single blinded study, evaluated the difference between lidocaine/methylprednisolone injections compared with BTX-A injections in affected myofascial trigger points within the psoas, piriformis, or scalenus anterior muscles; 80 to 150 units of toxin were used. Each group received benefit, but the toxin-treated patients experienced a greater duration of relief.[61] De Andres and colleagues have also confirmed the benefit of treatment of myofascial pain with BTX-A in an open-label study.[62] Opida has presented 31 patients with posttraumatic neck pain who he has treated with BTX-B injections in an open-label study. Of his patients, 71 percent noted significant reductions in pain and headache frequency and severity.[63] Taqi et al. have shown in two separate open-label studies that either type of botulinum toxin may be effective in the treatment of myofascial pain.[64,65] Several case reports of utilizing BTX-B injections in the management of chronic myofascial pain have suggested generally good results.[66-68]

Several other recent publications including a case report, an open-label study involving 77 patients, and one review have emphasized the benefit of botulinum toxin in the management of chronic myofascial pain.[69-71] One recently published review of the use of botulinum toxin for the treatment of musculoskeletal pain and muscle spasm concludes that, even if there is scientific evidence that botulinum toxin has analgesics qualities, these is currently a lack of sufficient clinical evidence of its efficacy in the treatment of chronic musculoskeletal disorders.[72]

The use of botulinum toxin in the management of chronic low back pain has also been explored. Foster and colleagues, in a randomized controlled study involving 31 patients with chronic low back pain, studied the effect of 200 units of BTX-A (five sites in the paravertebral levels L1 to L5 or L2 to S1, 40 units/site) compared with placebo injections. Pain and extent of disability were noted at baseline as well as at 3 and 8 weeks using the VAS scale as well as the Owestry Low Back Pain Questionnaire. At both 3 and 8 weeks, more patients who had received botulinum toxin injections (73.3 percent and

60 percent) experienced 50 percent or more pain relief compared with the placebo-treated group (25 percent and 12.5 percent). At 8 weeks there was less disability in the botulinum-toxin-treated group compared with the placebo-treated group.[73] A recent review by Porta and Maggioni has suggested similar outcomes.[74] Knusel and colleagues treated patients with low back pain associated with painful muscle spasm with different doses of type-A toxin and noted that only those treated with the highest doses (240 units) experienced greater relief than placebo-treated patients.[75]

There have been reports of the use of botulinum toxin for the treatment of piriformis muscle syndrome as well. Childers and colleagues concluded, following the completion of a randomized, controlled, crossover study of nine patients with piriformis muscle syndrome who were treated with both BTX-A (100 units) and placebo, that there was a trend toward greater pain relief for patients after receiving toxin as opposed to placebo. EMG and fluoroscopic guidance was utilized for the injections.[76] Fannucci et al. reported that 26/30 patients with piriformis syndrome who were injected with BTX-A under CT guidance obtained relief of their symptoms within 5 to 7 days.[77] Fishman has performed two studies looking at the use of botulinum toxin in patients with piriformis syndrome. In one noncontrolled study, Fishman and colleagues concluded that the injection of BTX-A may be a useful adjunctive measure to physical therapy in the management of this syndrome.[78] In a dose-ranging study with type-B toxin in the management of piriformis syndrome using EMG guidance, Fishman reported that patients experienced notable symptom improvement.[66] Lang has also recently concluded that BTX-B may be effective in the management of piriformis syndrome.[79]

Other recent reports suggest that the use of botulinum toxin injections may be helpful in the management of plantar fasciitis as well as lateral epicondylitis.[80-83]

THE USE OF BOTULINUM TOXIN IN THE MANAGEMENT OF NEUROPATHIC PAIN AND OTHER PAINFUL CONDITIONS

The use of botulinum toxin for the treatment of neuropathic pain remains novel, and there are only a few reports describing initial results in the management of postherpetic neuralgia, complex regional pain syndrome, and spinal cord injury pain.[84-86] Although reduction of pain is not the usual primary outcome measurement used in studies of botulinum toxin and spasticity, a study of patients treated with BTX-A for spasticity by Wissel has noted the analgesic benefit of this treatment for 54 of 60 patients treated.[87]

One recent randomized, controlled study suggests that BTX-A can be effective in reducing pain after an hemorrhoidectomy.[88] A recently published review suggests that botulinum toxin may be effective in the management of severe anorectal pain.[89]

REFERENCES

1. Settler PE. Therapeutic use of botulinum toxins: Background and history. *Clin J Pain* 2002;18:S19-S24.

2. Simpson LL. Identification of the characteristics that underlie botulinum toxin potency: Implications for designing novel drugs. *Biochemie* 2000;82:943-953.

3. Gobel H, Heinze A, Heinze-Kuhn K, Austermann K. Botulinum toxin A in the treatment of headache syndromes and pericranial pain syndromes. *Pain* 2001; 91:195-199.

4. Guyer BM. Mechanism of botulinum toxin in the relief of chronic pain. *Curr Rev Pain* 1999;3:427-431.

5. Hallet M. How does botulinum toxin work? *Ann Neurol* 2000;48:7-8.

6. Cui ML, Khanijou S, Rubino J, et al. Botulinum toxin A inhibits the inflammatory pain in the rat formalin model. *Soc Neurosci Abst* 2000;26:656.

7. Cui M, Li Z, You S, et al. Mechanisms of the antinociceptive effect of subcutaneous Botox®: inhibition of peripheral and central nociceptive processing. *Arch Pharmacol* 2002;365:33.

8. Aoki KR. Evidence for antinociceptive activity of botulinum toxin type A in pain management. *Headache* 2003;43(Suppl 1):S9-S15.

9. Borodic GE, Acquadro M, Johnson EA. Botulinum toxin therapy for pain and inflammatory disorders: Mechanisms and therapeutic effects. *Expert Opin Investig Drugs* 2001;10:1531-1544.

10. Blersch W, Sculte-Mattler WJ, Przywara S, et al. Botulinum toxin A and the cutaneous nociception in humans: A prospective, double-blind, placebo-controlled, randomized study. *J Neurol Sci* 2002;205:59-63.

11. Evans DM, Williams RS, Shone CC, et al. Botulinum neurotoxin type B: Its purification, radio iodination, and interaction with rat brain synaptosomal membranes. *Eur J Biochem* 1986;154:409-416.

12. Simpson LL. Kinetic studies on the interaction between botulinum toxin type A and the cholinergic neuromuscular junction. *J Pharmacol Exp Ther* 1980;212: 16-21.

13. Meunier FA, Schiavo G, Molgo J. Botulinum neurotoxins: From paralysis to recovery of functional neuromuscular transmission. *J Physiol (Paris)* 2002;96: 105-113.

14. Jurasinski CV, Lieth E, Dang Do AN, et al. Correlation of cleavage of SNAP-25 with muscle function in a rat model of botulinum neurotoxin type A induced paralysis. *Toxicol* 2001;39:1309-1315.

15. Tsui JKC. Botulinum toxin as a therapeutic agent. *Pharmacol Ther* 1996; 72:13-24.

16. Lew MF. Review of the FDA-approved uses of botulinum toxins, including data suggesting efficacy in pain reduction. *Clin J Pain* 18:S142-S146.

17. Binder WJ, Brin MF, Blitzer A, et al. Botulinum toxin type A (BOTOX®) for treatment of migraine headaches: An open-label study. *Otolaryngol Head Neck Surg* 2000;123:669-676.

18. Silberstein S, Mathew N, Saper J, et al. Botulinum toxin type A as a migraine preventive treatment. *Headache* 2000;40:445-450.

19. Brin MF, Swope DM, O'Brien C, et al. Botox® for migraine: Double blind, placebo-controlled, region-specific evaluation. *Cephalagia* 2000;20(abstract):421.

20. Barrientos N, Chana P. Efficacy and safety of botulinum toxin type A (Botox®) in the prophylactic treatment of migraine. Presented at the American Headache Society 44th Annual Scientific Meeting. Seattle, WA, 2002.

21. Eross EG, Dodick DW. The effects of botulinum toxin type A on disability in episodic and chronic migraine. Presented at the American Headache Society 44th Annual Scientific Meeting, Seattle, WA, 2002.

22. Mathew NT, Kallasam J, Kaupp A, et al. "Disease modification" in chronic migraine with botulinum toxin type A: Long-term experience. Presented at the American Headache Society 44th Annual Scientific Meeting, Seattle, WA, 2002.

23. Mauskop A. Long-term use of botulinum toxin type A (Botox®) in the treatment of episodic and chronic migraine headaches. Presented at the American Headache Society 44th Annual Scientific Meeting, Seattle, WA, 2002.

24. Opida C. Open-label study of Myobloc (botulinum toxin type B) in the treatment of patients with transformed migraine headaches. *J Pain* 2002;3(suppl 1):S10 (abstract).

25. Freund BJ, Schwartz M. A focal dystonia model for subsets of chronic tension headache. *Cephalagia* 2000;20(abstract):433.

26. Smuts JA, Baker MK, Wieser T, et al. Treatment of tension-type headache using botulinum toxin type A. *Eur J Neurol* 1999;6(suppl 4):S99-S102.

27. Relja M. Treatment of tension-type headache by local injection of botulinum toxin. *Eur J Neurol* 1997;4(suppl 2):S71-S73.

28. Wheeler AH. Botulinum toxin A, adjunctive therapy for refractory headaches associated with pericranial muscle tension. *Headache* 1998;38:468-471.

29. Schulte-Mattler WJ, Wieser T, Zierz S. Treatment of tension-type headache with botulinum toxin: a pilot study. *Eur J Med Res* 1999;4:183-186.

30. Zwart JA, Bovim G, Sand T, et al. Tension headache: botulinum toxin paralysis of temporal muscles. *Headache* 1994;34:458-462.

31. Gobel H, Lindner V, Krack PK, et al. Treatment of chronic tension-type headache with botulinum toxin. *Cephalagia* 1999;19(abstract):455.

32. Porta M. A comparative trial of botulinum toxin A and methylprednisolone for the treatment of tension-type headache. *Curr Rev Pain* 2000;4:31-35.

33. Ginies PR, Fraimout JL, Kong A, et al. Treatment of cluster headache with subcutaneous injection of botulinum toxin. Presented at the 8th World Congress on Pain, Vancouver, CANADA, 1996.

34. Freund BJ, Schwartz M. The use of botulinum toxin A in the treatment of refractory cluster headache: case reports. *Cephalagia* 2000;20:329-330.

35. Robbins L. Botulinum toxin for cluster headache. Presented at the 10th Congress of the International Headache Society, New York, NY, 2001.

36. Klapper JA, Klapper A. Use of botulinum toxin in chronic daily headaches associated with migraine. *Headache Q* 1999;10:141-143.

37. Silberstein SD, Starks SR, Lucas SM, et al. Botulinum toxin type A for the prophylactic treatment of chronic daily headache: A randomized, double-blind, placebo controlled trial. *Mayo Clin Proc* 2005;80:1126-1137.

38. Klapper JA, Mathew NT, Klapper A, et al. Botulinum toxin type A (BTX-A) for the prophylaxis of chronic daily headache. *Cephalagia* 2000;20 (abstract): 292-293.

39. Argoff C. Successful treatment of chronic daily headache with Myobloc. *J Pain* 2002;3(suppl 1, abstract):10.

40. Dodick DW. Botulinum neurotoxin for the treatment of migraine and other primary headache disorders: from bench to bedside. *Headache* 2003;43(suppl 1): 25-33.

41. Evers S. Is there a role for botulinum toxin in the treatment of migraine? *Curr Pain Headache Rep* 2003;7:229-234.

42. Evers S, Rahman A, Vollmer-Haase J, et al. Treatment of headache with botulinum toxin A—A review according to evidence-based medicine criteria. *Cephalagia* 2002;22:699-710.

43. Mauskop A. The use of botulinum toxin in the treatment of headaches. *Curr Pain Headache Rep* 2002;6:320-323.

44. Schwartz M, Freund B. Treatment of temporomandibular disorders with botulinum toxin. *Clin J Pain* 2002;18:S198-S203.

45. von Lindern JJ, Niederhagen B, Berge S, et al. Type A botulinum toxin in the treatment of chronic facial pain associated with masticatory hyperactivity. *J Oral Maxillofac Surg* 2003;61:774-778.

46. Freund B, Schwartz M, Symington J. Botulinum toxin: New treatment for temporomandibular disorders. *Br J Oral Maxillofac Surg* 2000;38:466-471.

47. Freund BJ, Schwartz M. Intramuscular injection of botulinum toxin as an adjunct to arthrocentesis of the temporomandibular joint: Preliminary observations. *Br J Oral Maxillofac Surg* 2003;41:351-352.

48. Nixdorf DR, Heo G, Major PW. Randomized controlled trial of botulinum toxin A for chronic myogenous orofacial pain. *Pain* 2002;99:465-473.

49. WE MOVE. Practical considerations for the clinical use of botulinum toxin type B: a self-study continuing medical education activity. February, 2002.

50. Lang AM. A preliminary comparison of the efficacy and tolerability of botulinum toxin serotypes A and B in the treatment of myofascial pain syndrome: A retrospective, open-label chart review. *Clin Ther* 2003;25:2268-2278.

51. Ferrante FM, Bearn L, Rothrock R, et al. Evidence against trigger point injection technique for the treatment of cervicothoracic myofascial pain with botulinum toxin type A. *Anesthesiology* 2005;103:277-283.

52. Graboski CL, Gray DS, Burnham RS. Botulinum toxin A versus bupivicaine trigger point injections for the treatment of myofascial pain syndrome—A randomized, double-blind, crossover study. *Pain* 2005;118:170-175.

53. Ojala T, Arokoski JP, Partanen J. The effect of small doses of botulinum toxin A on neck-shoulder myofascial pain syndrome—A double-blind, randomized, and controlled, crossover study. *Clin J Pain* 2006;22:90-96.

54. Wheeler A, Goolkasian P, Gretz S. Botulinum toxin A for the treatment of chronic neck pain. *Pain* 2001;94:255-260.

55. Freund B, Schwartz M. Treatment of whiplash-associated neck pain with botulinum toxin A: A pilot study. *Headache* 2000;40:231-236.

56. Juan FJ, Use of botulinum toxin A for musculoskeletal pain in patients with whiplash associated disorder. *BMC Musculoskeletal Disorder* 2004;13:5.

57. Cheshire WP, Abashian SW, Mann JD. Botulinum toxin in the treatment of myofascial pain syndrome. *Pain* 1994;59:65-69.

58. Wheeler AH, Goolkasian P, Gretz SS. A randomized, double blind, prospective pilot study of botulinum toxin injection for refractory, unilateral, cervicothoracic, paraspinal, myofascial pain syndrome. *Spine* 1998;23:1662-1666; discussion, 1667.

59. Lang A. A pilot study of botulinum toxin type A (BOTOX®), administered using a novel injection technique, for the treatment of myofascial pain. *Am J Pain Manage* 2000;10:108-112.

60. Ferrante M, Bearn L, Rothrock R, King L. Botulinum toxin type A in the treatment of myofascial pain. Presented at the annual meeting of the American Society of Anesthesiologists, 2002.

61. Porta M. A comparative trial of botulinum toxin type A and methylprednisolone for the treatment of myofascial pain syndrome and pain from chronic muscle spasm. *Pain* 2000;85:101-105.

62. DeAndres J, Gerda-Olmedo G, Valia JC, et al. Use of botulinum toxin in the treatment of chronic myofascial pain. *Clin J Pain* 2003;19:269-275.

63. Opida CL. Evaluation of Myobloc™ (botulinum toxin type B) in patients with post-whiplash headaches. Presented at the American Academy of Pain Medicine's 18th annual meeting, San Francisco, CA, 2002.

64. Taqi D, Gunyea I, Bhakta B, et al. Botulinum toxin type A (Botox®) in the treatment of refractory cervicothoracic myofascial pain. *Pain* 2002;3(suppl 1, abstract):16.

65. Taqi D, Royal M, Gunyea I, et al. Botulinum toxin type B (Myobloc™) in the treatment of refractory myofascial pain. *Pain* 2002;3(suppl 1, abstract):16.

66. Fishman LM. Myobloc™ in the treatment of piriformis syndrome—a dose finding study. Presented at the American Academy of Pain Medicine's annual meeting, San Francisco, CA, 2002.

67. Nalamachu S. Treatment with botulinum toxin type B (Myobloc™) injections in three patients with myofascial pain. Presented at the American Academy of Pain Medicine's annual scientific meeting, San Francisco, CA, 2002.

68. Smith H, Audette J, Dey R, et al. Botulinum toxin type B for a patient with myofascial pain. Presented at the American Academy of Pain Medicine's annual scientific meeting, San Francisco, CA, 2002.

69. Sheean G. Botulinum toxin for the treatment of musculoskeletal pain and spasm. *Curr Pain Headache Rep* 2002;6:460-469.

70. De Andres J, Cerda-Olmedo G, Valia JC, et al. Use of botulinum toxin in the treatment of chronic myofascial pain. *Clin J Pain* 2003;19:269-275.

71. Lang AM. Botulinum toxin therapy for myofascial pain disorders. *Curr Pain Headache Rep* 2002;6:355-360.

72. Saenz A, Avellanet M, Garreta R. Use of botulinum toxin type A on orthopedics: A case report. *Arch Phys Med Rehabil* 2003;84:1085-1086.

73. Foster L, Clapp L, Erickson M, Jabbari B. Botulinum toxin A and chronic low back pain: A randomized, double blind study. *Neurology* 2001;56:1290-1293.

74. Porta M, Maggioni G. Botulinum toxin (BoNT) and back pain. *J Neurol* 2004;251(suppl 1):I15-I18.

75. Knusel B, DeGryse R, Grant M, et al. Intramuscular injection of botulinum toxin type A (Botox®) in chronic low back pain associated with muscle spasm. Presented at the American Pain Society annual scientific meeting, San Diego, CA, 1998.

76. Childers MK, Wilson DJ, Gnatz SM, et al. Botulinum toxin type A use in piriformis muscle syndrome: A pilot study. *Am J Phys Med Rehabil* 2002;81:751-759.

77. Fannucci E, Masala S, Sodani G, et al. CT-guided injection of botulinum toxin for percutaneous therapy of piriformis muscle syndrome with preliminary MRI results about denervation process. *Eur Radiol* 2001;11:2543-2548.

78. Fishman LM, Anderson C, Rosner B. BOTOX® and physical therapy in the treatment of piriformis syndrome. *Am J Phys Med Rehabil* 2002;81:936-942.

79. Lang AM. Botulinum toxin type B in piriformis syndrome. *AM J Phys Med Rehab* 2004;83:198-202.

80. Placzek R, Deuretzbacher G, Meiss AL. Treatment of chronic plantar fasciitis with Botulinum toxin A: Preliminary clinical observations. *Clin J Pain* 2006;22:190-192.

81. Babcock MS, Foster L, Pasquina P, et al. Treatment of pain attributed to plantar fasciitis with botulinum toxin type A: A short-term, randomized, placebo-controlled, double-blind study. *Am J Phys Med Rehab* 2005;84:649-654.

82. Wong Sm, Hui AC, Tong PV, et al. Treatment of lateral epicondylitis with botulinum toxin- a randomized, double-blind, placebo controlled trial. *Ann Intern Med* 2005;11:793-797.

83. Hayton MJ, Santini AJ, Hughes PJ. Botulinum toxin injections in the treatment of tennis elbow—A double-blind, randomized-controlled pilot study. *J Bone Joint Surg Am* 2005;87:503-507.

84. Dubin A, Smith H, Tang J. Evaluation of botulinum toxin type B (Myobloc ™) injections in a patient with painful muscle spasms. *Pain* 2002;3(suppl a, abstract):11.

85. Jabbari B, Maher N, Difazio MP. Botulinum toxin A improved burning pain and allodynia in two patients with spinal cord pathology. *Pain Med* 2003;4:206-210.

86. Argoff CE. A focused review on the use of botulinum toxins for neuropathic pain. *Clin J Pain* 2002;18:S177-S181.

87. Wissel J, Muller J, Dressnandt J, et al. Management of spasticity associated pain with botulinum toxin A. *J Pain Symptom Manage* 2000;20:44-49.

88. Davies J, Duffy D, Boyt N, et al. Botulinum toxin reduces pain after hemorrhoidectomy: results of a double-blind, randomized study. *Dis Colon Rectum* 2003;46:1097-1102.

89. Hawley PH. Botulinum toxin for severe anorectal pain. *J Pain Symptom Manage* 2002;24:11-13.

Chapter 17

Radiopharmaceuticals

Rahul Parikh
Howard S. Smith

INTRODUCTION

Pain was reported as the most common complaint in more than 75 percent of patients with metastatic cancer to the bone.[1] Bone pain is a common symptom in patients with advanced solid tumors such as prostate, breast, lung, and kidney. Up to one-half of patients with cancer may develop metastases to bony sites, and about half of these patients will go on to suffer sequelae such as pain, pathological fractures, immobility, or hypercalcemia of malignancy (HCM).[2] Understanding the pathophysiology of cancer-related bone disease and potential treatment modalities may help treat painful bone metastases that up to 50 percent of breast cancer patients and up to 80 percent of advanced prostate cancer patients may experience.[1] During the course of their disease, up to 80 percent of patients with solid cancers go on to develop painful bone metastases to the vertebrae, pelvis, or extremities.[3] Within the patients with cancer spread to bone, 70 percent of these occur in the vertebrae and/or ribs, 40 percent have metastases in the pelvis, 25 percent occur in the femur, and 15 percent are found in the skull.[4] As the disease becomes more advanced, bone cancer pain can become more progressive and particularly difficult to treat. We have outlined in the following text the current understanding of oncology-related bone metastases, and will briefly discuss current approved and experimental treatment options available for these patients.

Clinical Management of Bone and Joint Pain
© 2007 by The Haworth Press, Inc. All rights reserved.
doi:10.1300/5771_19

Radiopharmaceuticals are extensively discussed as a potential treatment option for patients experiencing intractable pain from advanced cancer.

The approach to patients with bone metastases is complex—involving pharmacological and nonpharmacologic remedies, with frequent assessments of both symptomology and disease progression in a comprehensive approach.[5] Several factors that affect the complex process of cancer-mediated bone pain include hormonal, musculoskeletal, and hematological mechanisms discussed in further detail in the following sections. Conventional pharmaceutical therapy for treating painful metastases to the bone includes nonsteroidal analgesics and opiates. Oral analgesics such as nonsteroidal anti-inflammatory drugs (NSAIDs) and/or corticosteroids are effective in these situations as first-line therapy. In patients with progressive disease or increasing tolerance to pain, medication may respond to later stages of pharmacologic intervention (e.g., addition of mild to strong opiods). Local field external beam radiotherapy (EBRT) has been widely accepted as the mainstay of treatment for osseous metastases for palliation of bone pain, because it allows for maintenance of skeletal structure while preserving function.[6] Significant efficacy has been reported in the literature with local radiotherapy, ranging from a single fraction of 8 to 30 Gy in ten fractions.[7] While radiotherapy is a significant treatment modality for single or limited areas of disease, other treatment strategies for managing painful bone metastases include bisphosphonates, hormonal therapy, and surgery.[3] In addition to the guidelines of the World Health Organization's three-step analgesic ladder of drugs used for pain management, an emerging option for painful osseous metastases is the use of bone-seeking radiopharmaceuticals. These bone-targeted radionuclides may offer meaningful palliation/treatment for bony metastatic disease, especially when multiple sites are involved. Adding radiation therapy in the form of gamma- or beta-emitting radiopharmaceuticals to current treatment modalities may delay the onset of further metastatic disease and significantly improve quality of life and functional status with minimal side effects when compared with chronic analgesic use alone.[8]

Radiopharmaceutical therapy as palliative intent for bone pain has been effectively employed for more than 30 years.[9] Historically, radiopharmaceuticals are not a "new age" medicinal therapy; this therapeutic modality dates back to 1950, when radioactive phosphorus was used to treat "osteoblastic lesions" from metastatic breast cancer.[10] Newer data suggests that radiopharmaceuticals can effectively better a patient's quality of life, limit progression of disease, and prevent pathologic fractures.[11,12]

PATHOPHYSIOLOGY OF PAINFUL OSSEOUS METASTASES

The pathophysiology of bone metastasis and the sequelae of pain, pathological fracture, and bone marrow infiltration are complex. Disease complications are mainly based on three basic mechanisms of disease progression: direct malignant extension, tumor seeding, and hematogenous flow (i.e., retrograde venous flow).[13] Pain that is secondary to osseous metastasis may be due to direct tumor extension into bone and expansion of periosteal membranes that are richly innervated with nociceptors.[13] Mechanical nerve entrapment and mechanical stretch can also modulate the sensation of pain. Tumor seeding from bone to contiguous structures such as spinal cord, nerve roots, or nerve plexia can also contribute to pain. The mechanically unstable, "tumor-weakened" bones are highly susceptible to the release of "algesic chemical mediators" consisting of mainly inflammatory characters.[13] Current investigation agrees that metastases of most cancers usually begin in the marrow and spread via hematogenous routes rather than direct extension into bone.[14] This concept of tumor metastasis has significantly been expanded on since Stephen Paget's proposal of the "seed and soil" theory.[15] This is the foundation of the model system by which we explain how malignancies use molecular mechanisms to evade host factors and survive—some of which can manifest as painful spread of disease.

Pain intensity in metastatic oncologic disease is known to poorly correspond to the extent of tissue damaged and can be highly variable. According to Pandit-Taskar et al., while pain of neuropathic or inflammatory origin may be due to upregulation of *glial fibrillary acidic protein* found in the spinal cord,[2] pain from bone metastasis is actually of unknown etiology. There is speculation that osseous metastasis conveys pain by sensitizing the afferent nervous system via tumor-derived factors. Possible mechanisms that explain pain secondary to advanced malignancies infiltrating bone conclude that it involves both osteoblast and osteoclast recruitment via receptor activator for nuclear factor-κB (RANK).[16] Animal bone cancer models have substantiated that bony destruction is mediated by RANK ligand-induced osteoclastogenesis.[16] Immunocytochemical markings of neurotransmitters and central receptors in animal cancer models imply that certain signals, such as substance P, lower the threshold of pain at the level of the dorsal horn.

Bony metastasis sets the stage for several different biochemical interactions between host cells and tumor cells at the local and systemic levels. Multiple growth and regulatory factors between bone and particular tumors (especially prostate, breast, and lung) may directly promote carcinogenesis and indirectly support osteoclastic activation, leading to pain at synergistic levels that respond only to a multimodality treatment approach.

Both advanced malignancies and metastatic lesions in bone can be attributed to disturbances in cell-matrix and cell-cell adhesions, and the loss of growth factor regulation (see also Chapter 22). The chemotactic factors and cytokines implicated in the increased mobility of tumor cells include growth factors, hyaluronians, cytokinins (autotoxin and hepatoctye growth factor), and other tumor-secreted factors.[17] The properties of transforming growth factor-α (TGF-α) secreted from nearby cells and found in the bony matrix may encourage activation of osteoclasts, thereby promoting bony spread of disease.[18] Bone resorption has also been attributed to interleukin-1 (IL1) and interluekin-6 (IL6),[19] while expression of matrix metalloproteinases (MMPs) appears to promote degradation of extracellular matrix components of bone and allow formation of bone metastases by breaching of the basement membrane.[20] Calcitonin gene-related peptide (CGRP), fibroblast growth factor (FGF), bone morphogenetic proteins (BMPs), CD44, and endothelin 1 are some of the cytokines and growth factors that contribute to this process. Metastatic growth is further stimulated by growth factors and cytokines from lymphocytes and the bone matrix, which in turn, stimulate tumor cell repopulation.[18] It has also been postulated that lowered intracellular and extracellular pH levels in solid tumors may result in elevated levels of substance P and sensitized nocireceptors in bone.[21] Therefore, tumor-derived growth factors support osteoclast activation and subsequent bony resorption.

Bone physiology is a complex process by which osteoclasts resorb bone and osteoblasts replace bone to create a stable osteoid matrix. Directly and indirectly through local factors such as tumor-derived growth factors and cytokines, or systemic factors such as parathyroid hormone and steroids, this balance between bone destruction and formation can be disturbed. This may occur through several natural or unnatural processes, substances, or iatrogenic treatments (e.g., steroids, chemotherapy). Bone metastases can be predominately osteolytic in nature (e.g., lung and renal), osteoblastic (e.g., prostate), or mixed (e.g., breast). Just as "lytic" lesions can go on to become "blastic" in behavior, the mixed pattern that is most commonly found represents a *dynamic balance* between bone resorption, osteoblastic differentiation, and osteoid formation (Ref-PMID: 16172192). The increased blood flow to sites of more reactive, osteoblastic activity and increased surface are of calcium phosphate salts may be why there is greater uptake of radiopharmaceuticals in these areas of interest.[7]

Primarily radiation therapy has been shown to be effective for bone pain reduction even with single-site treatments totaling 5 to 10 Gy.[4] According to Silberstein,[4] the pain relief achieved from radiation treatment at lower doses is probably not due to a decreased population of malignant cells in the bone marrow but rather a consequence of several factors. It has been observed from external beam irradiation studies that the radiation dose needed for palliation of painful symptoms is significantly less than the radiation dose needed for effective cancer cell killing.[22] Therefore, pain palliation is not solely dependent on radiosensitivity and subsequent tumor cell population killing but rather based on radiation-induced changes in cytokine and growth factor release mechanisms in the normal bone environment. Also, the neurons that participate in afferent stimulation are actually radioresistant at such low doses of radiation.[9] Osseous metastatic pain relief may be sought by destroying lymphocytes via energetic beta-emitting radiation, even at low doses. As implied earlier, these lymphocytes could thereby no longer produce the cytokine-induced pain mechanism that is present in metastatic disease.

Metastatic lesions likely to advance as osteolytic problems *(most commonly lung)* can be best addressed with treatment that inhibits osteoclastic activation or impedes the attachment and downstream function of osteoclasts. For the past 10 years, the emergence of bisphosphonates has revolutionized metastatic disease palliation and has become an important treatment modality for symptomatic bone metastases. On the contrary, treatment modalities, such as radiopharmaceuticals, which inhibit or delay osteoblastic activation and reactive bone matrix that is stimulated by tumor-mediated growth factors, should be used to best manage "blastic" lesions.

CURRENT TREATMENT OPTIONS

Current management of bone pain from metastatic disease involves a multifaceted approach using one or more of the following: analgesic medications such as NSAIDs, opiates, analgesic adjuvants, chemotherapy, radiation, hormonal therapy, or surgery. Within the hierarchy of analgesic drug use, with respect to the recommended three steps of the WHO analgesic ladder system, the initial step is to use NSAIDs, including aspirin, naproxen, or ibuprofen, for mild to moderate pain relief.[23] The second step usually requires the addition of weak opioids such as hyrdrocodone or codeine. Higher doses and more powerful opioids may be necessary to achieve optimal analgesia from chronic, persistent pain. The medications used as the third-line treatment (WHO analgesic ladder) include morphine, fentanyl, hydromorphone, or methadone. All of these drugs are not without significant side effects including constipation, possible addiction, lethargy, cognitive dysfunction, and respiratory depression.

Bisphosphonates, an osteoclast inhibitor, are potent agents that can repair bony destruction from metastatic disease by interfering with osteoclast-mediated bone resorption and also stimulate osteoblastic differentiation.[24] Specifically, some of the more popular bisphosphonates include pamidronate, zoledronate, and clodronate. Bisphosphonates have been proven to significantly reduce skeletal sequelae, prevent painful events, as well as delay progression of disease in breast cancer and multiple-myeloma patients.[25] Since its main role in treatment for advanced cancer bone pain is based on interruption of stimulated osteoclasts, these drugs are mainly used bone lesions that have a "lytic" component, such as lung, breast, and myeloma.[26]

Surgical treatment modalities may be useful in cases where bone metastases has created pathologic fractures, involving the long or weight-bearing bones or collapsed vertebral bodies. Vertebroplasty is a popular procedure whereby polymethylmethacrylate (PMM) is percutaneously injected into the collapsed vertebral body to alleviate pain and provide stabilization in bone that has endured significant osteolysis (e.g., osteoporosis, metastatic cancer to bone, or multiple myeloma).[27] When PMM is injected into osteolytic lesions anywhere besides the vertebrae, it is called cementoplasty and is also another mode of rapid relief from compression fractures.

Other interventions for pain palliation in advanced metastatic bone disease is the use of EBRT as focal treatment sites or wider, hemibody radiation for multiple sites. Often times, the WHO pain ladder system, which is the prescription standard for analgesics, is followed by EBRT in single fractions for symptomatic relief of persistent pain.[28] Local field EBRT has provided significant analgesia (complete and partial responses) in about 80 to 90 percent of patients and a complete pain response in 50 to 60 percent of those patients.[29] The National Comprehensive Cancer Network on Cancer Pain, Ontario Guidelines for Palliative Pain, and the Second Workshop on Palliative Radiotherapy and Symptom Control, all encourage the use of EBRT for palliation of local bony metastases. They also agree that, if there are multiple metastatic lesions in bone, it may be well palliated via hemibody radiation or bone-targeted radiotherapy.[5] A study by the Radiation Therapy Oncology Group (RTOG), consisting of 949 patients with painful bone metastases from either prostate or breast cancers, was randomized to assess degree of palliation between groups exposed to 8 Gy, single-fraction EBRT, versus 30 Gy in ten fractions.[30] Although the single 8 Gy fraction group was two times as likely to receive retreatment, there was no significant difference between the groups in terms of pain relief, use of other narcotic analgesics, and pathologic fractures. Pain relief after one dose of radiation treatment usually occurs within 4 to 6 weeks in about 80 percent of patients.[31] Hemibody radiation for the treatment of diffuse, symptomatic bone metastases is not routinely performed because of significant toxicity (e.g., radiation pneumonitis, gastrointestinal toxicity, and bone marrow suppression), and has been largely replaced by radiopharmaceuticals.[32]

It is often assumed that the patients treated in several trials involving radiopharmaceuticals with palliative intent are of advanced disease and therefore are the only applicable patients to this treatment. However, it is evident that pain reduction can be achieved at even better rates with longer duration when multiple painful sites have not yet developed.[33] This is an attempt to explain a clinician's reluctance to use these agents and the current underutilization of radiopharmaceuticals for palliation of osseous cancer pain.

In sum, treatment modalities such as chemotherapy, radiopharmaceuticals, and hormonal therapy are best used for multiple, diffuse bony metastatic sites, while EBRT and surgery are more efficient modes of treatment for focal, limited metastatic disease.[34] Hence, there has been substantial elaboration upon the concept of a three-step ladder for cancer pain relief.

RADIOPHARMACEUTICAL AGENTS—OVERVIEW

Radiation has long been delivered to osseous metastases via external beam radiotherapy. Intravenous administration of radiopharmaceutical agents has transformed the way successful radiation therapy is provided at the sites of osseous metastases. Radiotherapy involves the use of ionizing radiation to cause DNA damage and subsequent "reproductive death" of malignant cells, even those that have gained access to bony sites.

An important consideration in radiotherapy as a treatment modality is to optimize delivery of effective treatment to meet certain goals of palliation or cure. In both scenarios, goals of such therapy should be the following: primary alleviation of pain, improve quality of life, improve survival if possible (mainly in curative regimens), and reduce the dependence on other treatment modalities that may be more toxic and nontolerable (e.g., chemotherapy and opioids). The boundaries of toxicity with radiation treatment may limit its use as systemic therapy (e.g., hemibody radiation), but radiopharmaceuticals can take advantage of the successful mechanism of radiotherapy against metastatic malignancies and provide less-toxic, more-targeted therapy.

Even with the long known analgesic effects of external beam radiotherapy, the past decade has seen increasing clinical use of alternative means for delivering radiation to osseous metastases. Aside from and sometimes in conjunction with external beam,[8] radiation is now commonly delivered to osseous metastases through intravenous administration of radiopharmaceuticals. A radiopharmaceutical (RP) is a complex combination of a radionuclide (RN) with a pharmaceutical (P) agent (RP = RN + P).

Radionuclides ("radioactive nuclides") are unstable atomic species that change naturally into other atomic species by altering their nuclear structure. Through this change, ionizing radiation is released, a mechanism reflecting the disintegration process (radioactive decay).[12] Traditionally, radiotherapy involves mechanisms of nuclear reactions known as alpha, beta, and gamma emissions.[35] Alpha emission is the emission of an alpha particle (helium nucleus, ^{4}He, which is found in decay of plutonium-239) that travels in a decay pathway through which a radioactive isotope becomes a stable isotope. Secondary reactions can occur in molecules that are affected by the helium nucleus, but this form of radiation travels only a short distance and has no invasive effect with considerable skin toxicity (ref. same as previous). Beta radiation involves the emission of beta particles— the release of a very energetic electron from the atom's nucleus. Beta-type radioactive decay of particles such as carbon-14 have much more invasiveness when compared with alpha radiation. Highly energetic beta emissions may lead to increased bone marrow toxicity. and very-low-energy beta emissions may not penetrate enough for effective malignant cell killing.[12] The third form of emission is the release of high-energy photons not involving the emission of particles. Since the nucleus can lose excess energy by means of gamma radiation, this can occur concurrently with both alpha and beta emissions. Physiologically, gamma radiation is highly energetic and highly invasive, so purely gamma-emitting radionuclides make poor therapeutic agents, but are useful for imaging.

If the radionuclide is a pure beta emitter, diagnostic imaging cannot be performed, but metastatic lesions can still receive therapeutic radiation. If the radionuclide is a pure gamma emitter, imaging may be possible, but radiation of bone metastases will not be effective. If the radionuclide is both beta and gamma emitter with an appropriate keV, then both treatment and imaging may be possible. Radiopharmaceuticals can be easily administered intravenously and provide advantages over conventional external beam radiotherapy since multiple/diffuse sites can be treated with a single injection. This is usually at the expense of mild bone marrow depression and may avoid potential nausea/vomiting, diarrhea, and tissue insult associated with external beam radiotherapy.

Pharmaceutical agents used for palliation of painful osseous metastases are essentially the same agents used for imaging in "bone scans" for nuclear medicine. These agents [e.g., methylene diphosphonate (MDP)] are phosphonates and are "bone-seeking" agents. Phosphonates are also used to treat pain and hypercalcemia of bony metastases.[24] The "attachment" of the radionuclide (RN) to the bone-seeking agents (P) enables the radiation to be emitted at the sites of bone metastases. These are the spots that generally "light up" or "take up" radiopharmaceuticals on a bone scan. What makes these agents "bone-seeking" is their biochemical similarity to the area of interest.[4] This is based on chemisorption by the phosphate moiety of phophonate chelates, formation of insoluble salts with bone, and the direct substitution into hydroxyapatite.[12] In order to follow images on bone scans, a radiopharmaceutical agent should have optimal photon emission with moderately energetic beta emissions.

The effort to create the optimal radiopharmaceuticals for palliation of painful bone metastases also requires consideration of the dose rate and proper, controlled dosimetry. The variability in dosimetry between radiopharmaceuticals depends on the speculation of the patient's bone marrow, uptake, and distribution of drug within the infiltrating malignancy.[36] The half-life ($T_{1/2}$) of a radionuclide determines the initial dose rate and, therefore, the total amount of radioactivity that can be administered.[12] A moderate $T_{1/2}$ can avoid an excessive initial dose rate that may lead to insult of normal cells and limit further initial tissue toxicity. An exceedingly long $T_{1/2}$ may lead to problems with environmental safety (e.g., in case of spills), while a very short $T_{1/2}$ can pose problems with shipping, shelf life, and increased requirement for total of required administered activity.[12] Nevertheless, there is a need to use radiopharmaceuticals with the knowledge of the balance between efficacious penetration and cell killing of bone metastases while preserving adequate bone marrow and surrounding tissues. As previously discussed, since the depth of soft tissue penetration is directly related to the energy of the electrons, the appropriate radionuclide is determined by these characteristic emissions.

RADIOPHARMACEUTICAL AGENTS

The United States Nuclear Regulatory Commission labels these radiopharmaceuticals as "unsealed sources," as opposed to "teletherapy" used in external beam radiation. Table 17.1 shows the seven radiopharmaceuticals that have been investigated by multiple examiners. According to Silberstein, tumoricidal effect is dependent on beta emission of the particular source and is not dependent on the gamma emission.[37] More energetic beta particle energy can provide greater malignant cell killing but only at the price of greater myelosuppression. In addition, isolated gamma emission can be used to trace the sites of reactive bone formation with minimal to no cell killing.[37] For example, ^{99}Tc-labeled bisphosphonate bone scan can identify bone metastases that are osteoblastic and can also aid in computing dosimetry of radiopharmaceuticals.[38] Although there are individual differences in half-life, beta MeV, and gamma MeV, all of the listed radiopharmaceuticals in Table 17.1 are not significantly different with respect to pain relief in bone metastases.[4]

The only radiopharmaceuticals that are Food and Drug Administration (FDA) approved and currently available in the United States for clinical administration are strontium-89 (^{89}Sr, Metastron), phosphorus-32 (^{32}P, orthophosphate), and samarium-153-ethylene diamine tetramethylene phosphonate (^{153}Sm-EDTMP, Samarium Sm153 Lexidronam, and Quadramet). Other non-FDA-approved radionuclides currently under investigation include: rhenium-188 hydroxyethylidene (HEDP), rhenium-186 HEDP, 117mSn-DTPA (diethylenetriaminepentacetic acid), strontium-85 (^{85}Sr), and ^{186}Re-CTMR. The reasons why specific radiopharmaceuticals are approved for use in the United States and other radiopharmaceuticals are not remain somewhat speculative and are probably related to industry decisions of which radiopharmaceuticals to attempt approval in the United States.

All three of the available radiopharmaceuticals emit beta particles at therapeutic levels but with variable physical properties such as half-life, and degree of beta and gamma particle emission (see Table 17.1). The energetic beta particles (mean E_B in MeV) released from ^{153}Sm-EDTMP is considerably lower than that of ^{32}P and ^{89}Sr. As discussed previously, tissue invasiveness is proportional to the beta energy of the decayed radionuclide, and in this case, ^{153}Sm-EDTMP

TABLE 17.1. Therapeutic radiopharmaceuticals: Physical characteristics and treatment expectations.

Radiopharmaceutical	Half-life (days)	Max. energy (MeV)	Mean energy (MeV)	Maximum range (mm)	Gamma-emission (KeV)	Response time (days)	Response duration (weeks)	Retreatment interval (months)
89 Sr-chloride*	50.5	1.46 (β)	0.58 (β)	7.00	None	14-28	12-26	>3
32 P-phosphate*	14.3	1.7 (β)	0.69 (β)	7.90	None	14	10	>3
153 Sm-EDTMP*	1.9	0.81 (β)	0.23 (β)	2.50	103	2-7	8	>2
186 Re-HEDP	3.8	1.07 (β)	0.33 (β)	4.50	137	2-7	8-10	>2
188 Re-HEDP	0.7	2.12 (β)	0.73 (β)	11.00	155	2-7	8	Not established
117 mSn-DTPA	13.6	0.127 & 0.152 (conversion electrons)	None	0.27	159	5-19	12-26	>2
223 RaCl2	11.4	5.78 (α)	5.78 (α)	<0.1	154	<10	Not established	Not established

Source: Compiled from Silberstein, 2005 and Lewington, 2005.

*FDA-approved, available in US.

would be less likely to reach deeper tissues, but may tend to spare the bone marrow. Myelosuppression from highly energetic, highly penetrating particles such as ^{32}P is an unappealing side effect not recommended in advanced solid tumor patients.

Another important variation amongst the clinically accessible radiopharmaceuticals is half-life. Dose delivery time can be shortened with radionuclides such as ^{153}Sm-EDTMP, which has a half-life of 1.9 days, allowing 75 percent of the radiation dose to be delivered within 3.8 days. A drug like ^{89}Sr may be unfavorable because 75 percent of the beta radiation is delivered in 100+ days, ultimately delaying the onset of pain relief. In addition to the degree of beta emission and half-life, gamma emission also varies among the drugs. ^{153}Sm-EDTMP is the only drug that is FDA approved for both treatment of bone metastases and for diagnostic imaging studies such as radionuclide bone scans. This is due to its significant gamma emission (103 keV) coupled with a moderately energetic beta component (0.81 MeV). Importantly, no radiopharmaceutical used alone has ever been observed to prolong survival of such treated patients,[39] with the exception of a handful of limited studies involving ^{89}Sr with chemotherapy.

In 1998, Ben Josef et al. surveyed 2,500 members of the American Society for Therapeutic Radiology and Oncology (ASTRO),[32] with questions about the clinical approach to radiotherapeutic management. They found that local field radiotherapy in long fractionation schemes was the most common modality utilized (54 percent of patients alone and 74 percent in combination with other therapy). 11 percent used radiopharmaceuticals alone for therapy of painful osseous metastases from prostate cancer and 79 percent used radiopharmaceuticals in combination with local field irradiation.[32] Systemic radionuclides were used more often in prostate cancer patients versus breast cancer patients (1.2 percent versus 0.1 percent). ^{89}Sr was by far the most common radiopharmaceutical in use (99 percent).[32] The standard administered doses are 4 mCi (73 percent) and 10.8 mCi (26 percent).[32] Hemibody radiation therapy (HBI) was used in only 1 to 2 percent of patients. A recent ASTRO survey revealed that systemic radiopharmaceutical therapy has essentially replaced half-body irradiation.[32]

Strontium-89 (^{89}Sr-Chloride, Metastron)

As discussed earlier, ^{89}Sr is reported as the most common radionuclide administered at doses 148 MBq (4 mCi) or 1.48 MBq/kg (40 µCi/kg). The reasons why ^{89}Sr remains so popular is speculative and unclear; however, it may be due to the perception of significant hematologic depression from ^{32}P as well as the fact that ^{89}Sr was approved for use in the United States well before ^{153}Sm-EDTMP. It has the most U.S. literature/experience/clinical use of any radiopharmaceutical for therapy of osseous metastases. In addition, perceptions of ^{89}Sr include: good preferential accumulation at perimetastatic sites,[40-42] with good retention at these sites as once incorporated into metastatic lesion; ^{89}Sr is not metabolized and may remain for 100 days.[40] In addition normal bone takes up only a small fraction of ^{89}Sr with a significantly shorter retention time.[40]

^{89}Sr-chloride decays by beta emission with the longest half-life ($T_{1/2}$ = 50.5 days) of the radiopharmaceutical agents clinically available for treatment of painful osseous metastases. It has a very-low-yield gamma emission, which makes it unsuitable for imaging. It is rapidly cleared from the blood by renal excretion and incorporation into bone mineral.[43,44] The suggested dose is 0.04 mCi/Kg or 4 mCi per patient.[43,44] Pain relief usually begins within 2 weeks of treatment with maximal benefit by 6 weeks lasting about 4 to 15 months.[43,44] Mild thrombocytopenia and/or leukopenia may occur in up to 80 percent of patients.[43,44] Platelets decline about 15 to 30 percent below pretreatment levels and usually completely recover in 2 to 3 months, enabling repeat treatment at that time.[43,44] Occasionally, recovery of platelet count to baseline may take about 6 months.[43,44] In addition, 15 to 20 percent reductions in white blood cells have also been seen following ^{89}Sr administration.[43,44] A transient flushing sensation immediately after ^{89}Sr injection has been noted and is self-limited.

^{89}Sr is a calcium analog, which is preferentially deposited, in osseous tissue.[45] Approximately tenfold more ^{89}Sr is absorbed by bone metastases than by marrow.[45] In addition, ^{89}Sr has a much longer biological half-life (>50 days) at sites of bone metastases compared with normal bone (approximately 14 days), which further increases its therapeutic specificity.[45,46] Up to 88 percent of the injected ^{89}Sr dose is retained at 100 days post treatment.[45]

Multiple clinical trials have reported that intravenous ^{89}Sr administration yields pain relief for the majority of patients with bone metastases secondary to breast or prostate cancer, with about 10 to 20 percent[47,48] of patients becoming pain free and some investigators reporting improved quality of life.[45,48-50]

A small study (n = 26) by Lewington et al. compared a single injection of ^{89}Sr at 4.0 mCi to placebo in symptomatic men with bone scan confirmed hormone-positive prostate cancer.[51] There was subjective, "substantial improvement" in pain, but there was no objective evaluation of the actual analgesic benefit from [89]Sr. Laing et al. reported overall response rate of 75 percent at 12 weeks post treatment (22 percent dramatic improvement—effectively pain free, 33 percent with substantial improvement—over 50 percent, and 20 percent with some improvement).[49] Although improvement was primarily in pain assessment/analysis and therefore reflected pain relief, other parameters assessed were analgesic intake, mobility and general conditions (e.g., mood, appetite, and sleep patterns).[49]

In a study by McEwan et al. an overall response rate of 77 percent was reported with [89]Sr (parameters assessed included pain, analgesic requirements, mobility, and Karnofsky index).[50] Robinson et al. reported an overall response rate of 80 percent[45] and confirmed this in 1993 analyzing 240 patients with prostate cancer and 47 patients with breast cancer. Parameters assessed included pain, sleep, analgesic use, activity, and quality of life.[47] Robinson et al. also noted over half the patients experienced a dramatic improvement in pain and quality of life with 15 percent becoming pain free.[47]

The United Kingdom Metastron Investigators' Group compared ^{89}Sr with hemibody radiotherapy.[52] Patients treated with ^{89}Sr had a reduced rate of appearance of new sites of pain. In this study, ^{89}Sr delayed the progression of pain.[52] This is postulated to be secondary to the pharmacokinetics of strontium, which is taken up by and retained at all sites of sclerotic metastases, even if they are asymptomatic.[40,52] In addition to the use of radionuclides as a single agent of palliative radiation, ^{89}Sr has been found to be a useful adjunct to local field radiation treatment.[8] Another UK trial compared 284 men with symptomatic hormone-responsive prostate cancer ^{89}Sr versus traditional radiotherapy in the form of EBRT or HBI.[53] They also found significant reduction in new painful metastases and significantly minimized the need for repeat radiotherapy with ^{89}Sr compared with focal EBRT.

A Canadian prospective multicenter, randomized controlled trial by Porter et al. conducted with 126 patients with endocrine-resistant advanced prostate cancer.[54] All patients received external beam radiotherapy and either a placebo or a single dose of 400 MBq of [89]Sr. [89]Sr significantly improved overall pain control, reduced analgesic requirements, delayed disease progression, and on certain measures enhanced quality of life.[54] Overall, treatment costs may have been reduced in the ^{89}Sr group as well as larger improvements in scores reflecting improved fatigue and overall quality of life.[54]

In another phase III study by Porter et al., doses of ^{89}Sr at 400 MBq (10.8 mCi) were administered to endocrine-resistant prostate cancer patients. There was a significant reduction in pain as well as a significant biochemical decrease in PSA and prostatic acid phosphatase.[8] However, there were also significantly greater incidences of grade 3 and 4 hematologic toxicity, precluding such dose-escalated injections of [89]Sr.

Molina et al. evaluated the effects of ^{89}Sr treatment on fibrinolysis and coagulation in prostate cancer patients in response to a recent warning/alert to physicians to closely monitor for the progression of disseminated intravascular coagulation (DIC) in prostate cancer patients to be treated with [89]Sr.[55] They found no major alterations on fibrinolysis or coagulation caused by ^{89}Sr therapy. However, the potential cytopenias which could occur in these patients secondary to the myelosuppressive effects of ^{89}Sr and/or by tumor bone marrow invasion may be "adding insult to injury" in patients with a pre-existing low-grade ("subclinical") DIC. As patients with prostate cancer are "at risk" of disordered fibrinolysis, it may be prudent to screen hematologic parameters (e.g., D-dimer, fibrinsplit products, plasma fibrinogen, and PTT/PT INR) and examination of peripheral smear in all patients with advanced prostate cancer who are soon to undergo therapy with [89]Sr.

In its history, there have been two accounts of acute myeloid leukemia several months (17 and 26) after ^{89}Sr treatments for advanced prostate cancer.[56] The chain of causation to ^{89}Sr was difficult to determine because both patients had undergone several different investigational drugs, ultrahigh doses of chemotherapy, and several rounds of external beam radiotherapy. Nevertheless, the benefit of long-term pain palliation significantly outweighs the risk of acute leukemic crisis in these patients.

The aforementioned results have been encapsulated into a practice guideline by the Cancer Care Ontario Practice Guidelines Initiative that advocates the use of ^{89}Sr in patients with endocrine-refractory prostate cancer with symptomatic, multiple intractable sites of bone metastases.[57] There is maximum benefit from ^{89}Sr when the patient is suffering from bone metastases on both sides of the diaphragm, maximal analgesic remedy is already prescribed, presence of sufficient hematologic reserve, and external beam radiation therapy is contraindicated. Multiple metastatic bone lesions must be validated with a diagnostic radionuclide bone scan before radionuclide administration.

Phosphorus-32 (^{32}P, Orthophosphate)

Phosphorus-32 is a purely beta-emitting (1.71 MeV) radioactive isotope of phosphorus that has a half-life of 14.3 days. More than 60 years ago (in 1942), Friedell and Storaasli began treating patients with widespread painful osseous metastases with ^{32}P and found that 83 percent had significant palliation of pain[10] uptake of ^{32}P in bone is avid and as phosphorous is a component of the hydroxyapatite crystal together with calcium and the hydroxyl moiety. The average tissue penetration is 2 to 3 mm (max 7.9 mm) after IV administration.[58] It is excreted mainly in the urine with 5 to 10 percent removed in the first day and 20 percent over 7 days.[58] Although at least 25 studies document its use, ^{32}P has not gained widespread use nowadays because the studies are generally poor and do not clearly support efficacy.[58] For example, there is a reported response rate up to 87 percent of the 46 patients with advanced prostate cancer to bone when given 200 to 800 MBq of ^{32}P in fractions of 20 to 80 MBq, but only after hormonal, androgen priming therapy.[59] Since it is possible that exogenous androgen administration may alter and possibly under-represent the myelosuppresive nature of ^{32}P, interpreting the efficacy of this radionuclide alone is difficult.

In addition, ^{32}P is a pure beta emitter, and therefore cannot be imaged well.[58] Most importantly, its high maximum energy of beta emission offers the greatest risk of myelotoxicity and hematologic depression. However, at doses 12 mCi/month or less and if given in fractionated doses with no more than 3 mCi per day, bone marrow depression is considered to be clinically insignificant.[58]

In general, the trials of ^{32}P suffer from small numbers of patients, patients treated with varing histologies, patients treated with varying doses and regimens of ^{32}P, poorly defined response criteria, and variable entry criteria.[60] In addition, no randomized clinical trial has evaluated the use of differing ^{32}P carriers, or the use of hormonal manipulation compared with ^{32}P alone in efforts to determine if these management strategies improve response rate or reduce toxicity.[60]

While pain relief takes place within the 14th day ($T_{1/2}$ = 14.3 days), significant bone marrow suppression is documented to occur during the fourth and fifth week after administration.[58] Although bone marrow suppression is dose dependent,[58] there is no dose dependence with ^{32}P activity in breast cancer patients.[58] Nevertheless, dose-limiting pancytopenia is actually quite rare even with cumulative doses up to 444 MBq.[2]

Samarium-153-Ethylene Diamine Tetramethylene Phosphonate ([153]Sm-EDTMP, Samarium Sm153 Lexidronam, and Quadramet)

[153]Sm-EDTMP was originally described by William Goeckler in 1984 and approved by the FDA in 1997 for relief of pain in patients with osteoblastic bone metastases.[61] It is a stable complex of radioactive samarium-153 and ethylene diamine tetramethylene phosphonic acid (EDTMP).[62-65] Favorable features of [153]Sm-EDTMP include a short physical half-life ($T_{1/2}$ = 1.9 days) allowing for efficient handling and possibility of fractionated dosing, gamma emission of 103 KeV, which is appropriate for scintigraphic imaging, low tissue penetration decreasing radiotoxicity to bone marrow, no measurable *in vivo* degradation, and no liver or other soft tissue uptake seen.[62,64] The recommended dose is roughly 1.0 mCi/Kg IV administered over 1 min.[62-65] The onset of analgesia is about 48 hours to 7 days.[62-65] Repeated dosing may be used if necessary but should wait at least 6 to 8 weeks.[62-65] The maximally tolerated dose is 2.5 mCi/kg.[62-65]

[153]Sm-EDTMP has a total skeletal uptake of about 50 percent of the IV administration dose with the advantage of the amount of

radiation absorbed by bone being five times that absorbed by the bone marrow.[62-64,66] It is cleared rapidly from the blood with 5.2 percent remaining at 2 hours post injection, 2.1 percent remaining at 4 hours, and less than 1 percent of the administered dose remains in the blood at 5 hours post injection.[62-64,66] The significant forms of toxicity that has been observed is thrombocytopenia and neutropenia with increased doses showing increased marrow suppression.[61,63,64] Generally a 2-week delay was seen before a rapid decrease in platelet count that then remained stable for 2 weeks before returning to pretreatment levels within 2 to 4 weeks.[61,63,64] For white blood cells (WBCs), the nadir occurred at an average of 24 days post injection with a median time of 44 days to recovery to pretreatment levels.[61,63,64] Hematologic recovery to baseline occurred in 87 percent of patients.[61,63,64] Those who did not recover had marrow replacement with cancer or radiation therapy for progressive diseases.[61,63,64] Significant analgesia was seen in 65 to 95 percent of those treated with a duration of pain palliation ranging from 1 to 11 months.[63-65]

The bone marrow radiation dose should be limited to 1.5 Gy. A standard administered activity of 37 MBq/Kg may lead to significant myelotoxicity in some patients. Prospective individual dosimetry by urine collection and counting can enable clinicians to limit the bone marrow radiation dose to 1.5 Gy but this method is cumbersome and requires meticulous care to ensure that all urine is collected. Cameron et al. actually developed a simple and reliable whole-body scintigraphic technique, to prospectively calculate a safe and effective dose of [153]Sm-EDTMP in individual patients to palliate bone metastases without myelotoxicity.[67] As seen in Table 17.1, the retreatment interval observed with [153]Sm-EDTMP use is >2 months.

The efficacy of [153]Sm-EDTMP has been compared with placebo in two prospective, randomized, double-blind phase III trials. Sartor et al. compared 152 symptomatic males with hormone-refractory prostate cancer (HRPC) metastatic to bone with radioactive [153]Sm versus nonradioactive [153]Sm.[68] If a patient in the placebo group was a "nonresponder," the patient was allowed to receive radioactive [153]Sm-EDTMP. Within 1 to 2 weeks of [153]Sm-EDTMP administration, pain was significantly reduced as per visual analog scales and pain descriptor scales.[68] Also, the placebo group had significantly fewer reductions in analgesic consumption at about 3 to 4 weeks. Since no grade

4 thrombocytopenia or neutropenia was encountered and blood counts in most patients had improved by 8 weeks, this study found that 1.0 mCi/kg of [153]Sm-EDTMP is safe and effective for painful metastases from HRPC.[68]

Serafini et al. studied [153]Sm-EDTMP in a double-blind, randomized, placebo-controlled study in 118 symptomatic patients (68 percent prostate cancer patients) with bone metastases from different primary cancers.[69] Similar to the study performed by Sartor et al., the open-label method was utilized to make the drug available to placebo-treated patients who did not respond by 4 weeks. This study involved three groups of patients—those receiving [153]Sm-EDTMP at 1.0 mCi/kg or 0.5 mCi/kg, or placebo.[69] Pain relief was assessed by physician and patient evaluations and opioid medication changes. Response rates of those subjects receiving 1.0 mCi/kg of radioactive [153]Sm-EDTMP ranged from 62 percent to 72 percent by the end of the first 4 weeks.[69] Pain relief and reduction in opioid use was extended through 16 weeks after intravenous drug administration of 1.0 mCi/kg [153]Sm-EDTMP in 43 percent of patients Just as the previously mentioned study, bone marrow toxicity with [153]Sm-EDTMP was limited and tolerable with no grade 4 toxicities noted.[69]

Rhenium-186 HEDP ([186]Re-Etidronate)

Rhenium-186 hydroxyethylidene ([186]Re-HEDP) is a beta emitter (E_{max} = 1.07 MeV) with a maximum range of penetration of 5 mm and a physical half-life of 89 hours (3.7 days). It also emits gamma photons (137 KeV) suitable for imaging.[70,71] [186]Re-HEDP is rapidly cleared from the blood by urinary excretion and skeletal uptake with 14 percent of the administered activity remaining in the blood at 30 min post injection.[70,71] The dose administered is generally 35 mCi and the myelosuppressive dose is higher than ^{89}Sr, so that patients taking [186]Re-HEDP may be treated as outpatients.[70,71] Brenner et al. have described a new method of quantifying total bone uptake of [186]Re-HEDP and [153]Sm-EDTMP using 24 hour urinary excretion of radiopharmaceuticals.[72] The method allows for calculation of bone uptake and soft tissue retention separately, thus providing a means of obtaining detailed kinetic data to potentially improve the assessment of the radiation dosage to bone and bone marrow.[72]

Significant pain relief can be achieved with [186]Re-HEDP. Although pain relief may begin within 2 weeks, 75 percent of responders have some effect within 1 week, giving it a faster onset than other currently available radiopharmaceuticals,[70,71] probably due to its half-life of 3.7 days (see Table 17.1). Pain palliation typically lasts 8 to 10 weeks (Table 17.1). Mild thrombocytopenia and/or leukopenia may occur with usually spontaneously recover in 6 to 8 weeks, allowing for retreatment after 2 months.[70,71] Reports suggest that additional pain relief can occur on retreatment.[70,71] In addition, Kolesnikov-Gauthier et al. concluded that [186]Re-HEDP provided safe, symptomatic relief of pain in prostate cancer patients with painful bone metastases. On the basis of pain reduction, analgesic use, and performance status, two-thirds of prostate cancer patients achieved palliation of pain symptoms.[73] They also evaluated breast cancer patients with painful bone metastases, but benefit was less dramatic.[73] This may have been due to the breast cancer patients having advanced disease.[73] The investigators concluded that further studies should be carried out especially earlier in the course of breast cancer.[73]

There have been varying degrees of success with [186]Re-HEDP in clinical models. Just as Kolesnikov-Gauthier et al. had implied in 2000, Sciuto et al. further studied this in breast cancer patients in 2001. They calculated a response rate and overall pain palliation in about 92 percent of symptomatic breast cancer patients treated with [186]Re-HEDP.[74] In another study in breast cancer patients with metastatic bone pain, Han et al. achieved a less impressive 58 percent response rate for significant pain reduction with half of patients also demonstrating reduced analgesic usage.[75]

INVESTIGATIONAL RADIOPHARMACEUTICALS

Rhenium-188 HEDP

This investigational radionuclide is similar to rhenium-186 HEDP but may have slight advantages for same-day, on-demand outpatient therapy.[76,77] It has the advantage of ready and on-demand availability of [188]Re from a generator.[78] Although commercial kits are not currently available and is not approved in the United States, Schmaljohann et al. have shown that a simplified two-component kit is possible with sufficient complex stability for at least 4 hours after preparation.[78] In addition, [188]Re-HEDP may be significantly more efficacious than other agents like hormonal, therapy, EBRT, and chemotherapy alone.[76,77] Liepe et al. have suggested that [188]Re-HEDP represents an attractive agent for radiopharmaceutical therapy with suitable properties for palliative treatment.[78] They studied the radiation dose/kinetics of [188]Re-HEDP in bone metastases, finding rapid urinary excretion resulting in a low whole-body dose with a high radiation dose in bone metastases.[78] Beta emission reaches a maximum at 2.12 MeV and can reach tissue depths up to 11 mm (see Table 17.1), thereby providing generous cancer cell death. Administration of 1110 MBq (30 mCi) of [188]Re-HEDP significantly improved quality of life with 67 percent of subjects being able to reduce their analgesic intake.[79]

More recently, in a randomized phase II trial with [188]Re-HEDP was conducted by Palmedo et al., 64 symptomatic HRPC patients were treated with either single injection or repeated injections of [188]Re-HEDP and assessed for pain palliation and clinical outcome until death.[80] Progression-free survival and pain relief was significantly greater in those patients treated with multiple injections of this radionuclide, justifying the need for larger-scale evaluation of this drug.

117mSn-DTPA
(117mSn-Diethylenetriaminepentaacetic Acid)

117mSn-DTPA is another experimental radionuclide with a half-life of 13.6 days, emits conversion electrons at 0.127 and 0.152 MeV (rather than beta emission), and decays by highly abundant (86 percent) gamma emission at 159 keV (see Table 17.1). Although not well studied, it may potentially be advantageous because of its relative low potential for myelotoxicity and tissue penetration of 0.2 to 0.3 mm as per Table 17.1.[81] Its efficacy may be equal or somewhat less than other currently used radiopharmaceuticals.[81] Skeletal distribution appears similar to the Tc-labeled diphosphonates. 117mSn-DTPA has several other advantages such as it can be imaged, can be administered for outpatient therapy, has an intermediate physical half-life (<2 weeks), and is reasonably stable resulting in easy storage and shipping.[82]

Srivastava et al. performed a detailed analysis of the clinical data to assess the long-term safety and efficacy of 117mSn-DTPA for the treatment of metastatic bone pain.[82] They concluded that at up to 10.6 MBq/Kg dose, 117mSn-DTPA shows much less hematologic toxicity than beta-emitting bone pain palliation agents ($p < 0.01$).[82] In addition, overall response rates (75 percent) were similar and time to onset of pain relief was shorter at higher doses ($p < 0.05$).[82] In a subsequent study, Srivastava et al. ascertained effective pain relief with 117mSn-DTPA in 78 percent of the patients at single doses of 10 to 20 mCi per 70 kg body weight, with much less myelosuppression compared to another agents.[83] They hypothesized that decreased marrow toxicity might allow safe administration of 117mSn-DTPA as an adjuvant following radiotherapy and/or chemotherapy for the treatment of primary/metastatic cancer in bone.[83] Srivastava et al. concluded that both [117]Sn citrate as well as high-pressure liquid chromatography (HPLC)-purified 117mSn-DTPA are promising for radionuclide therapy of primary/metastatic cancer in bone.[84]

Bishayee et al. used a mouse femur model and concluded that the short-range conversion electron emitter, such as 117mSn, offers a large dosimetric advantage (i.e., can use higher doses) over energetic beta particle emitters for alleviating bone pain from osseous metastases while ultimately minimizing marrow toxicity.[85] Despite several gains in researching 117mSn-DTPA, the development of this drug has been largely arrested due to financial issues.

^{223}Ra-Cl2 (^{223}Ra-Chloride)

Radium, an extremely radioactive decay product of uranium, has been long known (since 1930s) to cause sores, anemia, and certain primary bone malignancies. The body consumes the causative agent, radium, as if it were calcium and becomes deposited into bone matrix. Subsequently its radioactivity can destroy bone marrow and stimulate bone cell proliferation—arguably the cause of Marie Curie's premature death in 1934. A medical expert from Geneva diagnosed Curie with an aplastic pernicious anemia that was probably injured by cumulative radiation exposure.[86] By directing the radioactivity of radium into active osteoblastic cells and limiting stimulated cell burden, it has the potential to be used as a therapeutic radionuclide.

^{223}Ra-Cl2 is primarily an alpha particle emitter with a half-life of 11.4 days. Henriksen et al. compared this mode of radioactive attack to metastatic osseous lesions to ^{89}Sr in mice. The total decay energy of the four alpha-particles via daughter isotopes is 28 MeV.[87] Taking into advantage the short-range of alpha-emitting particles as discussed earlier, there may be less irradiation to bone marrow when compared with highly energetic beta-emitting particles like ^{89}Sr. Preclinical animal studies revealed that there is no limiting toxicity to healthy bone marrow while treating the surface of bone lesions effectively.[87]

It is important to note that expensive, large-scale studies have not been performed to evaluate radiopharmaceuticals side-by-side to ascertain relative efficacy among the available agents.[4] Therefore, the radionuclide with the most superior response rate has not been established and selection of the appropriate agent should limit side effects such as myelosuppression and provide the most available pain relief.[4] As discussed subsequently, this suggests that other modalities of palliation may be used in conjunction with radiopharmaceuticals with significant benefit.

Strontium-85 (^{85}Sr)

This investigational drug has been shown to be effective and well tolerated for the palliative treatment of refractory metastatic bone pain in one study.[88] Like ^{89}Sr, ^{85}Sr is a bone-seeking radionuclide that decays by electron capture, with a gamma emission of 514 keV and a physical half-life of 64 days.[88] It can be imaged and it allows a macroscopic estimation of the absorbed dose to lesions. Studies indicate that approximately three in four patients received benefit, lasting up to 3 years with few serious side effects.[88] Patients with an early stage of metastatic disease and/or prostate cancer seem to have the best results with this experimental radionuclide.[88]

^{186}Re-CTMR

Kothari et al. have developed and evaluated a novel cyclic-tetraphosphonate-derivative complexed with ^{186}Re to achieve similar therapeutic efficacy. The ligand, CTMP, is made of a cyclic array of tetra-aminomethylphosphonate groups, and was synthesized using orthophosphorus acid, 1,4,8,11-tetraazacyclotetradecane, and formaldehyde.[89] Testing mainly consisted of biodistribution studies in Wistar rats and monitored activity in the femur. The initial results in this animal model are promising and suggest that [186]Re-CTMP be considered for further evaluation in higher animals for symptomatic bone pain.[90]

PATIENT SELECTION CRITERIA AND TREATMENT GUIDELINES

Patients referred to radiopharmaceuticals for palliation of osseous metastases are most commonly prostate cancer and, less commonly, breast and lung cancer patients.[11] It is recommended that treatment by this modality be optimized by a multidisciplinary approached including medical oncology, radiation oncology, nuclear medicine, and palliative care.

Classically, candidates for palliative treatment with radiopharmaceutical therapy have had recurrent bone pain due to metastatic prostate or breast cancer.[2] Such cases have typically failed standard treatments, such as hormonal manipulation. However, pain from bone metastases due to other cancers (e.g., lung) can also be palliated effectively with radiopharmaceuticals. Radiopharmaceutical agents are typically appropriate for multiple painful osteoblastic osseous metastases. They are especially compelling in cases of widespread or diffuse bony metastasis, but may also be effective early in disease progression with limited painful metastatic sites. They have limited efficacy in cases of soft tissue metastases because of their targeted absorption mainly at sites of bony metastases. Likewise, these agents are usually not of great utility in spinal cord or peripheral nerve invasion by adjacent metastases or when pain arises from sources other than bone metastases, such as in nerve root compression or musculoskeletal problems.[47] They are also not usually of great utility in acute pathologic fractures.[37] Although not useful for pure osteolytic lesions, radiopharmaceutical agents may be helpful if lesions have a significant osteoblastic component (i.e., mainly breast malignancies to bone).

Treatment usually requires platelet count greater than 60,000 (some investigators have accepted as low as 40,000) and WBC count greater than 2,400.[43] It is recommended that complete blood counts be performed within 1 week of treatment since these advanced caner patients may be experiencing significant myelosuppression from concurrent chemotherapy or radiotherapy. Continuous monitoring with interval blood counts every other week for 3 months after injection or until recovery to baseline is necessary.

Choosing between traditional external beam radiotherapy versus "internal beta emitters" may be decided based on pain response, adverse effects, and the actual indications otherwise.[4] Although radiotherapy is indicated for acute spinal cord compression, there is a dose-limiting criterion that may limit its use for noncompressive skeletal metastasis and indicate radiopharmaceuticals use for further retreatment. Cumulative doses of EBRT exceeding 45 Gy in 22 to 25 fractions to single vertebral lesions may lead to considerable spinal cord toxicity and preclude the further use of external teletherapy.[91] Therefore, since radioactive uptake on a bone scan of multiple metastatic lesions in bone is representative of osteoblastic lesions, "internal electron emitters" may especially be indicated.

On the basis of the preceding discussion, a bone scan is imperative upon assessment of the nature of the patient's metastatic bone lesions. Histological criteria, doses of agents used, length of treatment, and comparison of different treatment arms were varied in most of the studies, and therefore the data was not pooled for review. Based on limited clinical, randomized controlled trials, the current recommendations include the use of strontium-89 and samarium-153 for the palliation of multiple sites of bone pain from metastatic prostate cancer. This is delineated because HRPC patients were approximately 80 percent of the responding patients in several clinical trials.[57] Also, strontium-89 and samarium-153 may be considered for metastatic lesions in symptomatic patients with breast and lung primary malignancies, since the remaining 20 percent of the patients fit this criteria.

As per the current guidelines, careful selection of patients for radionuclide therapy for pain palliation should be based on patient's performance status, recent use of chemotherapy or radiotherapy with potential marrow suppression, and patient's marrow functional status. A complete history and physical exam with a thorough neurological assessment is warranted prior to treatment considerations. Also, the patient should be considered ineligible for chemotherapy, wide or local field external beam radiotherapy, hormonal therapy, and bisphosphonates.[57]

Major indications for radiopharmaceutical use are multiple painful osseous metastases despite analgesics and skeletal metastasis to

>1 site positive on bone scintigraphy. Absolute contraindications for using radiopharmaceuticals include pregnancy, breastfeeding, women of child-bearing age, and patient refusal. Also, acute spinal cord compression (external beam radiotherapy is indicated), acute or chronic renal failure, or glomerular filtration rate < 30 ml/min. Relative contraindications always require including careful consideration of risks versus potential benefits within the context of the patients wishes. Significant limitations to treatment include pre-existing severe bone marrow depression or reason to believe the patient may develop bone marrow depression in near future, such as immediately after some chemotherapy or radiotherapy treatments. Therefore, limitations would include hemoglobin < 90 g/l, total white blood cell count < 3.5 × 19^9/l, absolute neutrophil count < 1500/l, platelets < 60,000/l, or urea < 12 mmol/l and creatinine < 200 mmol/l. Severe renal insufficiency is a significant limitation since the clearance of intravenous radiopharmaceuticals is mainly renal. Other relative contraindications include the inability of the patient to follow radiation safety precautions such as a patient at home with dementia and urinary incontinence, as well as impending spinal cord compression or pathologic fracture. Therefore, ureteric stents or urinary catherization can be considered before treatment. Significant bone marrow suppression is a risk if chemotherapy and/or external beam radiation is to be used shortly after radiopharmaceutical administration.[43] Further assistant with guidelines regarding the use of radiopharmaceuticals set forth by the Therapeutic Radiopharmaceutical Guidelines Group can be found at www. guideline.gov.

ADMINISTRATION OF RADIOPHARMACEUTICALS AND FOLLOW-UP

According to Silberstein, administration of radiopharmaceuticals, or "unsealed beta emitters," requires a careful workup including radiographs, a bone scan corresponding to the symptomatic area, and close monitoring of the patient's blood counts.[4] Once the patient's has met the required qualifications that indicate radionuclide use, the patient is educated about radiation safety precautions and informed consent is obtained. Before administration of the desired agent, a proper intravenous line is made certain to prevent extravasation of tracer and to limit exposure to the physician. It is recommended that the injecting physician utilize a finger dosimeter to monitor exposure to the physician's fingers.[4] Since there is considerable electromagnetic radiation, known as bremsstrahlung radiation, especially released from radionuclides at higher atomic numbers, a plastic syringe shield (rather than a lead syringe shield) should be utilized. Overall, there is no need to accommodate for expensive, high-technology equipment when administering radiopharmaceuticals.

It is prudent to ensure adequate hydration prior to administration in order to have minimal bladder wall exposure, and a minimum of 500 ml of fluids is recommended provided the patient has no contraindications to such a fluid challenge. The recommended dose for strontium-89 is 148 mBq (4 mCi) by slow intravenous injection (1 to 2 min), accompanied by intravenous or oral hydration (at least 500 ml). The recommended dose for samarium-153 is 37 mBq/kg (1 mCi/kg) by slow intravenous injection (1 to 2 min), accompanied by intravenous or oral hydration (at least 500 mL) (57). Rapid injection of ^{89}Sr can cause vasodilation or arrythmias because of its similarity to calcium, whereas calcium chelators like samarium-153 and ^{186}Re can cause symptoms of hypocalcemia.[4] Patients treated with samarium-153 should be followed-up with a bone scan within 24 hours to compare with the initial diagnositic image.

The patient should be advised to void as often as possible after administration of radiopharmaceuticals. Analgesics should continue throughout treatment as pain relief may be delayed 2 to 7 days. Pain relief can be attained in 2 to 7 days, and can last for up to several months.[3] In addition, about 10 percent of patients may experience an initial "flare" in pain. This pain exacerbation usually lasts for 2 to 3 days and is usually mild and self-limited. It generally responds well to modest short-term increases in analgesics. Repeated injections may be needed if symptoms recur or if there is partial response in degree of pain relief. This may be appropriately performed only after sufficient recovery of bone marrow constituents.

Because of the unpredictability of myelosuppression associated with each individual agent, careful follow-up of patients treated with radionuclides includes complete blood counts every other week, up to 3 months after the injection or until recovery to baseline counts (generally the usual hematological response is a 20 to 30 percent decrease in platelet count with nadir about 5 to 6 weeks and recovery by 12 weeks). Subjective measurements of symptomatic progression can be monitored with daily entries in a medical diary during the postinjection period. The criteria evaluated include pain score from 0/10 to 10/10 and side effects such as nausea, vomiting, diarrhea, constipation, headache, and evening temperature. Close patient follow-up post injection is ultimately required for successful therapy.

FUTURE WORK

Future refinements of the use of radiopharmaceuticals for palliation of painful metastases may include selective therapy with radiopharmaceuticals "attached" to monoclonal antibodies against tumor cells (to improve analgesia and/or diminish tumor burden), the use of sensitization agents (e.g., chemotherapy, hormonal therapy) in conjunction with radiopharmaceutical therapy, and the use of cytokines with radiotherapy to attempt to protect the bone marrow and/or modulate the effects of radiopharmaceutical therapy. Potential "cocktails" utilizing matrix metalloproteinase (MMP) inhibitors, antiinflammatory agents, chemotherapeutic agents, hormonal agents/cytokines, and/or convention external radiotherapy are being developed and may improve current efficacy or safety.

Brenner et al. studied the myeloprotective effects of amifostine, a scavenger of free radicals, after treatment of rabbits with high-dose ^{153}Sm-EDTMP or ^{186}Re-HEDP.[92] Amifostine was shown to significantly reduce the toxic effects to platelets after high-dose treatment with ^{153}Sm-EDTMP or ^{186}Re-HEDP.[72] It was concluded that amifostine may be able to either decrease the damage to the bone marrow and/or allow for higher dose regimens in order to improve the therapeutic efficacy of bone pain palliative therapy.[92] In addition, whole body mild hyperthermia, which may enhance the therapeutic effects of radioimmunotherapy,[93] may also enhance the therapeutic effectiveness of radiopharmaceutical therapy.

Preliminary clinical data suggest that combining chemotherapy and radiopharmaceutical therapy in the treatment of hormone-escaped metastatic prostate cancer may yield additive or possibly synergistic effects in term of efficacy.[46,94,95] Geldof et al. studied the *in vitro* effects of chemotherapy and radiopharmaceutical agents used together.[96]

It was concluded that combination [186]Re-HEDP therapy with cisplatin-based chemotherapy could enhance the effects of each in eliminating proliferating tumor cells. These supra-additive/synergistic effects may have implications for future uses of radiopharmaceutical agents in palliation of osseous metastases.

There are several *in vivo* studies experimenting the use of standard chemotherapy agents with radiopharmaceuticals in novel regimens for HRPC patients. In a nonrandomized, multicenter, phase II study by Akerley et al., estramustine and vinblastine were combined with ^{89}Sr in 44 patients with symptomatic bone metastases. The combined efficacy failed to reveal significant survival benefit, but hinted at possible palliative benefit.[97] In another study, 72 patients with HRPC to bone were randomized to single agent doxorubicin with either [89]Sr (4 mCi) or placebo after induction chemotherapy was given. There was limited difference in biochemical response (serum PSA level). The group treated with ^{89}Sr experienced significantly longer time to progression (13 versus 7 months) and significantly longer median survival (28 versus 17 months).[98] Albeit in combination with standard chemotherapy, this is one of the few studies demonstrating prolonged survival with radiopharmaceuticals. Aside from symptomatic relief, this suggests tumoricidal behavior from radionuclides when partnered with chemotherapy agents.

In addition, potential future therapies for osseous metastases may include adjuncts to radiopharmaceuticals, aimed against cytochemical changes in bone metastases. These could include antagonists to MMPs, antagonists to CGRP, and antagonists to endothelin-1. According to Papatheofanis et al., serum procollagen type IC terminal peptide (PICP) is a marker of bone turnover and reduced levels of PICP have corresponded to a favorable clinical response to ^{89}Sr in HRPC patients.[99] It was also observed that patients treated with ^{89}Sr have a decreased secretion of cell adhesion molecules such as E-selectin, an established criterion of metastatic potential.[100]

Lenarczyk et al. concluded that a noninvasive *in vivo* assay for determining micronuclei in peripheral blood reticulocytes can potentially be useful as a biologic dosimeter, measuring absorbed dose rate and absorbed dose to bone marrow form incorporated radionuclides.[101] Although this was done in preclinical models (mice), it may have future implications to help optimize radiation delivery to metastases and minimize marrow dose with various radiopharmaceuticals for different patients. The need for future trials to utilize dosimetry, similar to teletherapy, may be encouraged with the use of short-range electrons such as 117mSn-DTPA or alpha-emitting radiopharmaceuticals such as ^{223}Ra-Cl2. These agents are less likely to cause cumulative myelosuppressive side effects found with highly energetic beta particles, and therefore can be used for repeated, fractionated doses.

Currently, there is insufficient evidence to conclude significant benefit with palliation therapy when combining radiopharmaceuticals with chemotherapy or radiotherapy. There may be some gain in delay in time of more numerous symptomatic bone metastases or in duration of pain relief as shown in the aforementioned studies.[97,98]

CONCLUSION

Much work still needs to be done. Outcome studies are required to better define: (a) optimal radiopharmaceuticals for various clinical situations, (b) optimal administered activity for these radiopharmaceuticals, (c) optimal dosing (i.e., single dose versus divided dosages), (d) the efficacy of treating currently asymptomatic osteoblastic metastasis (e.g., will this prolong the asymptomatic period), and (e) the use of "adjuvants" for synergistic effects.[80] Radiopharmaceuticals have shown to be of benefit for those appropriately selected for treatment. Good performance status, adequate bone marrow reserve, and short-term life expectancy are just some of the selection criteria used for optimal outcomes in these patients.

The goals of systemic administration of radiopharmaceuticals is to palliate pain, better quality of life, improve survival when possible, and decrease the need for opioids, chemotherapy, and external radiation therapy. The initial steps that allow effective management of pain in the cancer patient involves conducting a comprehensive assessment, competently providing analgesic drugs, and communicating with the patient and family as a whole.

Ultimately, radiopharmaceutical agents offer a reasonably safe and effective therapeutic analgesic option for patients with cancer and painful osseous metastases. Nonetheless, the use of radiopharmaceutical agents for the treatment of "multisite metastatic pain" remains underutilized. Although no definite "niche" or "step" in a treatment algorithm currently exists, the use of radiopharmaceutical agents, either alone or as an adjunct to other therapy, should be considered amongst all of the current choices for optimal treatment of painful osseous metastases.

REFERENCES

1. Nielsen OS, Munro AJ, Tannock IF. Bone metastases: pathophysiology and management policy. *J Clin Oncol* 1991;9:509-524.

2. Pandit-Taskar N, Batraki M, Divgi CR. Radiopharmaceutical therapy for palliation of bone pain from osseous metastases. *J Nucl Med* 2004;45:1358-1365.

3. Silberstein EB. Systemic radiopharmaceutical therapy of painful osteoblastic metastases. *Semin Radiat Oncol* 2000;10:240-249.

4. Silberstein EB. Teletherapy and radiopharmaceutical therapy of painful bone metastases. *Semin Nucl Med* 2005;35:152-158.

5. Benedetti C, Brock C, Cleeland C, Coyle N, Dube JE, Ferrell B, et al. NCCN Practice Guidelines for Cancer Pain. Oncology (Williston Park) 2000 Nov; 14(11A):135-150.

6. Poulsen HS, Nielsen OS, Klee M, Rorth M. Palliative irradiation of bone metastases. *Cancer Treat Rev* 1989;16:41-48.

7. Rose CM, Kagan AR. The final report of the expert panel for the radiation oncology bone metastasis work group of the American College of Radiology. *Int J Radiat Oncol Biol Phys* 1998;40:1117-1124.

8. Porter AT, McEwan AJ, Powe JE, Reid R, McGowan DG, Lukka H, et al. Results of a randomized phase-III trial to evaluate the efficacy of strontium-89 adjuvant to local field external beam irradiation in the management of endocrine resistant metastatic prostate cancer. *Int J Radiat Oncol Biol Phys* 1993;25:805-813.

9. Lewington VJ. Bone-seeking radionuclides for therapy. *J Nucl Med* 2005;46 Suppl 1:38S-47S.

10. Friedell HL, Storaasli JP. The use of radioactive phosphorus in the treatment of carcinoma of the breast with widespread metastases to bone. *Am J Roentgenol Radium Ther Nucl Med* 1950;64:559-575.

11. Reisfield GM, Silberstein EB, Wilson GR. Radiopharmaceuticals for the palliation of painful bone metastases. *Am J Hosp Palliat Care* 2005;22:41-46.

12. Atkins HL, Srivastava SC. Radiopharmaceuticals for bone malignancy therapy. *J Nucl Med Technol* 1998;26:80-83.

13. Bennett A. The role of biochemical mediators in peripheral nociception and bone pain. *Cancer Surv* 1988;7:55-67.

14. Urch C. The pathophysiology of cancer-induced bone pain: current understanding. *Palliat Med* 2004;18:267-274.

15. Paget S. The distribution of secondary growths in cancer of the breast. 1889. *Cancer Metastasis Rev* 1989;8:98-101.

16. Clohisy DR, Mantyh PW. Bone cancer pain and the role of RANKL/OPG. *J Musculoskelet Neuronal Interact* 2004;4:293-300.

17. Mundy GR. Metastasis to bone: Causes, consequences and therapeutic opportunities. *Nat Rev Cancer* 2002;2:584-593.

18. Hauschka PV, Mavrakos AE, Iafrati MD, Doleman SE, Klagsbrun M. Growth factors in bone matrix. Isolation of multiple types by affinity chromatography on heparin-Sepharose. *J Biol Chem* 1986;261:12665-12674.

19. Mundy GR. Endothelin-1 and osteoblastic metastasis. *Proc Natl Acad Sci USA* 2003;100:10588-10589.

20. McCawley LJ, Matrisian LM. Matrix metalloproteinases: Multifunctional contributors to tumor progression. *Mol Med Today* 2000;6:149-156.

21. Mantyh PW, Clohisy DR, Koltzenburg M, Hunt SP. Molecular mechanisms of cancer pain. *Nat Rev Cancer* 2002;2:201-209.

22. Weichselbaum RR, Hallahan D, Fuks Z, Kufe D. Radiation induction of immediate early genes: Effectors of the radiation-stress response. *Int J Radiat Oncol Biol Phys* 1994;30:229-234.

23. Maltoni M, Scarpi E, Modonesi C, Passardi A, Calpona S, Turriziani A, et al. A validation study of the WHO analgesic ladder: A two-step vs three-step strategy. *Support Care Cancer* 2005;13:888-894.

24. Fulfaro F, Casuccio A, Ticozzi C, Ripamonti C. The role of bisphosphonates in the treatment of painful metastatic bone disease: A review of phase III trials. *Pain* 1998;78:157-169.

25. Body JJ, Bartl R, Burckhardt P, Delmas PD, Diel IJ, Fleisch H, et al. Current use of bisphosphonates in oncology. International Bone and Cancer Study Group. *J Clin Oncol* 1998;16:3890-3899.

26. Berenson JR, Rosen LS, Howell A, Porter L, Coleman RE, Morley W, et al. Zoledronic acid reduces skeletal-related events in patients with osteolytic metastases. *Cancer* 2001;91:1191-1200.

27. Dixon RG, Mathis JM. Vertebroplasty and kyphoplasty: Rapid pain relief for vertebral compression fractures. *Curr Osteoporos Rep* 2004;2:111-115.

28. Stjernsward J. WHO cancer pain relief programme. *Cancer Surv* 1988; 7:195-208.

29. Berk L. Prospective trials for the radiotherapeutic treatment of bone metastases. *Am J Hosp Palliat Care* 1995;12:24-28.

30. Hartsell WF, Scott CB, Bruner DW, Scarantino CW, Ivker RA, Roach M, III, et al. Randomized trial of short- versus long-course radiotherapy for palliation of painful bone metastases. *J Natl Cancer Inst* 2005;97:798-804.

31. Hoskin PJ. Radiotherapy for bone pain. *Pain* 1995;63:137-139.

32. Ben Josef E, Shamsa F, Williams AO, Porter AT. Radiotherapeutic management of osseous metastases: A survey of current patterns of care. *Int J Radiat Oncol Biol Phys* 1998;40:915-921.

33. Pons F, Fuster D. Under-utilization of radionuclide therapy in metastatic bone pain palliation. *Nucl Med Commun* 2002;23:301-302.

34. Payne R. Mechanisms and management of bone pain. *Cancer* 1997;80 (Suppl 8):1608-1613.

35. Kassis AI, Adelstein SJ. Radiobiologic principles in radionuclide therapy. *J Nucl Med* 2005;46 (Suppl 1):4S-12S.

36. Silberstein EB. Dosage and response in radiopharmaceutical therapy of painful osseous metastases. *J Nucl Med* 1996;37:249-252.

37. Silberstein EB. The treatment of painful osteoblastic metastases: What can we expect from nuclear oncology? *J Nucl Med* 1994;35:1994-1995.

38. Subramanian G, McAfee JG, Blair RJ, Rosenstreich M, Coco M, Duxbury CE. Technetium-99m-labeled stannous imidodiphosphate, a new radiodiagnostic agent for bone scanning: Comparison with other 99mTc complexes. *J Nucl Med* 1975;16:1137-1143.

39. Brundage MD, Crook JM, Lukka H. Use of strontium-89 in endocrine-refractory prostate cancer metastatic to bone. Provincial Genitourinary Cancer Disease Site Group. *Cancer Prev Control* 1998;2:79-87.

40. Blake GM, Zivanovic MA, McEwan AJ, Ackery DM. Sr-89 therapy: Strontium kinetics in disseminated carcinoma of the prostate. *Eur J Nucl Med* 1986; 12:447-454.

41. Breen SL, Powe JE, Porter AT. Dose estimation in strontium-89 radiotherapy of metastatic prostatic carcinoma. *J Nucl Med* 1992;33:1316-1323.

42. Ben Josef E, Lucas DR, Vasan S, Porter AT. Selective accumulation of strontium-89 in metastatic deposits in bone: Radio-histological correlation. *Nucl Med Commun* 1995;16:457-463.

43. Robinson RG, Preston DF, Spicer JA, Baxter KG. Radionuclide therapy of intractable bone pain: Emphasis on strontium-89. *Semin Nucl Med* 1992;22:28-32.

44. Silberstein EB, Williams C. Strontium-89 therapy for the pain of osseous metastases. *J Nucl Med* 1985;26:345-348.

45. Robinson RG, Blake GM, Preston DF, McEwan AJ, Spicer JA, Martin NL, et al. Strontium-89: Treatment results and kinetics in patients with painful metastatic prostate and breast cancer in bone. *Radiographics* 1989;9:271-281.

46. Mertens WC, Porter AT, Reid RH, Powe JE. Strontium-89 and low-dose infusion cisplatin for patients with hormone refractory prostate carcinoma metastatic to bone: A preliminary report. *J Nucl Med* 1992;33:1437-1443.

47. Robinson RG, Preston DF, Baxter KG, Dusing RW, Spicer JA. Clinical experience with strontium-89 in prostatic and breast cancer patients. *Semin Oncol* 1993;20(3 Suppl 2):44-48.

48. Tennvall J, Darte L, Lundgren R, el Hassan AM. Palliation of multiple bone metastases from prostatic carcinoma with strontium-89. *Acta Oncol* 1988;27: 365-369.

49. Laing AH, Ackery DM, Bayly RJ, Buchanan RB, Lewington VJ, McEwan AJ, et al. Strontium-89 chloride for pain palliation in prostatic skeletal malignancy. *Br J Radiol* 1991;64:816-822.

50. McEwan AJ. Use of radionuclides for the palliation of bone metastases. *Semin Radiat Oncol* 2000;10:103-114.

51. Lewington VJ, McEwan AJ, Ackery DM, Bayly RJ, Keeling DH, Macleod PM, et al. A prospective, randomised double-blind crossover study to examine the efficacy of strontium-89 in pain palliation in patients with advanced prostate cancer metastatic to bone. *Eur J Cancer* 1991;27:954-958.

52. Bolger JJ, Dearnaley DP, Kirk D, Lewington VJ, Mason MD, Quilty PM, et al. Strontium-89 (Metastron) versus external beam radiotherapy in patients with painful bone metastases secondary to prostatic cancer: Preliminary report of a multicenter trial. UK Metastron Investigators Group. *Semin Oncol* 1993;20(3 Suppl 2): 32-33.

53. Quilty PM, Kirk D, Bolger JJ, Dearnaley DP, Lewington VJ, Mason MD, et al. A comparison of the palliative effects of strontium-89 and external beam radiotherapy in metastatic prostate cancer. *Radiother Oncol* 1994;31:33-40.

54. Porter AT, McEwan AJ. Strontium-89 as an adjuvant to external beam radiation improves pain relief and delays disease progression in advanced prostate cancer: results of a randomized controlled trial. *Semin Oncol* 1993;20(3 Suppl 2):38-43.

55. Paszkowski AL, Hewitt DJ, Taylor A, Jr. Disseminated intravascular coagulation in a patient treated with strontium-89 for metastatic carcinoma of the prostate. *Clin Nucl Med* 1999;24:852-854.

56. Kossman SE, Weiss MA. Acute myelogenous leukemia after exposure to strontium-89 for the treatment of adenocarcinoma of the prostate. *Cancer* 2000; 88:620-624.

57. Bauman G, Charette M, Reid R, Sathya J. Radiopharmaceuticals for the palliation of painful bone metastasis-a systemic review. *Radiother Oncol* 2005;75: 258-270.

58. Silberstein EB. The treatment of painful osseous metastases with phosphorus-32-labeled phosphates. *Semin Oncol* 1993;20(3 Suppl 2):10-21.

59. Burnet NG, Williams G, Howard N. Phosphorus-32 for intractable bony pain from carcinoma of the prostate. *Clin Oncol (R Coll Radiol)* 1990;2:220-223.

60. Mertens WC, Filipczak LA, Ben Josef E, Davis LP, Porter AT. Systemic bone-seeking radionuclides for palliation of painful osseous metastases: Current concepts. *CA Cancer J Clin* 1998;48:321, 361-374.

61. Samarium-153 lexidronam for painful bone metastases. *Med Lett Drugs Ther* 1997;39:83-84.

62. Holmes RA. [153Sm]EDTMP: A potential therapy for bone cancer pain. *Semin Nucl Med* 1992;22:41-45.

63. Bayouth JE, Macey DJ, Kasi LP, Fossella FV. Dosimetry and toxicity of samarium-153-EDTMP administered for bone pain due to skeletal metastases. *J Nucl Med* 1994;35:63-69.

64. Collins C, Eary JF, Donaldson G, Vernon C, Bush NE, Petersdorf S, et al. Samarium-153-EDTMP in bone metastases of hormone refractory prostate carcinoma: A phase I/II trial. *J Nucl Med* 1993;34:1839-1844.

65. Alberts AS, Smit BJ, Louw WK, van Rensburg AJ, van Beek A, Kritzinger V, et al. Dose response relationship and multiple dose efficacy and toxicity of samarium-153-EDTMP in metastatic cancer to bone. *Radiother Oncol* 1997;43:175-179.

66. Eary JF, Collins C, Stabin M, Vernon C, Petersdorf S, Baker M, et al. Samarium-153-EDTMP biodistribution and dosimetry estimation. *J Nucl Med* 1993; 34:1031-1036.

67. Cameron PJ, Klemp PF, Martindale AA, Turner JH. Prospective [153]Sm-EDTMP therapy dosimetry by whole-body scintigraphy. *Nucl Med Commun* 1999; 20:609-615.

68. Sartor O, Reid RH, Hoskin PJ, Quick DP, Ell PJ, Coleman RE, et al. Samarium-153-Lexidronam complex for treatment of painful bone metastases in hormone-refractory prostate cancer. *Urology* 2004;63:940-945.

69. Serafini AN, Houston SJ, Resche I, Quick DP, Grund FM, Ell PJ, et al. Palliation of pain associated with metastatic bone cancer using samarium-153 lexidronam: a double-blind placebo-controlled clinical trial. *J Clin Oncol* 1998;16: 1574-1581.

70. Maxon HR, III, Schroder LE, Hertzberg VS, Thomas SR, Englaro EE, Samaratunga R, et al. Rhenium-186(Sn)HEDP for treatment of painful osseous metastases: results of a double-blind crossover comparison with placebo. *J Nucl Med* 1991;32:1877-1881.

71. Maxon HR, III, Thomas SR, Hertzberg VS, Schroder LE, Englaro EE, Samaratunga R, et al. Rhenium-186 hydroxyethylidene diphosphonate for the treatment of painful osseous metastases. *Semin Nucl Med* 1992;22:33-40.

72. Brenner W, Kampen WU, von Forstner C, Brummer C, Zuhayra M, Muhle C, et al. High-dose treatment with (186)Re-HEDP or (153)Sm-EDTMP combined with amifostine in a rabbit model. *J Nucl Med* 2001;42:1545-1550.

73. Kolesnikov-Gauthier H, Carpentier P, Depreux P, Vennin P, Caty A, Sulman C. Evaluation of toxicity and efficacy of 186Re-hydroxyethylidene diphosphonate in patients with painful bone metastases of prostate or breast cancer. *J Nucl Med* 2000; 41:1689-1694.

74. Sciuto R, Festa A, Pasqualoni R, Semprebene A, Rea S, Bergomi S, et al. Metastatic bone pain palliation with 89-Sr and 186-Re-HEDP in breast cancer patients. *Breast Cancer Res Treat* 2001;66:101-109.

75. Han SH, Zonneberg BA, de Klerk JM, Quirijnen JM, het Schip AD, van Dijk A, et al. 186Re-etidronate in breast cancer patients with metastatic bone pain. *J Nucl Med* 1999;40:639-642.

76. Maxon HR, III, Schroder LE, Washburn LC, Thomas SR, Samaratunga RC, Biniakiewicz D, et al. Rhenium-188(Sn)HEDP for treatment of osseous metastases. *J Nucl Med* 1998;39:659-663.

77. Liepe K, Franke WG, Kropp J, Koch R, Runge R, Hliscs R. [Comparison of rhenium-188, rhenium-186-HEDP and strontium-89 in palliation of painful bone metastases]. *Nuklearmedizin* 2000;39:146-151.

78. Liepe K, Hliscs R, Kropp J, Runge R, Knapp FF, Jr., Franke WG. Dosimetry of 188Re-hydroxyethylidene diphosphonate in human prostate cancer skeletal metastases. *J Nucl Med* 2003;44:953-960.

79. Liepe K, Kropp J, Runge R, Kotzerke J. Therapeutic efficiency of rhenium-188-HEDP in human prostate cancer skeletal metastases. *Br J Cancer* 2003;89: 625-629.

80. Palmedo H, Manka-Waluch A, Albers P, Schmidt-Wolf IG, Reinhardt M, Ezziddin S, et al. Repeated bone-targeted therapy for hormone-refractory prostate carcinoma: Randomized phase II trial with the new, high-energy radiopharmaceutical rhenium-188 hydroxyethylidenediphosphonate. *J Clin Oncol* 2003;21: 2869-2875.

81. Atkins HL. Overview of nuclides for bone pain palliation. *Appl Radiat Isot* 1998;49:277-283.

82. Srivastava SC, Atkins HL, Krishnamurthy GT, Zanzi I, Silberstein EB, Meinken G, et al. Treatment of metastatic bone pain with tin-117m Stannic diethylenetriaminepentaacetic acid: A phase I/II clinical study. *Clin Cancer Res* 1998; 4:61-68.

83. Srivastava SC, Atkins HL, Krishnamurthy GT, et al. Long-term analysis of clinical data from patients treated with Sn-117 DTPA for metastatic bone pain. *J Nucl Med* 1999;40 (suppl):65P.

84. Srivastava SC, Meinken GE, Atkins HL, et al. New tin-117m formulations for therapy of cancer in bone. *J Nucl Med* 1999;40 (suppl):121P.

85. Bishayee A, Rao DV, Srivastava SC, Bouchet LG, Bolch WE, Howell RW. Marrow-sparing effects of 117mSn(4+) diethylenetriaminepentaacetic acid for radionuclide therapy of bone cancer. *J Nucl Med* 2000;41:2043-2050.

86. Mazeron JJ, Gerbaulet A. The centenary of discovery of radium. *Radiother Oncol* 1998;49:205-216.

87. Henriksen G, Fisher DR, Roeske JC, Bruland OS, Larsen RH. Targeting of osseous sites with alpha-emitting 223Ra: comparison with the beta-emitter 89Sr in mice. *J Nucl Med* 2003;44:252-259.

88. Giammarile F, Mognetti T, Blondet C, Desuzinges C, Chauvot P. Bone pain palliation with 85Sr therapy. *J Nucl Med* 1999;40:585-590.

89. Kothari K, Samuel G, Banerjee S, Unni PR, Sarma HD, Chaudhari PR, et al. 186Re-1,4,8,11-tetraaza cyclotetradecyl-1,4,8,11-tetramethylene phosphonic acid: a novel agent for possible use in metastatic bone-pain palliation. *Nucl Med Biol* 2001;28:709-717.

90. Kothari K, Pillai MR, Unni PR, Shimpi HH, Noronha OP, Samuel AM. Preparation, stability studies and pharmacological behavior of [186Re]Re-HEDP. *Appl Radiat Isot* 1999;51:51-58.

91. Schultheiss TE, Kun LE, Ang KK, Stephens LC. Radiation response of the central nervous system. *Int J Radiat Oncol Biol Phys* 1995;31:1093-1112.

92. Brenner W, Kampen WU, Brummer C, von Forstner C, Zuhayra M, Muhle C, et al. Myeloprotective effects of different amifostine regimens in rabbits undergoing high-dose treatment with 186rhenium-(tin)1,1-hydroxyethylidene diphosphonate (186Re-HEDP). *Cancer Biother Radiopharm* 2003;18:887-893.

93. Morris MJ, Pandit-Taskar N, Divgi C, Larson S, Scher AH. Targeting osseous metastases: rationale and development of radio-immunotherapy for prostate cancer. *Curr Urol Rep* 2005;6:163-170.

94. Mertens WC. Radionuclide therapy of bone metastases: prospects for enhancement of therapeutic efficacy. *Semin Oncol* 1993;20(3 Suppl 2):49-55.

95. Sciuto R, Maini CL, Tofani A, Fiumara C, Scelsa MG, Broccatelli M. Radiosensitization with low-dose carboplatin enhances pain palliation in radioisotope therapy with strontium-89. *Nucl Med Commun* 1996;17:799-804.

96. Geldof AA, de Rooij L, Versteegh RT, Newling DW, Teule GJ. Combination 186Re-HEDP and cisplatin supra-additive treatment effects in prostate cancer cells. *J Nucl Med* 1999;40:667-671.

97. Akerley W, Butera J, Wehbe T, Noto R, Stein B, Safran H, et al. A multi-institutional, concurrent chemoradiation trial of strontium-89, estramustine, and

vinblastine for hormone refractory prostate carcinoma involving bone. *Cancer* 2002;94:1654-1660.

98. Tu SM, Millikan RE, Mengistu B, Delpassand ES, Amato RJ, Pagliaro LC, et al. Bone-targeted therapy for advanced androgen-independent carcinoma of the prostate: a randomised phase II trial. *Lancet* 2001;357:336-341.

99. Papatheofanis FJ. Serum PICP as a bone formation marker in 89Sr and external beam radiotherapy of prostatic bony metastases. *Br J Radiol* 1997;70:594-598.

100. Papatheofanis FJ. Decreased serum E-selectin concentration after 89Sr-chloride therapy for metastatic prostate cancer bone pain. *J Nucl Med* 2000;41:1021-1024.

101. Lenarczyk M, Goddu SM, Rao DV, Howell RW. Biologic dosimetry of bone marrow: induction of micronuclei in reticulocytes after exposure to 32P and 90Y. *J Nucl Med* 2001;42:162-169.

Chapter 18

Muscle Relaxants

Gary McCleane

Muscle pain and spasm are common accompaniments of diseases of the bone and joints. Indeed, pain arising from muscle may be more intense and debilitating than that arising from the adjacent malfunctioning bone or joint. While adequate treatment of the causative bone or joint condition may ultimately be rewarded by an overall reduction in pain, a more rapid resolution may be achieved if the muscle pain or spasm is addressed concomitantly.

Where spasticity is encountered, upper motor neuron pathology can be expected. This is beyond the scope of our considerations. Where spasm or muscle pain arises, it is common for it to be the result of irritation or dysfunction of surrounding tissue rather than evidence of primary muscle dysfunction. However, on occasions, the cause of the muscle spasm or pain may not become clear until it is treated, when an underlying cause (for example, an arthritic facet joint or ligamentous irritation) may become apparent.

The diagnosis of muscle spasm is suggested when there is palpable hardness of the muscle under examination and there is stiffness on movement of the region supplied by that muscle. This is aided if the symptoms arising from the spasm are unilateral, when there is an opportunity to compare the muscle hardness on the affected and unaffected sides. If the muscle is also tender on palpation, then the supposition of muscle spasm and pain is supported. If there is definite tenderness over the enthesis (that is, where the muscle joins to bone), then this again can be taken as supportive evidence. For example, with muscle spasm and pain over one side of the neck suggested, a palpable difference in muscle tone over one side as compared with the other, resistance to movement that involves stretching of those muscle groups, and the presence of enthetic tenderness (mastoid process, occipital region, and spinous processes of cervical vertebrae) all support the diagnosis.

When muscle relaxant drugs are considered, a clear distinction between those drugs used to reduce muscle spasm and pain and those used in anesthetic practice must be made. The latter group is used to give complete muscle relaxation (including the respiratory muscles) and works by interfering with neuromuscular transmission. This has no place in the management of muscle pain.

Of the muscle relaxant drugs used in nonanesthetic practice, the majority achieve muscle relaxation by virtue of their effects on the central nervous system (CNS). Only dantrolene works on the muscle itself. Therefore, CNS side effects such as drowsiness are not uncommon with their use. The majority of drugs are intended for the short-term treatment of acute episodes of muscle spasm. Baclofen and tizanadine may be exceptions to this and are often used in the long-term management of muscle spasm and pain.

When muscle spasm and pain occur, they are commonly accompanied by inflammation, either of the muscle itself or the enthesis. Muscle relaxant drugs have no anti-inflammatory properties, and so when used alone often have a partial, rather than complete, effect. Their efficacy can be improved by the addition of a nonsteroidal anti-inflammatory drug (NSAID). Similarly, when a NSAID is used alone in the presence of muscle spasm and pain, its effect is again often incomplete. This effect can be enhanced by the addition of a muscle relaxant drug.

When muscle relaxants are used clinically, duration of therapy must be considered. When symptoms are acute, short-term use of a muscle relaxant is appropriate. When the patient suffers from long-standing muscle pain and spasm, long-term use of a muscle relaxant is required. The patient can be stabilized on a particular dose of the chosen relaxant and provided with instructions how to increase the dose of that relaxant or an alternate relaxant to add in during periods of flare up. When muscle pain and spasm are of intermediate duration (weeks to months), there is merit in using the relaxant chosen (often along with a NSAID) continuously for several months in the hope that, when treatment is stopped, there will be no return of symptoms. If symptoms do return at that stage, then treatment, if previously effective, can be reinstituted for several more months.

In this chapter a variety of muscle relaxant drugs will be considered. A clinically effective muscle relaxant treatment, namely the use of botulinum toxin, will not be considered as it is the subject of another chapter. Clearly pharmacological treatment is only one of the options for the treatment of muscle spasm and pain. Physical therapy, acupuncture, dry needling, massage, application of heat, and many other approaches can be effective, but the focus of this chapter is on the pharmacological treatments.

BACLOFEN

Baclofen is the *p*-chlorophenyl derivative of gamma-amino butyric acid (GABA). It achieves its effect by being a GABA-B agonist and includes among its side effects sedation and confusion. Abrupt cessation of long-term treatment can be associated with a withdrawal reaction. That said, baclofen is usually well tolerated, has a relatively quick onset of action, and is relatively effective in the treatment of muscle spasm. It is also used in the treatment of trigeminal neuralgia.

The exact mechanisms of action of baclofen are not known for certain but seem to involve both pre- and postsynaptic GABA-B receptor actions. At the presynaptic site, baclofen decreases calcium conductance with resultant decreased neurotransmitter and excitatory amino acid uptake. At the postsynaptic site, baclofen increases potassium conductance (with resultant neuronal hyperpolarization) and may also inhibit the release of substance P.

Baclofen is available in an oral formulation and also in a form used for intrathecal infusion in patients with refractory spasticity.

BENZODIAZEPINES

Benzodiazepines bind to benzodiazepine receptors located in the terminals of primary fibers, leading to increased chloride flux across the terminal membrane with resultant increase in membrane potential.

Side effects of the benzodiazepine group as a whole include sedation, cognitive impairment, and, with prolonged use, withdrawal reactions on discontinuation of the drug. Diazepam is frequently used as a muscle relaxant, but if so used, its use should be short term and only for acute flare-ups of muscle spasm. Clonazepam appears to possess analgesic and perhaps amnesic properties, but has a long half-life, and so drug accumulation may occur. Lorazepam, having a shorter half-life than diazepam or clonazepam, has some advantage from a pharmacokinetic perspective and may be used in preference, particularly in the elderly.

CARISOPRODOL

This agent is primarily metabolized in the liver with multiple metabolites including meprobamate. As metabolism is dependent on deacetylation via the liver microenzyme CYP 2C19, which a proportion of the population have a deficiency of, there exist "poor metabolizers" of this drug who are at increased risk of experiencing concentration-based side effects such as drowsiness, hypotension, and CNS depression at otherwise "normal" doses. There is some risk of respiratory depression with carisoprodol, this risk being increased by the coadministration of propoxyphene.

While the exact mode of action of carisoprodol is not established, it may be that flumazenil may have a role in reversing carisoprodol toxicity.

CYCLOBENZAPRINE

This compound has a tricyclic structure very similar to amitriptyline. Not surprisingly, therefore, it shares a propensity to cause anticholinergic side effects with the TCAs.

It can be of use in patients with acute and intermittent musculoskeletal conditions including low back pain, muscle spasm, and fibromyalgia.

DANTROLENE

This drug is unusual among the muscle relaxant drugs, in that it works directly on skeletal muscle. It achieves its effect by an action on calcium uptake by the sarcoplasmic reticulum. Dantrolene is used in the treatment of malignant hyperpyrexia, a condition occasionally triggered by anesthetic agents and in which intense muscle spasm is a predominant feature. In those individuals thought to be susceptible to malignant hyperpyrexia, dantrolene can be used in a prophylactic fashion.

When used in the treatment of muscle spasm and spasticity, a gradual escalation of dose to an effective level is used. Consequently, dantrolene is of little use in the immediate treatment of a flare-up of muscle spasm, but it rather has value in the longer-term management of muscle-based pain. Dantrolene can affect liver function, and so periodic blood sampling to assess liver function should be carried out.

METAXALONE

This oxazolidone derivative can have a muscle relaxant effect when there is a peripheral musculoskeletal condition but not when there is spasticity secondary to a neurologic disorder. It is generally well tolerated but shares the potential side effect of sedation with many other muscle relaxant drugs.

METHOCARBAMOL

Methocarbamol is a carbamate derivative of guaifenisin and is structurally related to mephenerin. It is available in both oral and parenteral formulations.

ORPHENADRINE

Orphenadrine is a monomethylated derivative of diphenhydramine. Centrally acting antihistamines such as this exhibit muscle relaxant and analgesic properties, although the muscle relaxant effect of orphenadrine may also be attributable to its modulating effect of the raphespinal serotinergic systems as well.

Orphenadrine also seems to exhibit the characteristics of an *N* methy-D-aspartate (NMDA) receptor antagonist, and this may also account for some of its possible analgesic effects.

Side effects associated with orphenadrine use are partially related to its anticholinergic action, and therefore include dry mouth, urinary retention, confusion, blurred vision, agitation, and restlessness.

Orphenadrine is often presented in combination with acetaminophen, aspirin, and NSAIDs.

TIZANADINE

Tizanadine is an imidazoline derivative that is structurally related to clonidine. Like clonidine, it is an α_2-adrenoreceptor agonist. Its effect, mediated by this receptor, is to cause a direct inhibition of release of excitatory amino acids and a concomitant inhibition of facilitatory coeruleospinal pathways. It is known that epidural and spinal administration of clonidine with local anesthetics opioid combinations is associated with enhanced analgesia, and it would therefore be expected that tizanadine may also have analgesic properties.

Somnolence is one of the most frequent side effects of tizanadine use. Its elimination half-life is between 1 and 3 hours, and so it can be administered up to four times daily with a greater proportion of the total daily dose being given at night to augment sleep both because of its hypnotic properties and because muscle relaxation and pain relief may allow a more uninterrupted nights rest.

MISCELLANEOUS

A variety of other agents are used by some in the treatment of muscle spasm and pain. The evidence that supports their use is anecdotal:

- Quinine sulphate (leg cramps)
- Diphenhydramine hydrochloride
- Procainamide
- Phenytoin, gabapentin, pregabalin
- Propoxyphene

- Tricyclic antidepressants
- Magnesium sulphate
- Cyproheptadine
- Chlorpromazine
- Dronabinol
- L-Threonine (a precursor of glycine)
- Cannabinoids

SUGGESTED CLINICAL USE OF MUSCLE RELAXANT DRUGS

Acute Muscle Spasm and Pain

In this scenario, a rapidly acting muscle relaxant is required. Baclofen fits this requirement and can be initiated at a dose of 10 mg three times daily (adjusted to a lower dose in the elderly and infirm) along with a NSAID provided no contraindications exist for their use. Effect from baclofen is usually apparent within 24 hours. In those intolerant of this dose level, reduction to 5 mg three times daily can reduce side effects and still maintain effect (Table 18.1).

TABLE 18.1. Commonly used muscle relaxant drugs (suggested doses for fit, healthy adults).

Proprietary name	US generic	UK generic	Suggested dose
Baclofen	Lioresal	Lioresal	10 mg tid
Carisoprodol	Soma	Carisoma	350 mg tid
Clonazepam	Klonopin	Rivotril	1 to 2 mg nocte
Cyclobenzaprine	Flexeril		10 mg tid
Dantrolene	Dantrium	Dantrium	25 mg daily, increasing by 25 mg weekly to 25 mg tid
Diazepam	Valium Valrelease	Valium	2 mg tid
Metaxalone	Skelaxin		200 mg qid
Methocarbamol	Robaxin Robaxisal	Robaxin	1.5 g qid
Orphenadrine	Norflex	Biorphen Disipal	100 mg qid or BID
Tizanidine	Zanaflex	Zanaflex	2 mg tid, 6 mg nocte

Chronic Muscle Spasm and Pain

Baclofen is also a viable option for the management of longer-term muscle spasm and pain. Should it fail to be effective, other options are worthy of thought. If sleep disturbance is present, then tizanadine can be used with a greater proportion of the total daily dose being given at night since sedation is a not infrequent accompaniment of its use. Therefore, muscle relaxation and sleep may be promoted. Where sedation is not acceptable, dantrolene 25 mg daily, increased to 25 mg twice daily after 1 week, and by further 25 mg increments on a weekly basis to 25 mg four times daily, can be tried. If this is effective but the patient still experiences intermittent flare-ups, then the total daily dose of dantrolene can be increased to 150 mg to counteract these flare ups.

Where muscle spasm is concentrated to one muscle group, consideration to the use of botulinum toxin injected into these muscles can be given.

BIBLIOGRAPHY

Muscle Spasm

Chou R, Peterson K, Helfand M. Comparative efficacy and safety of skeletal muscle relaxants for spasticity and musculoskeletal conditions: a systematic review. *J Pain Symptom Manage* 2004.
Shapiro RT. Management of spasticity, pain, and paroxysmal phenomena in multiple sclerosis. *Curr Neurol Neurosci Rep* 2001; 1: 299-302.

Benzodiazepines

Cendrowski W, Sobczyk W. Clonazepam, baclofen and placebo in the treatment of spasticity. *Eur Neurol* 1997; 16: 257-262.
Roussan M, Terrance C, Fromm G. Baclofen versus diazepam for the treatment of spasticity and long-term follow-up of baclofen therapy. *Pharmatherapeutical* 1987; 4: 278-284.

Carisoprodol

Dalen P, Alvan G, Wakelkamp M, et al. Formation of meprobamate from carisoprodol is catalyzed by CYP2C19. *Pharmacogenetic* 1996; 6: 387-394.
Dougherty RJ. Carisoprodol should be a controlled substance. *Arch Fam Med* 1995; 4: 582.

Reeves RR, Pinkofsky HB, Carter OS. Carisoprodol: a drug of continuing abuse. *J AM Osteopathic Assn* 1997; 97: 723-724.

Roberge RJ, Lin E, Krenzelok EP. Flumazenil reversal of carisoprodol (Soma) intoxication. *J Emerg Med* 2000; 18: 61-64.

Cyclobenzaprine

Browning R, Jackson JL, O'Malley PG. Cyclobenzaprine and back pain: a meta-analysis. *Arch Internal Med* 2001; 161: 1613-1620.

Lofland JH, Szarlej D, Buttaro R, et al. Cyclobenzaprine hydrochloride is a commonly prescribed centrally acting muscle relaxant, which is structurally similar to tricyclic antidepressants (TCAs) and differs from amitriptyline by only one double bond. *Clin J Pain* 2001; 17: 103-104.

Reynolds WJ, Moldofsky H, Saskin P, et al. The effects of cyclobenzaprine on sleep physiology and symptoms in patients with fibromyalgia. *J Rheumatol* 1991; 18: 452-454.

Orphenadrine

Hunskaar S, Donnell D. Clinical and pharmacological review of the efficacy of orphenadrine and its combination with paracetamol in painful conditions. *J Intern Med Res* 1991; 19: 71-87.

Hunskaar S, Berge OG, Hole K. Orphenadrine citrate increases and prolongs the antinociceptive effects of paracetamol in mice. *Acta Pharmacol Toxicol* 1986; 59: 53-59.

Hunskaar S, Berge OG, Hole K. Antinociceptive effects of orphenadrine in mice. *Eur J Pharmacol* 1985; 111: 221-226.

Tizanadine

Cowards DM. Tizanadine: Neuropharmacology and mechanisms of action. *Neurology* 1994; 44S9: 6-11.

Milanov I, Georgiev D. Mechanisms of tizanadine action on spasticity. *Acta Neurol Scand* 1994; 89: 2724-2729.

Smith HS, Barton AE. Pharmaceutical update: tizanadine in the management of spasticity and musculoskeletal complaints in the palliative care population. *Am J Palliat Care* 2000; 17: 50-58.

Chapter 19

Other Options

Howard S. Smith
Mark Guerdan

Although there is not a wealth of publications on this topic, there exists an assortment of alternative medications other than conventional agents (e.g., local anesthetics, corticosteroids, glucosamine, hyaluronic acid, and opioids) for intra-articular pain and inflammation.

This chapter will deal with a potpourri of miscellaneous agents that have been utilized via intra-articular administration in efforts to diminish discomfort [e.g., achieve articular analgesia (arthranalgesia)], improve joint function, and subsequently increase function/activity level.

NSAIDS

Aspirin and all other nonsteroidal anti-inflammatory drugs (NSAIDs) are used to treat inflammation and pain in a variety of clinical applications; besides their anti-inflammatory and analgesic applications they also possess an antipyretic action. The Food and Drug Administration FDA has approved specific NSAIDs for designated disease states; however, all probably exhibit some degree of effectiveness in rheumatic arthritis and acute localized musculoskeletal syndromes (sprains and strains). Certain NSAIDs have been used as intra-articular injectables.[1]

Clinical Management of Bone and Joint Pain
© 2007 by The Haworth Press, Inc. All rights reserved.
doi:10.1300/5771_21

Since aspirin is the prototype for NSAID class, let us examine it more closely. Many home remedies used since the beginning of recorded time have depended on salicylates as an integral component. Over 100 years ago aspirin was formulated from salicylic and acetic acids. This synthesis helped to spur the entire modern pharmaceutical industry. Low-dose aspirin as a prophylactic agent in thrombotic events was first reported over 25 years ago. Since aspirin was synthesized, pharmacologists have made it a priority to search for other NSAIDs with decreased toxicity and increased potency. At the usual dosage, aspirin's main adverse effects are gastric upset (intolerance) and gastric and duodenal ulcers, while hepatotoxicity, asthma, rashes, and renal toxicity occur less frequently. Upper gastrointestinal bleeding associated with aspirin use is usually related to erosive gastritis. High-dose aspirin has been associated with increase in fecal blood loss and "salicylism"—vomiting, tinnitus, decreased hearing, and vertigo—reversible by reducing the dosage. Still larger doses of salicylates cause hyperpnoea through a direct effect on the medulla. At toxic salicylate levels, respiratory alkalosis followed by metabolic acidosis (salicylate accumulation), respiratory depression, and even cardiotoxicity and glucose intolerance can occur. Two grams or less of aspirin daily usually increases serum uric acid levels, whereas doses exceeding 4 g daily decrease urate levels. In the 1950s and 1960s this search for a better aspirin was undertaken by mainstream pharmaceutical industry, facilitating the development of ibuprofen in 1964. Ibuprofen was introduced as over-the-counter in the United Kingdom in 1966/1983 and in the United States in 1974/1984.

The NSAIDs are grouped in several chemical classes; this chemical diversity yields a broad range of pharmacokinetic characteristics. Although there are many differences in the kinetics of NSAIDs, they have some general properties in common. Most of the NSAIDs are weak organic acids with ionization constants (pKa) between 3 and 5. Therefore, at lower pHs, more of the drug becomes ionized, yielding higher membrane concentrations (Nabumetone is nonacidic). NSAIDs tend to be well absorbed, and food does not substantially change their bioavailability. Most of the NSAIDs are highly metabolized, some by phase I followed by phase II mechanisms and others by direct glucuronidation (phase II) alone. Metabolism of most NSAIDs proceeds, in part, by way of the CYP3A or CYP2C families of P450 enzymes in the liver. While renal excretion is the most important route for final elimination, nearly all undergo varying degrees of biliary excretion and reabsorption (enterohepatic circulation). In fact, the degree of lower gastrointestinal tract irritation appears to correlate with the amount of enterohepatic circulation. Most of the NSAIDs are highly protein bound (≥98 percent), usually to albumin. Some of the NSAIDs (e.g., ibuprofen) are racemic mixtures, while one, naproxen, is provided as a single enantiomer, and a few have no chiral center (e.g., diclofenac).[1]

All NSAIDs can be found in synovial fluid after repeated dosing. Drugs with short half-lives remain in the joints longer than would be predicted from their half-lives, while drugs with longer half-lives disappear from the synovial fluid at a rate proportionate to their half-lives.[1]

The anti-inflammatory activity of NSAIDs is mediated chiefly through inhibition of biosynthesis of prostaglandins. Various NSAIDs have additional possible mechanisms of action, including inhibition of chemotaxis, downregulation of interleukin-1 production, decreased production of free radicals and superoxide, and interference with calcium-mediated intracellular events. Aspirin irreversibly acetylates and blocks platelet cyclo-oxygenase (COX), while most non-COX-selective NSAIDs are reversible inhibitors. Selectivity for COX-1 versus COX-2 is variable and incomplete for the older members, NSAIDs. Highly selective COX-2 inhibitors have become available, and other highly selective coxibs are being developed. The highly selective COX-2 inhibitors do not affect platelet function at their usual doses. In testing using human whole blood, aspirin, indomethacin, piroxicam, and sulindac were somewhat more effective in inhibiting COX-1; ibuprofen and melclofenamate inhibited the two isozymes almost equally. The efficacy of COX-2-selective drugs equals that of the older NSAIDs, while gastrointestinal safety may be improved. On the other hand, some highly selective COX-2 inhibitors may increase the incidence of edema and hypertension.[1]

The NSAIDs decrease the sensitivity of vessels to bradykinin and histamine, affect lymphokine production from T-lymphocytes, and reverse vasodilation. To varying degrees, all newer NSAIDs are analgesic, anti-inflammatory, and antipyretic, and essentially all (except the COX-2-selective agents and the nonacetylated salicylates) inhibit platelet aggregation to some extent. NSAIDs are all gastric irritants as well; though, as a group the newer agents tend to cause less gastric irritation than aspirin. Nephrotoxicity has been observed for all NSAIDs, and hepatotoxicity can also occur with any NSAID.[1] Although these drugs effectively inhibit inflammation, there is no evidence that they alter the course of an arthritic disorder—in contrast to drugs such as methotrexate and gold.[1]

Ketorolac

Ketorolac is an NSAID that has primarily been used for its analgesic and not its anti-inflammatory effects. It is the only parenteral NSAID available in the United States. It has been successful in reducing postsurgical opioid requirements by 25 to 50 percent, however; its potential antithrombotic effects and renal toxicity have led to caution with its perioperative use.[1] Calmet and colleagues prospectively assessed the postoperative analgesic effect of intra-articular Ketorolac, morphine, and bupivacaine during arthroscopic outpatient partial meniscectomy.[2] Four groups of (n = 20) patients were randomized into 60 mg intra-articular Ketorolac, intra-articular bupivacaine 0.25 percent, 1 mg intra-articular morphine diluted in 10 ml saline, and (control group) only 10 ml saline.[2] Three parameters were measured: postoperative analgesia (period measured from the end of the surgery until further analgesia was demanded), postoperative pain (at 1, 2, 3, 12, and 24 hours postoperatively using visual analog pain scale), and additional pain medication (for 1 day after surgery).[2] The best analgesic effects were achieved with intra-articular Ketorolac. The statistically significant was apparent in postoperative analgesic effect and the need for additional pain medication immediately postoperatively and after 24 hours.[2] No complications were observed. Calmet and colleagues concluded that 60 mg intra-articular Ketorolac provides better analgesic effects than 10 ml intra-articular bupivacaine 0.25 percent or 1 mg intra-articular morphine.[2]

Piroxicam

Piroxicam, an oxicam, is a nonselective COX inhibitor, but at high concentrations also inhibits polymorphonuclear leukocyte migration, decreases oxygen radical production, and inhibits lymphocyte function. Its long half-life permits once-daily dosing.

Piroxicam can be used for the usual rheumatic indications. Toxicity includes gastrointestinal symptoms (20 percent of patients), dizziness, tinnitus, headache, and rash. When piroxicam is used in dosages higher than 20 mg/day, an increased incidence of peptic ulcer and bleeding is encountered. Epidemiologic studies suggest that this risk may be as much as 9.5 times higher with piroxicam than with other NSAIDs.

Izdes and colleagues conducted a double-blinded study in 90 patients undergoing elective arthroscopic knee surgery to determine whether there is a role of inflammation in the analgesic efficacy of intra-articular piroxicam.[3] At the end of the operation, after harvesting synovial biopsies, patients were randomized into three intra-articular groups equally.[3] Group 1 received 25 ml saline, Group 2 received 25 ml 0.25 percent bupivacaine, and Group 3 received 25 ml 0.25 percent bupivacaine and piroxicam 20 mg.[3] After microscopic examination of the synovial materials, the patients were divided into two subgroups, inflammation positive (I+) and inflammation negative (I−).[3] Preoperatively and postoperatively at 1, 2, 4, and 6 hours, pain levels, analgesic duration, and postoperative analgesic consumption were recorded.[3] Analgesic duration was significantly longer in the I+ subgroup than the I− subgroup of Group 3 ($p < 0.05$). Pain scores at 1, 2, and 4 hours postoperatively were significantly lower in the I+ subgroup than the I− subgroup of Group 3 ($p < 0.05$), whereas there were no significant differences among the subgroups of Groups 1 and 2.[3] Izdes and colleagues concluded that preoperative inflammation is an important determinant of analgesic efficacy for intra-articular piroxicam.[3]

Tenoxicam

Tenoxicam is an oxicam similar to piroxicam and shares its nonselective COX inhibition, long half-life (72 hours), efficacy, and toxicity profile. It is available abroad but not in the United States.

Colbert and colleagues utilized a prospective, double-blind, randomized trial design and compared the analgesic effect of intra-articular Tenoxicam 20 mg with intravenous Tenoxicam on postoperative pain in 88 patients undergoing knee arthroscopy.[4] Patients in group A received 20 mg Tenoxicam made up to 40 ml with normal saline intra-articularly (IA) and 2 ml normal saline IV. Patients in group B received 40 ml normal saline IA and 2 ml, 20 mg of Tenoxicam IV.[4] Patients receiving IA Tenoxicam had lower pain scores (at rest and upon movement) at 30, 60, 120, and 180 min postoperatively (0.8 ± 0.2 versus 2.5 ± 0.2 at rest and 1.24 ± 0.2 versus 3.4 ± 0.2 at movement at 60 min; $p < 0.0001$).[4] In addition, fewer patients required additional analgesia in the first four hours postoperatively (33 percent versus 84 percent; $p < 0.00001$) and the time to first analgesia (23.7 ± 11.2 versus 9.4 ± 0.6; $p < 0.02$) was longer in those receiving IA Tenoxicam.[4] Colbert and colleagues concluded that intra-articular Tenoxicam provides superior postoperative analgesia and reduces postoperative analgesic requirements compared with IV Tenoxicam in patients undergoing knee arthroscopy.[4]

BIOSYNTHETIC OPTIONS

Some of the most promising intra-articular therapies have been developed in the biosynthetic areas: Anakinra—recombinant form of nonglycosylated human interleukin-1 receptor antagonist, Orgotien—superoxide dismutase enzyme produced from beef liver as a copper-zinc (Cu-Zn) mixed chelate, Orthokine—interleukin-1 receptor antagonist and other anti-inflammatory mediators that are recovered in the serum, Somatastatin—somatotropin release-inhibiting factor (SRIF), is a natural cyclic peptide inhibitor of pituitary, pancreatic, and gastrointestinal secretion.

Individual Biosynthetic Agents

Anakinra

Anakinra is a recombinant form of nonglycosylated human interleukin-1 receptor antagonist expressed in *Escherichia coli*. The recombinant compound differs from naturally occurring nonglycosylated human interleukin-1 receptor antagonist by addition of one N-terminal methionine.[5] Natural interleukin-1 receptor antagonist is produced primarily by macrophages and activated monocytes in response to various stimuli. It competitively binds to both type I and type II interleukin-1 receptors, at least partially blocking cellular responses mediated by interleukin-1α and interleukin-1β. The binding affinity of natural interleukin-1 receptor antagonist is similar to that of interleukin-1. However, it lacks interleukin-1 agonist activity. In animal and *in vitro* studies, substantially higher concentrations of interleukin-1 receptor antagonist relative to interleukin-1 (up to 10,000-fold) have been required to completely inhibit cellular/hemodynamic effects of interleukin-1.[5] As only 5 percent receptor availability for interleukin-1 can initiate inflammatory responses, virtually all cellular receptors must be blocked for sufficient inhibition of systemic effects.[5] Anakinra has been investigated in several conditions considered mediated at least in part via interleukin-1 (mainly interleukin-1β); in most, the assumption is that endogenous levels of human interleukin-1 receptor antagonist (IL-1RA) are insufficient to counteract interleukin-1 pathogenic activity.[5] Mounting evidence suggests involvement of interleukin-1β in the pathogenesis of rheumatoid arthritis. In animal models of arthritis, intravenous Anakinra has improved clinical symptoms and suppressed cartilage and joint damage.[5]

Chevalier and colleagues examined the safety of intra-articular (IA) injections of recombinant human IL-1RA in patients with knee osteoarthritis (OA).[5] Six doses of IL-1RA were investigated ranging from 0.05 mg up to 150 mg in a prospective double-blinded (for dosing) multicenter trial of patients with symptomatic knee OA and without synovial fluid effusion.[5] Acute inflammatory reaction (the primary end point defining intolerance) was recorded if pain increased over 30 mm on a 100 mm visual analog scale and if synovial fluid effusion occurred within 72 hours after the IA injection.[5] As a secondary aim, efficacy was estimated (by total pain and Western Ontario and McMaster University OA functional index) until month 3.[5] One patient intentionally received 0.05 mg as an empirically derived no effect dose by study design because IA injections in humans had not yet been studied; 13 patients received 150 mg of IL-1RA.[5] No acute reaction occurred (one patient experienced postinjection joint swelling with no pain), and the 150 mg dose was considered the maximum tolerated dose (intolerance level 0 percent; confidence interval 0, 9.1 percent).[5] A significant improvement was still observed until month 3 in the 13 patients who received 150 mg IL-1RA: pain improved by -20.4 ± 23.3 mm ($p = 0.008$) and WOMAC global score by -19.5 ± 20.1 ($p = 0.005$).[4] Chevalier and colleagues concluded that an IA injection of IL-1RA in patients with knee OA was well tolerated and did not induce any acute inflammatory reaction.[5]

Orgotein

Orgotein is a superoxide dismutase enzyme produced from beef liver as a copper-zinc (Cu-Zn) mixed chelate.[6] This metalloprotein of 151 amino acids has a molecular weight of approximately 33,000 and a compact conformation maintained by about 4 gram-atoms of chelated divalent metals.[6] It should be noted that pharmaceutical versions of Cu-Zn superoxide dismutases obtained from bovine and other mammalian tissues are frequently referred to generically as Orgotein. The superoxide anion is a highly reactive form of oxygen that is formed when oxygen is reduced by a single electron. Superoxide anions are produced during the normal catalytic function of certain enzymes, by the oxidation of hemoglobin to methemoglobin and when ionizing radiation passes through water. They are also produced by phagocytizing cells (e.g., macrophages and polymorphonuclear cells), such as when granulocytes phagocytize bacteria or when the mitochondrial electron transport chain is impaired/inefficient. These oxygen-derived free radicals act as potent promoters of inflammation by degrading cell walls and subsequently causing the release of lysosomal enzymes, which further promote the inflammatory process. Superoxide dismutase (SOD) is an enzyme that acts as a powerful antioxidant in the body. There are three distinct types of SOD: Cu-Zn-SOD, the cytosolic SOD found in mammals; Mn-SOD, found in the mitochondria of eukaryotic cells and in prokaryotic cells; and Fe-SOD, found only in prokaryotic cells. SOD neutralizes the highly reactive and toxic oxygen-derived free radicals by catalyzing the conversion of two molecules of superoxide anion to one molecule of oxygen and one of hydrogen peroxide, eventually producing water. The anti-inflammatory properties of Orgotein may also depend on inhibition of phospholipase A2 activation [PLA2].[6] By reducing damage to cellular membranes, Orgotein appears to exert an effect on [PLA2], thereby impeding the release of arachidonic acid and its metabolic products (e.g., prostaglandins and leukotrienes).[6] In the synovial fluid of arthritic joints, superoxide radicals, produced by phagocytizing cells, induce cartilage deterioration by causing depolymerization of hyaluronic acid, alteration of collagen polymerization, degradation of proteoglycans, and an increase of prostaglandins. Intra-articular injection of superoxide dismutase may inhibit these processes.[6]

Orgotein (superoxide dismutase) for injection has been used in managing osteoarthritis for more than 7 years in Europe; however, well-controlled studies to establish an optimum dosage regimen have not been conducted.[6] McIlwain and colleagues evaluated three Orgotein dose/regimens compared with placebo in terms of efficacy, safety, and duration of effect in 139 patients with active osteoarthritis of the knee over 3 months.[6] Patients were randomized to receive one intra-articular injection of either placebo or Orgotein (8 to 32 mg) each week for 3 weeks.[6] Orgotein was effective in reducing symptoms of osteoarthritis for up to 3 months after treatment; 16 mg given twice was the most effective and best-tolerated regimen with transient minor discomfort at the injection site being the most frequent complaint, which may have been drug related.[6]

Orthokine

Orthokine is an alternative therapy, based on the intra-articular injection of autologous conditioned serum, which has been trialed in Europe. Orthokine is generated by incubating venous blood with etched glass beads.[7] In this way, peripheral blood leukocytes produce elevated amounts of the interleukin-1 receptor antagonist and other anti-inflammatory mediators that are recovered in the serum.[7] Considerable symptomatic relief has been reported in preliminary clinical trials of this product. Alternatively, instead of injecting a heterogeneous, incompletely characterized mixture of native molecules into the joint, it is possible to inject recombinant growth factors and cytokine antagonists.[7] None of these are in routine clinical use, but promising preliminary human trials have been performed with insulin-like growth factor-1 and the interleukin-1 receptor antagonist.[7] It is possible that sustained intra-articular production of such factors could be achieved by gene transfer.[7]

Somatostatin

Somatostatin, also known as SRIF, is a natural cyclic peptide inhibitor of pituitary, pancreatic, and gastrointestinal secretion. Somatostatin is a hormone produced by the hypothalamus, and is also found extensively outside the central nervous system. Its long-acting analogs are in clinical use for treatment of various endocrine syndromes and gastrointestinal anomalies. These analogs are more potent inhibitors of the endocrine release of GH, glucagon, and insulin than the native SRIF; hence, they do not display considerable physiologic selectivity. Octreotide is a somatostatin analog that is useful for the treatment of acromegaly, metastatic GRF-producing tumors, carcinoid syndrome and gastroenteropancreatic tumors. Somatostatin has been used in the management of hormone secreting tumors since the 1970s. However, the usefulness of natural somatostatin is limited by its extremely short duration of action that requires continuous infusion. Octreotide is a molecular form (octapeptide with two D-amino acid substitutions) that overcomes the problem of short duration of action. Octreotide can be given subcutaneously, usually peaks within 30 min, has a plasma half-life of about 100 min, and has a plasma duration of action of up to 12 hours (Sandostatin). Octreotide, like natural somatostatin, inhibits growth hormone secretion, insulin secretion, and glucagon secretion. After intravenous infusion, Octreotide lowers basal serum growth hormone, insulin, and glucagon levels more than natural somatostatin.[8]

Somatostatin has been considered for use in the treatment of phlogistic diseases of the joints by intra-articular administration. Russo et al. showed the results of a study conducted in 16 patients (athletes) with arthrosynovitis or tendonitis of the knee or of the ankle, in which somatostatin was administered (250 mg/treatment, one treatment/week). Somatostatin significantly reduced pain, improved movement/function, and decreased the effects of pain on activities of daily living. This therapy had no major side effects at the site of intra-articular injection or systemically.[8] Russo and colleague suggested that somatostatin may be potentially useful in the treatment of articular and tendoneous phlogistic diseases; however, more studies are needed.[8]

Others

Many other treatments have been developed to treat articular inflammation and pain via injection into the joint capsule. These treatments vary in there mechanisms of action and theoretical anti-inflammatory properties. Most have been discovered as other more accepted medical regimes.

Botulinum Toxin

Botulinum A toxin is a neurotoxin produced by *Clostridium botulinum,* a spore-forming anaerobic bacillus.[9] Seven distinct antigenic types of neurotoxins are generated by *Clostridium botulinum,* labeled A to G, however, only the A and B toxins are currently widely used clinically;[9] Botulinum B appears effective in the treatment of torticollis, particularly in patients who are immune to type A toxin. Botulinum A toxin is a double-chain protein with a molecular weight of approximately 900,000; the active portion of the molecule is the light chain, and the heavy chain is inactive, but is responsible for penetration into the synapse. The toxin appears to affect only one structure in humans, the presynaptic membrane of the neuromuscular junction, where it prevents calcium-dependent release of acetylcholine and produces a state of denervation. Following injection of the toxin into a muscle, the degree of resultant skeletal muscle weakness or paralysis is dependent on the dose administered; muscle inactivation persists until new fibrils grow from the nerve and form junction plates on new areas of the muscle cell walls. Botulinum A toxin has been characterized as a "long-term muscle relaxing agent," and is considered the first chemical entity available clinically that is capable of producing this effect.

In addition to exhibiting antinociception (in pain states due to "tight" spastic muscles or due to peripheral muscarinic dysafferentation[10]) via its traditional mechanisms (interfering with exocytic acetylcholine release), Botulinum toxin type A (BTX-A) may facilitate antinociceptive processes via direct inhibition of peripheral sensitization perhaps by attenuation of the exocytic release of neurotransmitters (e.g., glutamate, substance P, and calcitonin gene-related peptide) and/or by inhibiting the expression of specific receptors (e.g., TRPV1 and P2X3).[11] The direct inhibition of peripheral sensitization may also lead to an indirect inhibition of central sensitization.[11]

Botulinum toxin type A may possess analgesic utility via periarticular injection or possibly via intra-articular injection. Keizer et al. designed a pilot prospective randomized study that compared treatment with Botulinum toxin infiltration of the wrist extensor with a surgical wrist extensor release (a more invasive method) (Hohmann operation).[12] Forty patients with "tennis elbow" were randomized to two groups.[12] One group of patients had surgery (n = 20), the other group of patients was treated with Botulinum toxin (n = 20). Patients were evaluated after 3, 6, 12, and 24 months. One year after treatment, 13 (65 percent) patients in the Botulinum toxin group and 15 (75 percent) patients in the operative group had good to excellent results.[12] Two years after treatment 15 patients in the Botulinum toxin group (75 percent) had good to excellent results; four patients had been operated on after initial treatment with BTX-A.[12] Seventeen patients in the operative group scored good to excellent (85 percent) at 2 years.[12] When analyzed with an overall scoring system, no statistically significant differences were found between the two forms of treatment, and Keizer and colleagues suggested that Botulinum toxin infiltration may be an alternative for the surgical treatment of tennis elbow.[12]

Mikuzis reported a 73-year-old man (M1) and 79-year-old woman (F2) with chronic refractory knee joint pain secondary to osteoarthritis who received intra-articular BTX-A injections into the knees.[13] Neither patient received pain relief from multiple treatments of oral anti-inflammatory nonsteroidal and injectable steroids or viscoelastic supplementation with hyaluronic acid treatments.[13] Each patient received 50 U bilateral intra-articular injections per knee [100 U/ml of BTX-A (total per patient), reconstituted with 0.9 percent unpreserved saline].[13]

Pain reduction, visual analog scale (VAS) score (range 0-10), and clinical assessment of stride length and ambulation.[13] Prior to treatment, average VAS score was 7. Both patients had noticeable swelling and erythema in both knees, which worsened after activity. At 1-month follow-up, average VAS score was 0; and both achieved significant pain relief compared with baseline.[13] At follow-up at 4.5 months, VAS scores at rest were 0 (M1) and 0 to 2 (F2); after activity, it was

1 to 2 in both patients.[13] Improvements in stride length and ease of mobility were observed in both patients as determined by clinician subjective assessment.[13] M1, who had difficulty walking outside of his home prior to treatment, now reported walking 4 miles/hour and improved ability to play golf on a regular basis.[12] M1's use of 1000 mg of acetaminophen four times daily was decreased to 1000 mg as needed, and 100 mg of celecoxib twice daily was discontinued.[12] F2's use of 20 mg/day of valdecoxib was decreased to 10 mg three to five times per week.[13]

Singh and colleagues conducted a retrospective review of nine injections of 50 to 100 units of intra-articular BoNT/A (Allergan BOTOX) in six elderly patients with chronic refractory shoulder pain[14] (see Table 19.1). Pain intensity was assessed with an NRS-11 and function measured by upper extremity active flexion and abduction and compared using paired t-test.[14] A 71 percent maximum pain reduction was noted between 1 to 6 weeks after injection.[14] Pain reduction of > 50 percent was seen in seven patients and $\geq$ 33.3 percent in all injected joints.[14] Pain relief has lasted 6 to 11 weeks and two patients requested reinjection at week.[14] A clinically significant improvement in active flexion and abduction was noted at follow-up. No patient had increased joint swelling or pain, no new muscle weakness developed, and there were no systemic effects of fever or fatigue.[14]

TABLE 19.1. Effect of intra-articular injection of botulinum toxin on shoulder pain.

	Mean (SD)	Change
Age	75 (7.6)	
Time to onset of decreased pain (in days)	5.6 (3)	
Baseline pain (0-10 scale)	8.2 (1.1)	
Pain severity at time of maximum pain reduction	2.4 (1.9)	−5.8* (71% decrease)
Time to onset of maximum pain reduction (in days)	5.6 (3.0)	
Baseline flexion (in degress)	67.8 (27.6)	
Maximum flexion at follow-up (in degrees)	113.3 (46.6)	+45.6** degrees (67%↑)
Baseline abduction (in degrees)	50 (18.5)	
Maximum abduction at at follow-up (in degrees)	71.1 (2.3.1)	+21.2*** degrees (67%↑)

*p < 0.001; **p = 0.001; ***p = 0.01.

Dykstra and colleagues describe injecting BTX-A (Botox) into the sacroiliac joints, cervical/lumbar facets, C-2 roots, costosternal joint, and lumbar disc in nine patients with refractory pain.[15] Sacroiliac joints were injected in three patients with 50 units of BTX-A diluted in 2 cc normal saline via fluoroscopy.[15] One cervical and one lumbar facet joint, two cervical roots, one costosternal joint and one lumbar disc were injected with 25 units of BTX-A diluted in 0.5 cc normal saline via fluoroscopy.[15] Six of nine patients had benefited from steroid injections in the past. Data on reduction in pain severity, change in function (range of motion and improvement in activities of daily living), and adverse events were obtained.[15] Six of nine patients received a significant decrease in their pain (average of 3.7 points on a 0 to 10 pain scale) and improvement in function.[15] Beneficial effects lasted on average 3 months with no significant side effects observed.[15]

Mahowald and colleagues described injecting 25 to 100 units of BTX-A (BoNT/A) into multiple joints [15 joints (9 shoulder, 3 knees, 3 ankles] for refractory pain in 11 patients [2 female, 9 male] with ages ranging from 42 to 82 year and multiple diagnosis (5 with rheumatoid arthritis, 1 with psoriatic arthritis, and 5 with osteoarthritis).[15] Pain decrease began within 2 to 14 days post injection.[16] The mean maximum decrease in pain severity was 55 percent (6.8 ± 1.2 to 2.9 ± 2.3, $p = .018$) in LE joints and 71 percent (8.2 ± 1.1 to $2.41.9$ $p < .001$) in shoulders 4 to 12 weeks after injections.[16] And, 14/15 (93 percent) joints had a 30 percent pain reduction and 10/15 (67 percent) joints had a 50 percent or greater pain reduction. UE function improved +67 percent in active arm flexion ($p = .001$) and +42 percent in abduction ($p = .01$).[16] LE function improved by 43 percent—on 10× timed stands test (the time to perform sit to stand activity ten times) from 30 to 17 sec ($p = .038$).[16] There were no increases in joint inflammation, no periarticular muscle weakness, and no systemic effects of fever or fatigue. IA-BoNT/A effects lasted 3 to 12 months.[16] Patients requested reinjection of two shoulders at 3 months, two shoulders at 9 months, and a knee at 10 months—and experienced 42 percent to 100 percent reduction in pain severity after reinjection.[16] Two patients had sustained pain relief at 12 months, and three patients had slow increases in pain but not to the preinjection (baseline) pain severity and two patients were lost to follow-up.[16]

Although only anecdotal reports of the use of intra-articular Botulinum toxin exist at this point, it appears that randomized, double-blind, controlled, well-designed, large, multicenter studies may be worthwhile, especially if further pilot data supports this.

Chloroquine

Chloroquine is not recommended for the treatment of rheumatoid arthritis in patients in the United States because of the availability of safer alternative. Chloroquine has shown some benefit for the treatment of recent onset arthritis, palindromic rheumatism, or for bone damage associated with rheumatoid arthritis. Chloroquine has been used to treat rheumatoid arthritis, as well as treat or prophylax various parasitic infections, amebiasis, and malaria.[17]

Broll and colleagues investigated the influence of chloroquine diphosphate on protein synthesis in synovial fluid cells in eight patients suffering from rheumatoid arthritis.[17] Intra-articular injection of chloroquine diphosphate at a dose of 25 and 50 mg was followed by a small decrease in the incorporation of 3H-marked amino acids into the synovial fluid cells.[17] Above a dose of 100 mg, protein synthesis is significant reduced.[17] In a second experiment the supercoiled structure of DNA under C1Q was lost; however, after 2 hours the chain breaks were repaired.[17] There is no placebo-controlled data on intra-articular chloroquine.

Ketamine

Ketamine is an intravenous induction agent is also used as a sedative in certain settings and possess analgesic qualities. It is a phencyclidine that has one-tenth the potency of PCP and may cause disociative analgesia/anesthesia, functional and electrophysiological dissociation between the thalamoneocortical and limbic systems. Ketamine has been demonstrated to be an *N*-methyl-D-aspartate receptor antagonist, a subtype of the glutamate receptor. Other receptors may also contribute to the activity of Ketamine, such as norepinephrine, serotonin, and muscarinic cholinergic receptors.

The absorption of Ketamine is rapid when injected intramuscularly or IV its peak plasma level is reached in approximately 15 min.

Awakening from IV use is due to redistribution; Ketamine is more lipid soluble and less protein bound than thiopental, although it is equally ionized at physiological pH. Biotransformation occurs via the liver and end products of biotransformation are excreted renally.[18] Ketamine has a short half-life approximately 2 hours.[18]

The use of intra-articular Ketamine has no produced impressive analgesic results[19,20] and may not be significantly better than intra-articular saline.[21]

Neostigmine

Neostigmine is commonly used to reverse nondepolarizing muscle relaxants via its anticholinesterace activity. By inhibiting the destruction of the cholinesterace enzyme there is an increase in acetylcholine at the neuromuscular junction which leads to a competitive reversal of the nondepolarizing muscle relaxant if enough quantity of relaxant has dissipated. Muscarinic side effects are minimized by prior or concomitant administration of an anticholinergic agent. Neostigmine is also used to treat myasthenia gravis, urinary bladder atony, and paralytic ileus. All these effects are attributed to the increase in acetylcholine at its site of action. This increase in acetylcholine has been used for the analgesic effects in localized areas of pain and inflammation.[18]

Although epidural neostigmine may provide reasonable analgesic efficacy,[22] that analgesic results for intra-articular neostigmine as a sole agent are not impressive.[22,23]

Clonidine

Clonidine is an α_2-agonist that may result in multiple effects including sedation, analgesia, and muscle relaxation. Clonidine has been administered via multiple routes including topical, sublingual, oral epidural, intrathecal, intravenous, and intra-articular. Analgesic results for intra-articular clonidine as a sole agent have been disappointing;[23,24] however, it may still find a niche as an "intra-articular adjunct" combined with other analgesics (e.g., morphine).[25]

Mucopolysaccharide Polysulfuric Acid

Graf and colleagues performed a 6-week single-blind, randomized clinical trial comparing both the efficacy and safety of IA hyaluronic acid (HA) with that of IA mucopolysaccharide polysulfuric acid ester (MPA) in patients with osteoarthritis of the knee joint.[26] Patients received either seven injections of HA or 13 injections of MPA.[26] Joint function, range of motion, severity of pain, the general condition of the bony structure and soft tissue of the joint area, and the global clinical efficacy and safety of the medication were assessed.[26] The mean improvement in the modified total Larson rating score was 22 percent (SD = 28) after HA treatment and 7 percent (SD = 17) after treatment with MPA (analysis of variance: $p = 0.02$) thought to be predominantly from a reduction of pain with the onset of pain relief more rapid in the HA group.[26] During this interval, lasting 6 months after the start of treatment, a further reduction of pain and an improvement of knee joint function could be observed.[26] At the end of the study, 25 out of 33 (76 percent) patients in the HA group and 11 out of 24 (46 percent) patients in the MPA group were symptom-free or markedly improved (Chi-square test: $p = 0.02$).[26] Therefore, since both agents were equally well tolerated, there appears to be no advantages to using MPA over HA.

Radiopharmaceuticals

Small amounts of intra-articular "targeted radiation" may have therapeutic potential for treatment approaches to moderate to severe active synovitis. A radiopharmaceutical (RP) is a complex combination of a radionuclide (RN) with a pharmaceutical (P) agent (RP = RN + P). Radionuclides (radioactive nuclides) are unstable atomic species that change naturally into other atomic species by altering their nuclear structure. During the process of radioactive decay, ionizing radiation is released.

Clunie and colleagues reported that Samarium-153 particulate hydroxyapatite knee synovectomy is well tolerated and may be an effective treatment for carefully selected patients with persistent rheumatoid knee synovitis.[27] Lee and colleagues studied radiation synovectomy using 188 Rhenium (Re)–tin colloid for patients with rheumatoid arthritis.[28] Twenty-two knees from 21 RA patients refractory to conservative therapy and intra-articular corticosteroid injection were evaluated after 1, 4, 6, 9, and 12 months post treatment.[28] Pain intensity on a VAS decreased significantly 1 year after treatment (mean $\pm$ 23.4 mm; $p = 0.0001$ by the paired t-test).[28] Pain decreased in 19 cases (86.3 percent), joint tenderness improved in 14 cases (63.6 percent), and joint swelling was reduced in all cases (100 percent).[28]

Lee and colleagues reported that radiation synovectomy using 188Re–tin colloid for patients with rheumatoid arthritis was well tolerated and resulted in improvement of the arthritis and.[28] Kraft and colleagues assessed the efficacy and safety of 166-holmium-boro-macroaggregates (HMBA) for radiation synovectomy of the knees.[29] Roughly, half of the patients exhibited improved joint motion, and approximately 73 percent had significantly reduced pain (with about 13 percent being pain free) 6 to 8 weeks post treatment.[29] Only insignificant leakage from the joint cavity occurred into the inguinal notes with no sequel.[29]

In addition, nonradiopharmaceutical agents are being investigated for safety and efficacy of intra-articular administration for arthritis.

Paclitaxel, a chemotherapeutic agent which possesses anti-inflammatory properties is being studied for potential intra-articular use (this is the same agent which is one of the substances used to "coat" drug-eluting stents for placement across coronary artery stenosis in efforts to diminish the restenosis rate).

Liggins and colleagues studied the intra-articular administration of microsphere formulations of paclitaxel in healthy rabbit joints for biocompatibility as well as of arthritis for efficacy.[30] Studies revealed that 20 percent (35 to 105 µm size range) paclitaxel-loaded microspheres of poly(lactide-co-glycolide) (PLGA), poly(L-lacyic acid) (PLA), and poly(caprolactone) (PCL) were biocompatible (smaller microspheres produced an inflammatory response) and significantly reduced all study measures of inflammation.[30] The injection of 35 to 105 µm paclitaxel-loaded microspheres significantly reduced both the joint swelling and the number of cells in the joint (synovial) fluid roughly by about half relative to controls.[30] In addition, paclitaxel-loaded microspheres ameliorated the proteoglycan loss (an indicator of cartilage degradation) from animal arthritis models by roughly one-half or more.[30] The injection of control PLA microspheres in diseased animals revealed no effect on either proteoglycan loss or chondrocyte necrosis.

The synovial tissues from knees with arthritis induced by administration of albumin in complete Freund's adjuvant (CFA) demonstrated significant proteoglycan loss down to the bottom third layer of cartilage, which was scored as heavy loss with a poor score of 3 out of 4 (¾-4 being the worst possible) proteoglycan at the only slight loss of proteoglycan at the surface layer of cartilage with an relatively intact surface (score 1/4).[30] The synovial tissues from knees with carrageenan induced arthritis revealed severe loss of proteoglycans throughout all layers of cartilage (score 4/4), except the surface layer, which was only mildly affected.[30] Knees treated with paclitaxel microspheres showed much less proteoglycan loss (score 2/4), though the protective effects were not as dramatic as observed in the albumin in CFA model.[30]

Thakkar and colleagues studies microsphere formulations of celecoxib using a natural polymer, chitosan, as a carrier for intra-articular administration to in efforts to extend the retention of celecoxib in the knee joint.[31] Rats treated with celecoxib loaded chitosan microspheres were significantly improved ($p < 0.005$) compared celecoxib solution.[31]

Another intra-articular agent that may have potential therapeutic utility in the future is a type of water-soluble carboxymethyl chitosan (O-CMC) prepared by using chloracetic acid to react with C6-OH of chitosan.[32] O-CMC was evaluated in rabbits' knee joints and appeared to have potential to increase lubrication in the knee joint, inhibit proliferation of fibroblast cells in the joint, and facilitate repair of pathologic articular cartilage, which may yield beneficial effects for a human knee with active synovitis secondary to rheumatoid arthritis.[32]

THE FUTURE

Gene Therapy

The future treatment of joint pain and inflammation may exist in "gene therapy," which may offer solutions on the basis of molecular repair and regeneration of inflamed capsular tissues. Enhanced gene transfer to arthritic joints may be induced using adeno-associated virus type 5.

Gene therapy of the joint has great potential as a new therapeutic approach for the treatment of rheumatoid arthritis. The vector chosen is of crucial importance for clinical success. Adriaansen and colleagues investigated the tropism and transduction efficiency in arthritic joints *in vivo,* and in synovial cells *in vitro,* using five different serotypes of recombinant adeno-associated virus (rAAV) encoding β-galactosidase or green fluorescent protein genes.[33] Intra-articular injection of the rAAV5 serotype resulted in the highest synovial transduction, followed by much lower expression using rAAV2.[33] There was a minimal humoral immune response to rAAV5 compared with rAAV2.[33] It was found that both rAAV2 and rAAV5 can efficiently transduce human fibroblast-like synoviocytes obtained from patients with rheumatoid arthritis,[33] and Adriaansen and colleagues suggested that intra-articular rAAV mediated gene therapy in rheumatoid arthritis might be improved by using rAAV5 rather than other serotypes.[33]

Zhang and colleagues confirmed that foreign genes can be transferred to articular chondrocytes in primary culture.[34] Furthermore, Zhang and colleagues injected chitosan-DNA nanoparticles containing IL-1RA directly into the knee joint cavities of rabbits with osteoarthritis.[34] Expression of IL-1RA was detected in the knee joint synovial fluid, indicating *in vivo* transfer availability of chitosan vectors.[34] Zhang et al. suggested that this approach may represent a promising future treatment for osteoarthritis since significant reduction was observed in the severity of histologic cartilage lesions in the group that received the chitosan IL-1RA injection.[34]

Biological agents that suppress the activities and signaling of proinflammatory cytokines have shown efficacy as antiarthritic drugs, but generally require frequent administration and may exhibit systemic toxicities. Gene transfer approaches are being developed as an alternative approach for targeted, more efficient and sustained delivery of inhibitors of inflammatory cytokines as well as other therapeutic agents.[35] The efficacy of gene transfer for the treatment of arthritis has been demonstrated in mouse, rat, rabbit, and horse models of disease, whereas the feasibility of the approach has been demonstrated in Phase I clinical trials.[35] Robbins et al. reviewed the current status of both preclinical and clinical arthritis gene therapy including the advantages and disadvantages of different types of vectors, target cells, and therapeutic genes being developed for the treatment of arthritis as well as future directions of the field of arthritis gene therapy.[35]

SUMMARY

Intra-articular analgesia is very much in it infancy. The literature is sparse, sprinkled with case reports, retrospective descriptions, pilot studies, and anectology discussions. There are little to no well-designed studies; therefore, no firm conclusions can be made. Large, multicenter, well-designed, prospective, randomized, double-blind, placebo-controlled studies for persistent pain are needed, and currently do not exits. The future, however, is exciting in that it is conceivable "analgesic intra-articular cocktails" can be studied perhaps with combinations of biosynthetic agents and conventional analgesics (conceivably delivered via gene-therapy-type technology).

REFERENCES

1. Wagner W, Khanna P, Furst DE. Nonsteroidal Anti-inflammatory Drugs, Disease-Modifying Antirheumatic Drugs, Nonopioid Analgesics, and Drugs used in Gout. Chapter 36. In: *Basic & Clinical Pharmacology*, 9th Edition. (Ed) Katzung BG; 2004, Mc-Graw-Hill Publishing Co., New York, NY. Pages 576-603

2. Calmet J, Esteve C, Boada S, et al. Analgesic effect of intra-articular Ketorolac in knee arthroscopy: comparison of morphine and bupivacaine. *Knee Surg Sports Traumatol Arthrosc* 2004; 12: 552-555

3. Izdes S, Orhun S, Turanli S, et al. The effects of preoperative inflammation on the analgesic efficacy of intra-articular piroxicam for outpatient knee arthroscopy. *Anesth Analg* 2003; 97: 1016-1019

4. Colbert ST, Curran E, O'Hanlon DM, et al. Intra-articular Tenoxicam improves postoperative analgesia in knee arthroscopy. *Can J Anaesth* 1999; 46: 653-657

5. Chevalier X, Giraudeau B, Conrozier T, et al. Safety study of intra-articular injection of interleukin 1 receptor antagonist in patients with painful knee osteoarthritis: a multicenter study. *J Rheumatol* 2005; 32: 1317-1323

6. McIlwain H, Silverfield JC, Cheatum DE, et al. Intra-articular Orgotein in osteoarthritis of the knee: A placebo-controlled efficacy, safety, and dosage comparison. *Am J Med* 1989; 87: 295-300

7. Evans CH. *Orthokine* Novel biological approaches to the intra-articular treatment of osteoarthritis. *BioDrugs* 2005; 19: 355-362

8. Russo S, Mangrella M, Vitagliano S, et al. Local administration of somatostatin in joint diseases in athletes. *Minerva Med* 1997; 88: 265-270

9. Tsui JK, Eisen A, Calne DB. Botulinum toxin in spasmodic torticollis. *Adv Neurol* 1988; 50: 593-597

10. Smith HS, Quanzhi H. The Peripheral Muscarinic Dysafferentation (PMD) theory of neuropathic pain. *J Neur Pain Symptom Palliation* 2005; 1: 19-26

11. Aoki KR. Review of a proposed mechanism for the antinociceptive action of botulinum toxin type A. *Neurotoxicology* 2005; 26: 785-793

12. Keizer SB, Rutten HP, Pilot P, et al. Botulinum toxin injection versus surgical treatment for tennis elbow: a randomized pilot study. *Clin Orthop Relat Res* 2002; 401:125-131

13. Mikuzis J. Treatment of chronic refractory knee joint pain with botulinum toxin type A: A report of 2 cases. Poster presented at American Academy of Physical Medicine and Rehabilitation 65th Annual Assembly, October 7-10, 2004, Phoenix, AZ. *Arch Phys Med Rehabil* 2004; 85(9): EL3 ABS-Poster 6

14. Singh IA, Mahowald ML, Dykstra DD. Intra-articular Botulinum A Toxin for chronic shoulder pain in the elderly. Presented at a 2004 American Federation for Medical Research (AFMR) meeting. *J Invest Med* 2004; 52: S380 ABS 19

15. Dykstra DD, Stucky M, Schimpff S, et al. Effects of intra-articular botulinum toxin type A for sacroiliac, cervical/lumbar facet and costosternal joint pain and C-2 root and lumbar disc pain. Presented at Basic and Therapeutic Aspects of Botulinum and Tetanus Toxins International Conference 2005 (Toxins 2005), June 23-25, 2005, Denver CO. Toxins Meetings 2005, (Online): ABS-25

16. Mahowald ML, Singh JA, Dykstra DD. Long term effects of intra-articular botulinum A toxin for refractory joint pain. Presented at 66th Annual Scientific Meeting of the American College of Rheumatology (ACR) and 38th Annual Scientific Meeting of the Association of Rheumatology Health Professionals (ARHP), San Antonio, Texas, October 17-21, 2004. *Arthritis Rheum* 2004 Sep; 50(Suppl 9): S454 ABS-1147

17. Broll H. Effect of chloroquine diphosphate on the superhelix structure of DNA and protein synthesis in synovial cells in chronic polyarthritis. *Wien Klin Wochenschr* 1983; 95: 877-880

18. Nonvolatile Anesthetic Agents. Chapter 8. In: *Clinical Anesthesiology.* Fourth Edition. (Eds) Morgan GE, Mikhail MS, Murray MJ. Lange Medical Books 2006; Mc-Graw-Hill Publishing Co., New York, NY. Pages 576-603

19. Batra YK, Mahajan R, Bangalia SK, et al. Bupivacaine/Ketamine is superior to intra-articular Ketamine analgesia following arthroscopic knee surgery. *Can J Anaesth* 2005; 52: 832-836

20. Dal D, Tetik O, Altunkaya H, et al. The efficacy of intra-articular Ketamine for postoperative analgesia in outpatient arthroscopic surgery. *Arthroscopy* 2004; 20: 300-305

21. Rosseland LA, Stubhaug A, Sandberg L, Breivik H. Intra-articular (IA) catheter administration of postoperative analgesics. A new trial design allows evaluation

of baseline pain, demonstrates large variation in need of analgesics, and finds no an-algesic effect of IA Ketamine compared with IA saline. *Pain* 2003; 104: 25-34

22. Lauretti GR, de Oliveira R, Perez MV, Paccola CA. Postoperative analgesia by intra-articular and epidural Neostigmine following knee surgery. *J Clin Anesth* 2001; 13: 576-581

23. Gentili M, Enel D, Szymskiewicz O, et al. Postoperative analgesia by intra-articular clonidine and Neostigmine in patients undergoing knee arthroscopy. *Reg Anesth Pain Med* 2001; 26: 342-347

24. Tan PH, Buerkle H, Cheng JT, et al. Double-blind parallel comparison of multiple doses of apraclonidine, clonidine, and placebo administered intra-articularly to patients undergoing arthroscopic knee surgery. *Clin J Pain* 2004; 20: 256-260

25. Buerkle H, Huge V, Wolfgart M, et al. Intra-articular clonidine analgesia after knee arthroscopy. *Eur J Anaesthesiol* 2000; 17: 295-299

26. Graf J, Neusel E, Schneider E, Niethard FU. Intra-articular treatment with hyaluronic acid in osteoarthritis of the knee joint: a controlled clinical trial versus mucopolysaccharide polysulfuric acid ester. *Clin Exp Rheumatol* 1993; 11: 367-372

27. Clunie G, Lui D, Cullum I, et al. Clinical outcome after one year following samarium-153 particulate hydroxyapatite radiation synovectomy. *Scand J Rheumatol* 1996; 25: 360-366

28. Lee EB, Shin KC, Lee YJ, et al. 188Re-tin-colloid as a new therapeutic agent for rheumatoid arthritis. *Nucl Med Commun* 2003; 24: 689-696

29. Kraft O, Kasparek R, Ullmann V, et al. Our first clinical experience with radiosynoviorthesis by means of (166) Ho-holmium-boro-macroaggregates. *Nucl Med Rev Cent East Eur* 2005; 8: 131-134

30. Liggins RT, Cruz T, Min W, et al. Intra-articular treatment of arthritis with microsphere formulations of paclitaxel: Biocompatibility and efficacy determina-tions in rabbits. *Inflamm Res* 2004; 53: 363-372

31. Thakkar H, Sharma RK, Mishra AK, et al. Celecoxib incorporated chitosan microspheres: in vitro and in vivo evaluation. *J Drug Target* 2004; 12: 549-557

32. Hu Q, Zhang Z, Zhang M, et al. Study on a new antarthritic injection-O-carboxymethyl chitosan. *Sheng Wu Yi Xue Gong Cheng Xue Za Zhi* 2004; 21: 25-27

33. Adriaansen J, Tas SW, Klarenbeek PL, et al. Enhanced gene transfer to arthritic joints using adeno-associated virus type 5: implications for intra-articular gene therapy. *Ann Rheum Dis* 2005; 64: 1677-1684

34. Zhang X, Yu C, Xushi, et al. Direct chitosan-mediated gene delivery to the rabbit knee joints in vitro and in vivo. *Biochem Biophys Res Commun* 2006; 341: 202-208

35. Robbins PD, Evans CH, Chernajovsky Y. Gene therapy for arthritis. *Gene Ther* 2003; 10: 902-911

PART III

Chapter 20

Joint Pain

Gary McCleane

While individual pharmacological agents are discussed in previous chapters, this section attempts to give practical options for the management of joint pain. Specifically, this chapter will discuss options for pain relief from joint conditions that produce pain rather than those conditions in which pain is experienced over a joint but where the precipitating condition affects elsewhere. These other causes, such as, for example, in the case of referred or radiated pain, are discussed in other chapters.

To aid clarity, joint pain will be subdivided into monoarticular and polyarticular pain. In some senses this classification is somewhat false as not unusually patients identify one or a few joints as being most painful even when many other joints are sore. A list of options will be presented for both scenarios rather than treatments being placed in any order of preference. From a practical perspective such a list will allow further pharmacological options to be explored even if the initial choice fails to give the relief desired. Consideration also needs to be given as to whether therapy is used for short-term management or whether it is continued in the longer term. While ideally one option is tried at a time, ultimately treatment may involve use of a number of treatment modalities.

This chapter will focus on the treatment of pain arising in joints, not on the pathological processes initiating this pain.

Clinical Management of Bone and Joint Pain
© 2007 by The Haworth Press, Inc. All rights reserved.
doi:10.1300/5771_22

MONOARTICULAR PAIN

Topical/Transdermal Options

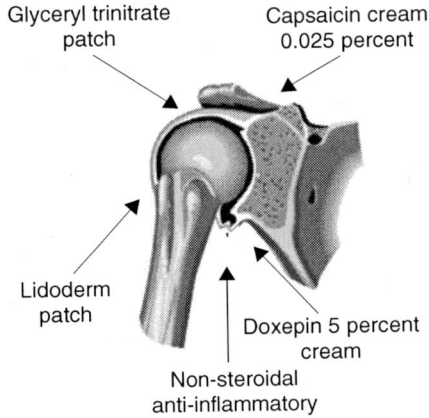

Glyceryl trinitrate patch

Capsaicin cream 0.025 percent

Lidoderm patch

Doxepin 5 percent cream

Non-steroidal anti-inflammatory

Transdermal Application (Not Necessarily Over Painful Joint)

Buprenorphine patch   Fentanyl TDDS

Intra-Articular Options

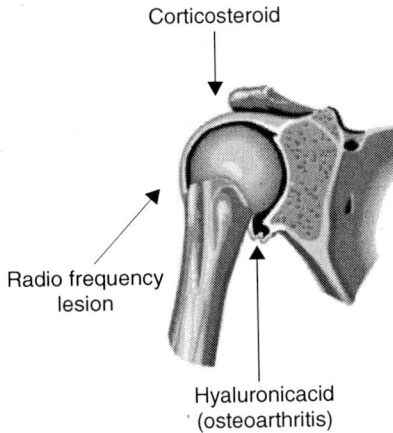

Corticosteroid

Radio frequency lesion

Hyaluronicacid (osteoarthritis)

Oral and Parenteral Options

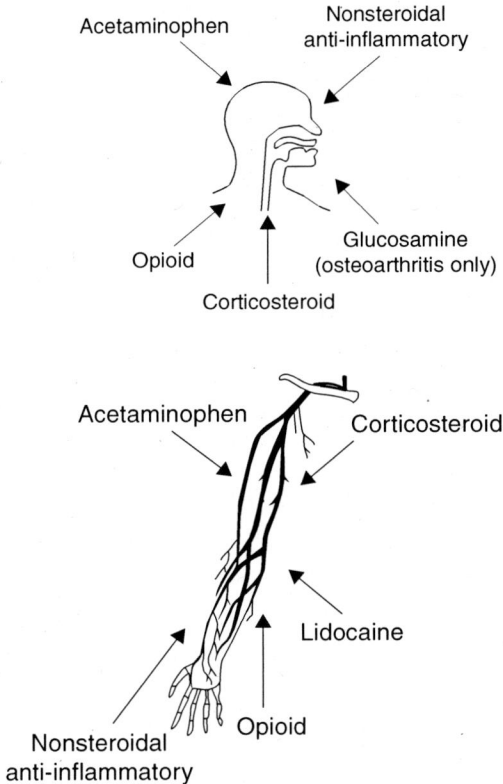

Perineural options
Nerve block (e.g., suprascapular nerve block)

POLYARTICULAR OPTIONS

All of the topical options listed here can be used on individual joints even when the pain affects multiple joints. Even with such polyarticular pain, patients will often identify one or a small number of joints as producing the worst pain: these can be targeted with the topical options, those agents with a more systemic effect being used for background pain relief for the other joints.

Transdermal Options *(Not Necessarily Over Painful Joint)*
Buprenorphine patch   Fentanyl TDDS

Oral and Parenteral Options

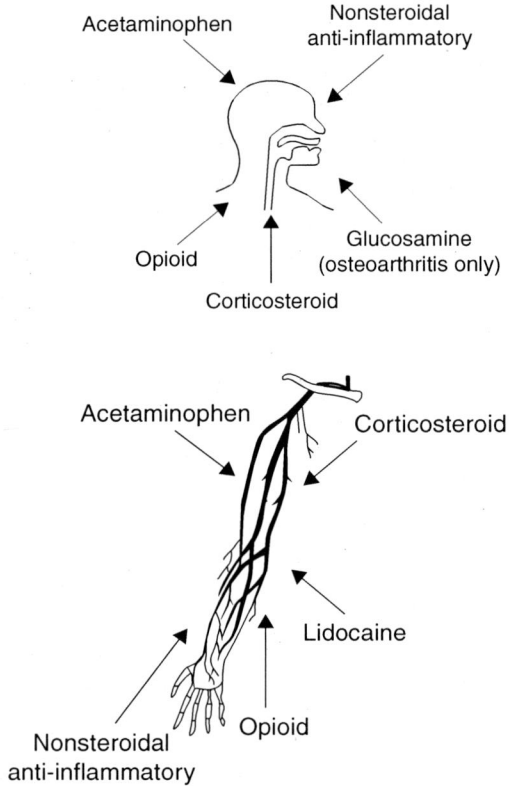

Acetaminophen   Nonsteroidal
                       anti-inflammatory

Opioid   Glucosamine
                       (osteoarthritis only)

Corticosteroid

Acetaminophen   Corticosteroid

                       Lidocaine

Nonsteroidal   Opioid
anti-inflammatory

Chapter 21

Fracture Pain

Gary McCleane

It goes without saying that the optimal treatment of pain emanating from a bone fracture is stabilization of the fracture with either surgical or nonsurgical methods. However, under some circumstances such stabilization is delayed, inadequate, or not possible and there is then a need for pharmacological intervention. In isolated cases stabilization is rarely undertaken, and in these situations management is almost entirely pharmacological. For example, treatment of rib fractures involves pain reduction by drug treatment and not stabilization.

The surgical management of bone fractures is beyond the scope of this book. The management of bone pain arising from infiltration of bone by tumor deposits is addressed in Chapter 22, although to some extent the methods outlined there will have relevance in this section as well. Simple pharmacological treatment of fracture pain revolves around use of acetaminophen, nonsteroidal anti-inflammatory drugs (NSAIDs), and mild opioid analgesics. There seems little merit discussing these options, which are covered elsewhere. Indeed, if pain relief were guaranteed by these options then this chapter would be superfluous. The lack of consistent pain relief when used for fracture pain treatment, however, dictates a consideration of other methods of analgesic management. Again, none of these other options to be considered has universal efficacy, and so an awareness of a range of alternate treatments is of greater use than an in depth understanding of single treatment options.

Clinical Management of Bone and Joint Pain
© 2007 by The Haworth Press, Inc. All rights reserved.
doi:10.1300/5771_23

IS FRACTURE PAIN ADEQUATELY TREATED?

Those that have witnessed a patient who has suffered from a bone fracture, or indeed have personal experience of having suffered from a fracture, can testify to the pain experienced. While stabilization can do much to reduce pain, it may not remove it completely.

Morgan-Jones (1996) undertook an audit of 100 consecutive patients who had suffered from an acute injury. He found that in the first 24 hours after hospital admission, 9 percent of patients received no analgesia whatsoever. In a further 14 percent, analgesia was prescribed, but not actually given. Further inadequacies were revealed by the narrow range of analgesics offered along with inappropriate routes of administration and dosing interval.

White and colleagues (2000) studied the Emergency Medical Services call reports of patients requiring hospital admission with extremity fractures over a 13 month period. The records of 1,073 patients were considered. Only 18 patients (1.8 percent) received analgesia (16 nitrous oxide and 2 morphine) prior to hospital admission.

Even when admitted to hospital, provision of analgesia is far from universal. Brown and colleagues (2003) considered 2,828 patients admitted to an emergency department with extremity or clavicular fractures. Overall 64 percent received an analgesic that was a narcotic in 42 percent. In those with moderate to severe pain, 73 percent received an analgesic that was a narcotic in 54 percent of the cases. The frequency with which analgesia was given to children was lower than with adults.

Proportion of Patients with Extremity or Clavicular Fracture Given Analgesics According to Age

Age	Proportion given any analgesic (percent)	Proportion given narcotic analgesic (percent)
0-3	54	21
4-8	63	30
9-15	60	27
16-29	67	47
30-69	68	51
≥70	58	41

Various interpretations of this data are possible. Among these are that there may be a prescription bias against using analgesics in the young and elderly or that the fractures in the young and more elderly patients may induce less pain.

PHARMACOLOGICAL OPTIONS

Inhalational

Nitrous Oxide

Inhaled nitrous oxide has a long tradition in fracture pain management and is often used to facilitate patient transfer, fracture reduction, and splint application. However, those from an anesthesiological background will point out that the analgesia provided by nitrous oxide is inconsistent. Some patients derive quick and effective pain relief while others seem resistant to its use. Nitrous oxide should never be administered on its own but in conjunction with oxygen to avoid a potentially hypoxic mixture.

Topical Skin

Glyceryl Trinitrate

As previously described, topically applied nitrates, such as glyceryl trinitrate, can have a local analgesic and anti-inflammatory effect. The only major side effect is nitrate headache, the risk of which can be reduced by using a smaller dose patch. While usually not sufficient on its own to reduce the pain of an acute fracture, it can be utilized in combination with other treatment modalities or as a sole analgesic when a natural reduction in the fracture pain has begun.

Lidoderm

Despite its indication for the treatment of postherpetic neuralgia, Lidoderm patches can provide analgesia in a number of conditions. While probably inadequate to provide analgesia on its own after acute fracture, it becomes useful when used in combination with other analgesic interventions in the acute situation or on its own after the initial acute phase. Particularly useful in the treatment of pain from fractured ribs.

Fentanyl

Transdermal fentanyl (25, 50, or 75 µg/hour) can provide useful background analgesia. Each patch remains applied for 72 hours during which a steady state for the drug is achieved.

Topical Mucous Membrane

Diamorphine

Desirable characteristics of any analgesic used in fracture pain treatment are efficacy, speed of onset, and ease of administration. A widely used method of acute analgesic administration is by intramuscular injection of an opioid such as morphine. It could be well argued that an intravenous administration of that opioid would be more appropriate, but the reality is in clinical practice that intramuscular injection is more widely used and accepted by clinical staff than intravenous use. Despite which method is contemplated, some patients, and in particular children, dislike any form of injection. It is known that the nasal mucous membrane is a well-perfused structure and that a variety of drugs can be administered by application to this membrane.

In a randomized controlled trial of 404 patients aged 3 to 16 years who had suffered a bone fracture, Kendall and colleagues (2001) compared the analgesic effect of nasally inhaled diamorphine 0.1 mg/kg with 0.2 mg/kg of intramuscular morphine. Lower pain scores were observed in patients given nasal diamorphine at 5, 10, and 20 min after administration when compared with IM morphine. By 30 min pain scores were similar. Eighty percent of the patients given nasal diamorphine showed no obvious sign of discomfort as compared with 9 percent in the IM morphine group. A result was obtained by Wilson and colleagues (1997), who found that nasal diamorphine was rated as "acceptable" in all of the parents of children who had limb fractures as compared with only 55 percent of those in the IM morphine group.

Fentanyl

While transdermal fentanyl has use as a background treatment of fracture pain, it is unlikely to provide much relief when movement of a fracture is likely as during patient transfer or splint application. In these circumstances fentanyl lozenges/lollipops can provide rapid-onset, intense analgesia.

Oral

NSAIDs

These are one of the primary building blocks of fracture pain management. They are used either alone, or often with added value when used in combination with other agents. Selection of which NSAID to use is largely based on personal preference and experience.

Opioids

Opioid analgesics have much merit in the short-term management of fractures, but are better at reducing the background pain that accompanies a fracture rather than the acute pain associated with movement. Given their propensity to induce constipation, prophylactic measures to prevent this eventuality are advisable. Those analgesics that contain codeine are not universally effective as a proportion of the population lack the cytochrome P450 enzyme necessary to convert codeine to morphine and hence to activate it. The same difficulty does not occur with dihydrocodeine or tramadol.

For more severe pain, strong opioids may be necessary. For the most acute situations, immediate-release strong opioids should be selected, while for less acute situations, sustained-release preparations supplemented by immediate release for breakthrough pain.

Acetaminophen

When used at appropriate doses, oral acetaminophen is an effective analgesic with a relatively benign side-effect profile. Only in overdose does it become less safe. Regular dosing with acetaminophen, often with a NSAID, is an effective treatment that should be instituted early and only supplemented with other agents or techniques if therapeutic failure occurs.

Muscle Relaxants

Skeletal muscle relaxants have no analgesic effect for pure bone fracture pain. However, muscle spasm is a frequent accompaniment of any fracture and can be painful by itself, but most importantly increases fracture pain by compounding the malalignment of fractured bone. Fracture reduction and stabilization may by themselves reduce or remove muscle spasm, but where it remains troublesome, a skeletal muscle relaxant drug may be indicated. Baclofen has a fairly rapid onset of action and a favorable side-effect profile and can be used in adults at a dose of 15 to 60 mg daily in three divided doses. Where muscle spasm becomes chronic, other agents such as dantrolene or tizanadine may be considered. Alternatively, if the spasm is confined to a well-defined muscle or muscle group, then Botulinum toxin injection may become an option.

Parenteral

Opioids

Parenteral administration of strong opioids is appropriate in the acute situation after fracture, when flare-ups of pain are expected (movement, splint application, etc.) and in the face of failure with other analgesic interventions. Parenteral morphine or oxycodone may be preferable to shorter-acting opiates such as meperidine.

Acetaminophen

The recent availability of an intravenous formulation of acetaminophen offers a new alternative to fracture pain management. A 1 g infusion of acetaminophen has comparable analgesic effect to 10 mg morphine. Indeed, parenteral acetaminophen may be preferable to parenteral strong opioid as the risks of nausea, sedation, and respiratory depression are avoided.

Ketamine

The intramuscular or intravenous administration of ketamine at correct doses is associated with pain relief which can be profound. At greater doses it becomes anesthetic. Consequently, ketamine can be used to facilitate fracture reduction and splint application.

Ketamine has some merit in that it maintains blood pressure which contrasts it with other potentially anesthetic agents. However, excess salivation can occur and patients may experience unpleasant dreams and hallucinations when it is used, and so its utility is limited.

Lidocaine

Anecdotal evidence suggests that the intravenous administration of lidocaine can have a significant analgesic effect with a variety of fractures and most particularly with rib fractures. Indeed the pain relief apparent after IV lidocaine can far outlast the half-life of the drug. Lidocaine infusion is not associated with side effects of opioids such as nausea, sedation, or respiratory depression, and even cardiovascular side effects, which one would intuitively associate with lidocaine use, are rare. Clinically doses of 1000 to 1200 mg over a 24 hour period can be used with dose adjustment depending on the size, age, and health status of the patient.

Perineural

Nerve Blocks

Single-shot nerve bocks are of little value in all but the most acute of situations, where they may reduce the worst excesses of fracture pain until more definitive treatment is instituted. Examples of where these single-shot nerve bocks may be of value include femoral or "three in one" blocks for femoral fractures, intercostals, or paravertebral blocks for rib fractures and suprascapular nerve blocks for upper humeral fractures and shoulder dislocations. A longer-lasting local anesthetic such as bupivicaine is preferable to those with less prolonged durations of effect.

Nerve blocks can be used to allow fracture manipulation and splint application: brachial plexus block being used for upper limb fracture manipulation and femoral nerve block for femoral fracture interventions.

A further technique that can allow manipulation or intervention on upper limb fractures is the intravenous regional block ("Bier's block"), where lidocaine is given intravenously on the affected side after a cuff is inflated above systolic pressure on that limb proximally. Good practice suggests that in fact a double cuff is used to minimize the risk of systemic leakage of the lidocaine.

A more localized technique is the hematoma block, usually used for distal forearm fractures, where local anesthetic is injected into the fracture hematoma.

Epidurals

The major utilization of epidurally administered drugs is in the management of rib fractures and chest trauma. Given that no operated intervention is normally possible for rib fractures, pain relief is a fundamental goal in rib fracture management.

TREATMENT OF SPECIFIC FRACTURES

Rib Fractures

Even isolated rib fractures can be the cause of morbidity and mortality. The impairment of respiratory function that is the almost inevitable consequence of the pain associated with a rib fracture can be enough to induce respiratory failure in those with pre-existent respiratory disease. When these fractures are multiple, even those with previous good health can be pushed into respiratory failure. When major trauma is involved, rib fractures may be associated with lung contusion and injury, which increases the risk of complication.

By their nature, rib fractures are not normally amenable to surgical fixation. The basis of treatment is therefore adequate pain relief. The full range of treatment options outlined earlier can be utilized. Because of the close relationship between rib fractures and respiratory function, the adequacy of treatment can be measured by undertaking simple respiratory tests. For example, when the effect of intravenous fentanyl is compared with the extradural infusion of the same dose of fentanyl, the effect can be compared by measuring vital capacity, $PaCO_2$, PaO_2, SaO_2, and so on. When this is done, extradural infusion of fentanyl appears to improve these parameters more so than intravenous infusion of the same dose.

A variety of specific local anesthetic techniques have gained popularity in the management of rib fracture pain. Their principal appeal is that they allow a greater depth of inspiration and active events such as coughing to be undertaken in a more normal fashion. In contrast to the use of strong opioids, this effect is produced without significant sedation or respiratory depression. While single-shot blocking procedures, such as the intercostal nerve block, often produce pain relief, their duration of effect is only as long as the duration of action of the local anesthetic used. Therefore, infusion techniques a more appropriate.

One such technique is the intrapleural infusion of a local anesthetic such as bupivicaine. An epidural type catheter is inserted intercostally and bupivicaine infused. In terms of results obtained, Haenel and colleagues (1995) found that this technique was effective in their group of patients who had failed to respond to intravenous opioids provided with a patient-controlled analgesia device. Not all reports of this technique are of positive results. Short and colleagues (1996) studied 16 patients with chest wall trauma. Their patients had a 24 hour infusion of both saline (placebo) and a lidocaine/bupivicaine combination at differing times and found no differences in the pain relief obtained.

A second local anesthetic technique involves the insertion of a catheter into the paravertebral space and the infusion of a local anesthetic with the most popular choice being bupivicaine. When rib fractures are unilateral this is a viable option. When they are bilateral, it is not.

Perhaps the most common local anesthetic intervention is the thoracic epidural infusion. Utilization of this technique has become the norm when simple interventions fail and when signs of respiratory impairment become apparent. In many instances the insertion of a thoracic epidural catheter and the infusion of a local anesthetic, usually in combination with an opioid, can prevent the need to institute mechanical ventilation because of the respiratory impairment caused by the pain from the fractured ribs. Even when ventilation is required, a thoracic epidural allows a lower level of sedation to be used and aids in weaning from ventilation.

A less common local anesthetic intervention is the intravenous infusion of lidocaine. When lidocaine is given intravenously, pain relief is often produced without the expected complication of numbness. Cardiovascular side effects are in reality rare. Clinical practice suggests that in a healthy adult a dose of 1000 mg of lidocaine infused over 24 hours has a reasonable chance of producing pain relief.

In the case of a sternal, as opposed to rib fracture, an additional local anesthetic technique exists. A catheter can be inserted subpereiostally in the sternum, close to the fracture and local anesthetic, with or without an opioid infused.

Treatment of Rib Fractures

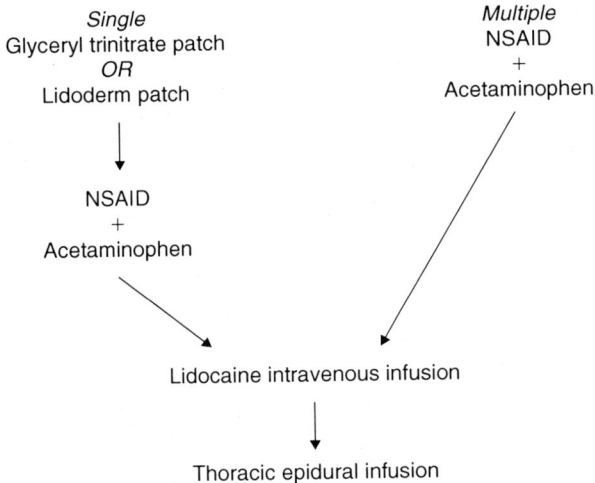

Single
Glyceryl trinitrate patch
OR
Lidoderm patch

↓

NSAID
+
Acetaminophen

Multiple
NSAID
+
Acetaminophen

Lidocaine intravenous infusion

↓

Thoracic epidural infusion

Femoral Fractures

It goes without saying that the pain from a major long-bone fracture is severe and that simple analgesic techniques are rarely sufficient to obtund this pain. Fortunately the nerve supply to the upper femur is relatively easily accessed and therefore amenable to local anesthetic techniques. Deposition of long-lasting local anesthetic, such as bupivicaine, around the femoral nerve can give partial relief. When a larger volume is used, a so-called "three-in-one block" can be achieved—the femoral, lateral cutaneous, and quadratus femoris nerves are all blocked. Alternatively a fascia iliaca compartment block can be used. While a variety of studies have suggested benefit of these blocks over use of strong opioid analgesics, the Cochrane Database Systematic Review by Parker and colleagues (2001) concluded that the studies available at that time failed to definitively show that any of these techniques offered advantage over other analgesic benefits, although these conclusions were generated by a small number of studies which included relatively few patients.

Vertebral Collapse Fractures

In the fit and healthy, considerable force is required to fracture a vertebra. In the patient with osteoporosis this can happen with forces that would otherwise be inconsequential. As with any fracture, immediate pain is normal after the fracture. What is more problematical is that pain can be a long-term consequence of such a fracture. When a vertebral body is traumatized to the extent that fracture occurs, its physical shape is often altered. A vertebral body exists in a dynamic structure/function relationship to its surrounding structures, and so with a change in shape, its architectural relationships change as well. The list of alterations that can occur is long (see Figure 21.1 for a graphic representation):

> Posterior longitudinal ligament
> Facet joint
> Interspinous ligament
> Paravertebral muscles
> Spinal cord
> Spinal nerve
> Intervertebral disc
> Anterior longitudinal ligament

Each one of these structures can give rise to pain. For example, unnatural stresses on an interspinous ligament can give rise to localized pain over the ligament with pain worse on back flexion. On occasions this is accompanied by a referred pain in the dermatomal distribution

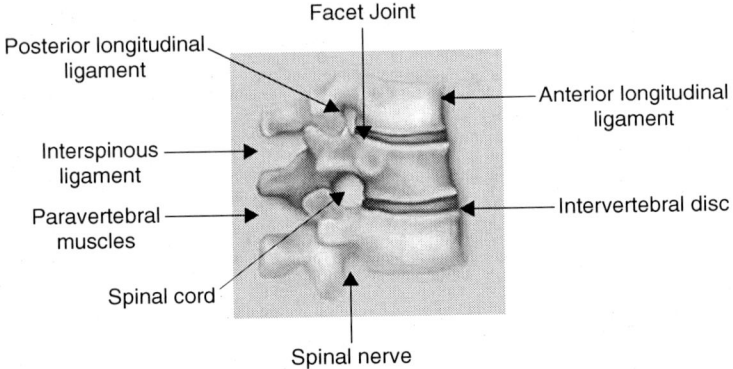

FIGURE 21.1. Examples of structures that can be disrupted by a vertebral fracture.

of the spinal nerves arising at that level. Being a midline structure, these ligaments often give rise to referred pain that is bilaterally experienced. More problematical is pain that arises from structures such as the anterior longitudinal ligament that has a sympathetic innervation and elements of the disc margin that have both somatic and sympathetic innervation. The quality and distribution of the pain arising from disruption of these structures is poorly defined.

When nerve impingement occurs, a radiated neuropathic pain is the consequence, and is suggested by the usually diagnostic symptoms and signs of neuropathic pain (e.g., paresthesia, numbness, allodynia, and lancinating pain). Therefore, adequate treatment of the longer-term pain that can occur with a vertebral collapse fracture requires a diagnosis as to which structure, or structures, are giving rise to the pain. Only then can there be significant hope of good-quality pain relief.

Alternatives for Treatment of Vertebral Fracture Pain— Medium and Long Term

<u>Interspinous ligament</u>
   NSAID
   Capsaicin
   GTN Patch

Lidoderm Patch
Local anesthetic/steroid injection
<u>Muscle spasm</u>
  Baclofen
  Methocarbamol
  Cyclobenzaprine
  Dantrolene
  Botulinum toxin
  NSAID
<u>Radiated/referred pain</u>
  Pregabalin
  Gabapentin
  Lamotrigine
  Oxcarbazepine
  Carbamazepine
  Tricyclic antidepressant

BIBLIOGRAPHY

Inadequate Treatment of Fracture Pain

Brown JC, Klein EJ, Lewis CW, Johnston BD, Cummings P. Emergency department analgesia for fracture pain. *Ann Emerg Med* 2003; 42: 197-205.
Morgan-Jones R. *Injury* 1996; 27: 539-541.
White LJ, Cooper JD, Chambers RM, Gradisek RE. Prehospital use of analgesia for suspected extremity fracture. *Prehosp Emerg Care* 2000; 4: 205-208.

Topical Options

Kendall JM, Reeves BC, Latter VS. Multicenter randomised controlled trial of nasal diamorphine for analgesia in children and teenagers with clinical fractures. *BMJ* 2001; 322: 261-265.
Wilson JA, Kendall JM, Cornelius P. Intranasal diamorphine for paediatric analgesia: assessment of safety and efficacy. *J Accid Emerg Med* 1997; 14: 70-72.

Oral Options—Codeine

Williams DG, Patel A, Howard RF. Pharmacogenetics of codeine metabolism in an urban population of children and its implications for analgesic reliability. *Br J Anaes* 2002; 89: 839-845.

Yu A, Kneller BM, Rettie AE, Haining RL. Expression, purification, biochemical characterisation, and comparative function of human cytochrome P450 2D6.1, 2D6.2, 2D6.10 and 2D6.17 allelic isoforms. *J Pharmacol Exp Ther* 2002; 303: 1291-1300.

Treatment of Specific Conditions—Rib Fractures

Duncan MA, McNicholas W, O'Keefe D, O'Reilly M. Periosteal infusion of bupivicaine/morphine post sternal fracture: A new analgesic technique. *Reg Anesth Pain Med* 2002; 27: 316-318.

Gabram SG, Schwartz RJ, Jacobs LM et al. Clinical management of blunt trauma patients with unilateral rib fractures: A randomized trial. *World J Surg* 1995; 19: 388-393.

Govindarajan R, Bakalova T, Michael R, Abadir AR. Epidural buprenorphine in management of pain in multiple rib fractures. *Acta Anaesthesiol Scand* 2002; 46: 660-665.

Haenel JB, Moore FA, Moore EE, Sauaia A, Read RA, Burch JM. Extrapleural bupivicaine for amelioration of multiple rib fracture pain. *J Trauma* 1995; 38: 22-27.

Karmakar MK, Chui PT, Joynt GM, Ho AM. Thoracic paravertebral block for management of pain associated with multiple fractured ribs in patients with concomitant lumbar spinal trauma. *Reg Anesth Pain Mang* 2001; 26: 169-173.

Karmakar MK, Critchley LAH, Ho AM, Gin T, Lee TW, Yim AP. Continuous thoracic paravertebral infusion of bupivicaine for pain management in patients with multiple fractured ribs. *Chest* 2003; 123: 424-431.

Mackersie RC, Karagianes TG, Hoyt DB, Davis JW. Prospective evaluation of epidural and intravenous administration of fentanyl for pain control and restoration of ventilatory function following multiple rib fractures. *J Trauma* 1991; 31: 443-449.

Short K, Scheeres D, Mlaker J, Dean R. Evaluation of intrapleural analgesia in the management of blunt traumatic chest wall pain: A clinical trial. *Am Surg* 1996; 62: 488-493.

Treatment of Specific Conditions—Femoral Fractures

Candal-Couto JJ, McVie JL, Haslam N, Innes AR, Rushmer J. Pre-operative analgesia for patients with femoral neck fractures using a modified fascia iliaca block technique. *Injury* 2005; 36; 505-510.

Chu RS, Browne GJ, Cheng NG, Lam LT. Femoral nerve block for femoral shaft fractures in a paediatric Emergency Department: Can it be done better? *Eur J Emerg Med* 2003; 10: 258-263.

Fletcher AK, Rigby AS, Heyes FL. Three-in-one femoral nerve block as analgesia for fractured neck of femur in the emergency department: A randomized, controlled trial. *Ann Emerg Med* 2003; 41: 227-233.

Lopez S, Gros T, Bernard N, Plasse C, Capdevila X. Fascia iliaca compartment block for femoral bone fractures in prehospital care. *Reg Anesth Pain Med* 2003; 28: 203-207.

Parker MJ, Griffiths R, Appadu BN. Nerve blocks (subcostal, lateral cutaneous, femoral, triple, psoas) for hip fractures. *Cochrane Database Syst Rev* 2001; 1: CD001159.

Van Leeuwen FL, Bronselaer K, Gilles M, Sabbe M, Delooz HH. The "three in one" block as locoregional analgesia in an emergency department. *Eur J Emerg Med* 2000; 7: 35-38.

Chapter 22

Pathophysiology and Analgesic Approaches to Painful Bone Metastasis

Howard S. Smith
Jennifer A. Elliott

INTRODUCTION

The mechanisms of bone pain in osseous metastatic lesions remain unclear but are almost certain to be multifactorial. Bone metastases may lead to pain via stimulation of nociceptors by algesic mediators (e.g., cytokines, PGE2, bradykinin, serotonin, and substance P). Involvement/invasion, stretching, or compression of pain-sensitive structures, such as nerves, vasculature, periosteum, various joint structures, and microfractures, may also lead to pain.

Pain from osseous metastatic lesions also may occur from mechanical instability of "weakened bone" or high intraosseous pressures (>50 mmHg).[1] In addition to osseous and tumor etiologies for the pain of bone metastases, proalgesic substances may contribute such as cytokines, inflammatory mediators, vasoactive intestinal peptide (VIP), matrix metallo proteinases (MMPs), endothelin 1, osteoclasts, and the acidic environment of bone resorption (e.g., protons activating the TRPV1 and/or acid-sensing ion channel [ASIC] receptors). See Figure 22.1 and Table 22.1.

The main culprit in bone destruction is the osteoclast. A second minor and later mechanism is tumor-mediated osteolysis. In addition, tumor involvement can compromise osseous vascular supply, leading

Clinical Management of Bone and Joint Pain
© 2007 by The Haworth Press, Inc. All rights reserved.
doi:10.1300/5771_24

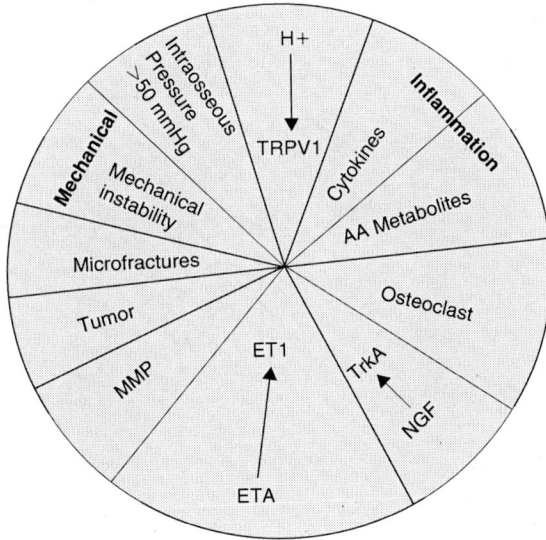

FIGURE 22.1. Potential mechanisms of pain in bone metastasis.

TABLE 22.1. Potential analgesic treatment strategies.

Mechanism	Treatment
Mechanical	Brace/Immobilize
	Steroids
	Radiation
	Surgery
Tumor	Chemotherapy
	Radiation
	Surgery
ET1	ETB AR Antagonist
AA Metabolites	Steroids
	NSAIDs (esp. if penetrate acid environment)
Inflammatory (Cytokines) Growth Factors	Steroids
	VIP
MMPs	TIMPs
	Tetracyclines

TABLE 22.1 *(continued)*

Mechanism	Treatment
	CMT (chemically modified tetracyclines)
	VIP
	Other
Osteoclasts	OPG (osteoprotegerin)
	Bisphosphonates
	Radiation
	Calcitonin
	Interferon—γ
H^+	TRPV2 1 antagonists (iodo-resiniferatoxin)
	ASIC
NGF	Anti-NGF antibody

to bone necrosis/destruction. Bone formation can occur by multiple mechanisms. Reactive bone formation (e.g., the usual response of bone to fracture) occurs commonly[2]; however, certain tumor cells may induce ossification of fibrous stroma (e.g., osteoblastic metastases with abundant stroma).

Widespread metastasis occurs after the primary tumor has "seede" the lymphatic and vascular channels to carry tumor cells to distant osseous sites. The tumor cells undergo endothelial attachment and are then able to make their way into the substance of the bone. Once the tumor cell is situated in bone and has "set up shop," growth can occur through tumor angiogenesis factors, attracting new vasculature.[2] Bone destruction takes place predominantly via vigorous osteoclast activity. Several tumors (e.g., breast, prostate, and lung) produce and secrete osteoclastic activators including transforming growth factor, prostaglandins, interleukins, tumor necrosis factor, and platelet-derived growth factor. Also, granulocyte-macrophage colony-stimulating factors, parathyroid hormone-related protein, procathepsin D, and 5-lipoxygenase metabolites (e.g., 5-hydroxyeicosatetraenoic acid and leukotrienes) stimulate isolated osteoclasts to resorb bone *in vitro*.

PATHOPHYSIOLOGY OF BONE RESORPTION

Although there are numerous contributing factors leading to the pain of osseous metastases, a significant portion of the pain seems to be related to osteoclastic bone resorption. Osteoclasts solubilize the mineral (e.g., hydroxyapatite) and degrade the organic matrix (e.g., type 1 collagen) with cysteine-proteinases. The bone resorption occurs in an acidic microenvironment produced by proton secretion via vacuolar H^+-ATPases in osteoclastic membranes. The first step in the process of bone resorption is that the osteoclast adheres to the bone surface. This adherence is mediated by specific membrane receptors. Podosomes are osteoclastic processes, which become the primary attachment sites to bone. The podosomes are made up of integrins and cytoskeletal proteins—actin microfilaments surrounded by vinculin and talin.[3] See Figure 22.2.

The predominant attachment sites are the vitronectin receptors (e.g., α and β_3 integrin), which recognizes the RGD (Arg-Gly-Asp) amino acid sequence in various bone matrix proteins (osteopontin, vitronectin, and bone sialoprotein).[3]

A highly convoluted membrane area termed the *ruffled border and sealing zone* appears in the osteoclast during bone resorption. The accumulation of podosomes at the bone surface occurs first with ligand

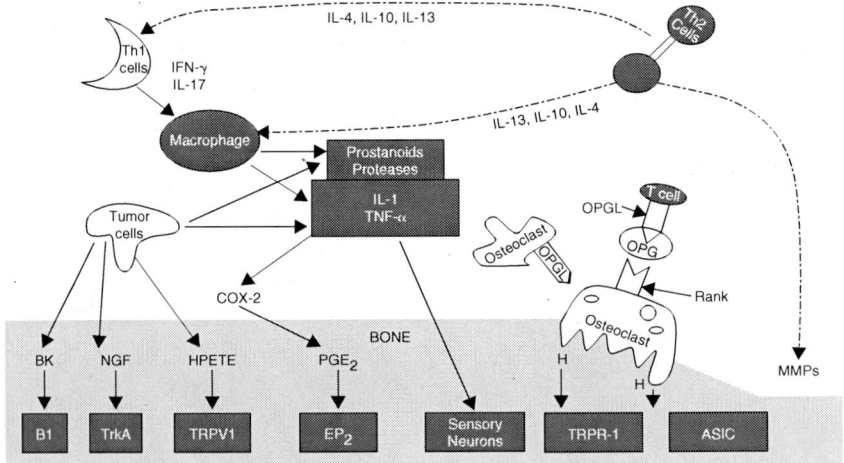

FIGURE 22.2. Algesic mediators of painful bone metastasis.

binding to the vitronectin receptor.[3] Subsequently a tight sealing zone is formed where osteoclastic acid and proteases are secreted to resorb bone. The sealing zone is completed as actively resorbing osteoclasts reorganize elements to form a "double circle" of vinculin and talin around a core of F-actin.[3]

c-Src-dependent tyrosine phosphorylation of PYK2 may be an important regulatory step promoting significant podosomal changes—with actin formation of a dense belt-like structure [involving vinculin, talin, vitronectin receptor (α_v and β_3 integrin)], leading to formation of the sealing zones.[4,5] PYK2, a member of the focal adhesion kinase family is the major adhesion-dependent kinase in osteoclasts.[5] Ligand binding or receptor clustering induces PYK2 phosphorylation of Src kinase in osteoclasts with c-Src, PYK2, and actin forming a stable complex on osteoclast adhesion.[5] PYK2 associates with p130 (an adaptor protein), and downstream signaling may involve recruitment of PI3-K to the cytoskeleton.[5]

Potential strategies, which may impair osteoclastic attachment and therefore function, include bafilomycin A1 (specific inhibitor of vacuolar and H^+-ATPase), or peptides with the RGD sequence, and/or other agents that may interfere with vinculin, talin, and/or F-actin (e.g., colchicine). Decoy RGD sequence peptides or agents adversely affecting vinculin, talin, or F-action may inhibit osteoclast attachment to the bone surface.

OSTEOCLAST OSTEOLYSIS

The osteoclast is affected by multiple influences. The first is a ryanodine receptor-like molecule on the cell surface, which acts as a divalent cation sensor.[3] A transient rise in cytosolic calcium results from this receptor-binding divalent cations, which then contributes to osteoclast regulation. Another means of osteoclast regulation is via its calcitonin receptor, which couples with G proteins. Osteoclasts are inhibited by phosphonates,[6] calcitonin,[7] and calcitonin gene-related peptide as well as multiple other factors.[7]

The interaction between osteoclasts and osteoblasts appears to result in osteoclast differentiation, a process that must occur to initiate osteoclastic activity. Tumor cells induce the interaction between osteoclasts and osteoblasts, and once the interaction occurs, osteoclasts increase in size, number, and activity. The accelerated bone destruction that occurs due to this process in patients with cancer may result in pain via several mechanisms. These include aberrant release of neurotransmitters such as substance P, causing stimulation of nerve fibers in the bone marrow, mineralized bone, and the periosteum. In addition, because osteoclasts destroy bone by forming an acidic compartment, nerve fibers sensitive to pH changes within the bone may be activated, resulting in pain (see Figure 22.2). Eventually, advanced bone destruction by osteoclastic activity may result in loss of mechanical strength in the bone, causing painful pathologic fractures that significantly limit patient mobility and quality of life. In addition to these mechanisms, it is apparent in animal models of advanced bone cancer pain that spinal cord changes and remodeling occur indicating the development of central sensitization (Figure 22.2).

MODULATION OF OSTEOCLASTIC ACTIVITY MODULATES NOCICEPTION

If much of the pain from metastatic bone lesions results from the effects of osteoclastic activity, then "shutting down" the osteoclasts is paramount to the analgesic treatment. Osteoclast bone-resorbing activity is dependent on the binding of the tumor necrosis factor (TNF) family molecule—osteoprotegerin ligand (OPGL),[8] which is expressed on activated T-cells and osteoblasts—to a receptor termed *receptor activator of nuclear kB* (NF-κB), abbreviated RANK.[8] RANK is expressed on osteoclast precursors and mature osteoclasts.[9] Any treatment that impedes the OPGL-RANK interaction will impair RANK activation and therefore impair osteoclastic activity and bone resorption. Osteoprotegerin (OPG) is a soluble TNF receptor molecule that is secreted and binds to the RANK-activating site of OPGL, acting as a "dummy" or "decoy" receptor, thereby preventing OPGL from binding to and activating the osteoclast RANK receptor (essentially by serving as a "lid or cap" covering the RANK-activating site of OPGL, Figure 22.2).[8,10,11]

Other terminology has been used for some of the aforementioned factors. Terms that have been used in the literature for OPGL include osteoclast differentiation factor and TNF-related activation-induced cytokine (receptor activator of nuclear factor κB ligand; RANKL).[12]

A term that has been used in the literature for RANK is osteoclast differentiation and activation receptor. Also, osteoprotegerin has been referred to as osteoclastogenesis inhibitor factor.

A series of elegant experiments demonstrated that OPG will "shut down" osteoclast activity, resulting in "analgesia" and significant improvement in pain behavior.[13-15] The mechanism by which osteoprotegerin appears to work is by preventing the interaction between osteoblasts and osteoclasts that is required for osteoclast differentiation/activity. In the absence of this interaction, the osteoclast precursor cells will die via apoptosis. Furthermore, it is conceivable that osteoclastic-induced algesia may in various situations be somewhat related to a RANKL-OPG imbalance with increased RANKL-OPG ratios (see Figure 22.3).

In a rat model of advanced bone cancer, osteoprotegerin administration halted further bone destruction, as confirmed radiographically. This occurred within 2 days of its administration. In this same animal model, an apparent decrease by 50 percent in ongoing and movement-evoked pain was found when testing the animals (a decrease in spontaneous flinches indicating decreased ongoing pain, and increased withdrawal threshold to palpation indicating decreased movement-evoked pain). Researchers have found that OPG may be effective in stabilizing bone destruction and reducing pain even in very advanced stages of bone destruction. It was also noted that, upon histologic examination, there was a reduction in the neurohumoral changes in the spinal cords of these animals as compared with those with bone cancer that did not receive OPG. This would appear to indicate a reduction in central sensitization related to OPG administration.[13-15]

Agents other than OPG may potentially contribute to "shutting down osteoclasts" include bisphosphonates[6] and interleukin-18 (IL-

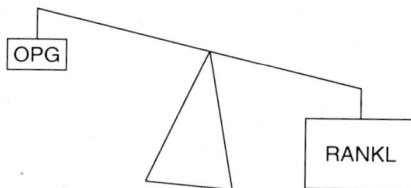

FIGURE 22.3. RANKL-OPG imbalance: RANKL-OPG ratio associated with increased osteoclastic-induced algesia.

18), which is a product of osteoblast-like cells and activated macrophages.[16] IL-18 inhibits osteoclast formation by inducing T-cells to produce granulocyte-macrophage colony-stimulating factor (G-MCSF).[16] Vasoactive intestinal peptide (VIP) may produce favorable analgesic effects in the treatment of painful osseous metastases via promoting Th-2 lymphocyte derived cytokines as well as boosting IL-4-mediated induction of OPG and suppressing TNF-α/IL-1.

Bisphosphonates may actually inhibit osteoclastic activity through stimulating OPG production (although that may only account for a small contribution part of bisphosphonate actions).[17] Of the bisphosphonates studied, zoledronic acid in particular may be of benefit in bone cancer. In an animal model of bone cancer, treatment with 30 mcg/kg of zoledronic acid on a repeated basis resulted in a significant reduction in bone destruction versus that seen in animals with bone cancer that were not given such treatment.[18] In addition to these radiographically observed findings, there was evidence of improvement in bone mineral density and bone mineral content in the zoledronic-acid-treated animals as compared with the untreated animals with bone cancer.[18] Mechanical allodynia and mechanical hyperalgesia were both attenuated in animals receiving zoledronic acid therapy, whereas use of celecoxib and pamidronate did not appear to provide benefit with regards to mechanical allodynia and hyperalgesia.[18] Thus, zoledronic acid may modify the course of bone cancer by minimizing tumor burden in bone and associated bone destruction, as well as pain from these lesions.[18]

Phytoestrogens (e.g., soy) may also stimulate OPG production and may be a "natural" alternative to inhibiting osteoclastic activities.[19]

Platelet products may stimulate osteoclast-like cells via prostaglandin/RANK-dependent mechanism,[20] thus making platelets a potential therapeutic target in certain situations of inflammatory bone pain.

Lumiracoxib, a highly selective COX-2 inhibitor, is in clinical trials and may be considered for the treatment of osteoarthritis, rheumatoid arthritis, and pain.[21,22] Compared with diclofenac, COX-189 has substantially reduced affinity for COX-1, being 300-fold less potent. The pKa of COX-189 is 4.3. COX-189 is predicted to be particularly effective in a low-pH environment. This may be beneficial for pain relief in sites of metastatic bone lesions where the local microenvironment is acidic in nature. In a rat model of bone cancer pain, chronic lumiracoxib treatment reduced mechanical hyperalgesia and allodynia, as well as significantly attenuating bone destruction induced by tumor cell injection.[23]

Furthermore, administration of matrix metalloproteinase inhibitors (e.g., chemically modified tetracyclines) may potentially have favorable analgesic effects for the treatment of painful osseous metatstases.

There may be other promising new therapeutic options for the treatment of painful osseous metastases in the future. The acid-sensing ion channel, TRPV1 receptor, appears to contribute to bone cancer pain, and mice administered RPV1 antagonists as well as TRPV1-knockout mice exhibited reduced pain behavior.[24] In a mouse model of bone cancer pain, pharmacologic blockade of the bradykinin B1 receptor appears effective in reducing bone-cancer-pain-related behaviors, suggesting that B1 antagonists might possess utility in alleviating suffering from painful osseous metastasis.[25] Furthermore, it appears that endothelin receptor activation and nerve growth factor (NGF) may contribute to painful osseous metastases, and therapy with endothelin receptor antagonists[26] as well as treatment with anti-NGF antibody[27] have been shown to reduce bone cancer pain.

In conclusion, by understanding some of the mechanisms leading to painful osseous metastases and launching a multifaceted treatment plan, we may be better equipped to achieve optimal analgesia.

REFERENCES

1. Hungerford DS. Bone marrow pressure and intromedullary venography, in Owen R, Goodfellow J, Bullough P (eds), *Scientific Foundations of Orthopedics and Traumatology.* London, England, Heinemann 1980; pp. 357-360

2. Garrett RI. Bone destruction in cancer. *Semin Oncol* 1993: 20: 4-9

3. Galasko CSB. Mechanisms of lytic and blastic metastatic disease of bone. *Clin Orthop* 1982; 169: 20-27

4. Duong LT, Rodan GA. The role of integrins in osteoclast function. *J Bone Miner Metab* 1999; 17: 1-6

5. Duong LT, Lakkakorpi P, Nakamura I, et al. Integrins and signaling in osteoclast function. *Matrix Biol* 2000; 19: 97-105

6. Coleman RE. Bisphosphonate treatment of bone metastases and hypercalcemia of malignancy. *Oncology* 1991; 5: 55-65

7. Houston SJ, Rubens RD. The systemic treatment of bone metastases. *Clin Orthop* 1995; 312: 95-104

8. Kong Y-Y, Felge U, Sarosi I, et al. Activated T cell regulate bone loss and joint destruction in adjuvant arthritis through osteoprotegerin ligand. *Nature* 1999; 402: 304-308

9. Hsu H, Lacey KL, Dunstan CR, et al. Tumor necrosis factor receptor family member RANK mediates osteoclast differentiation and activation induced by osteoprotegerin ligand. *Proc Natl Acad Sci USA* 1999; 996: 3540-3545

10. Simonet WS, Lacey DL, Dunstan CR, et al. Osteoprotegerin: A novel secreted protein involved in the regulation of bone density. *Cell* 1997; 89: 309-319

11. Thompson SWN, Tonge D. Bone cancer gain without the pain. *Nat Med* 2000; 6: 504-505

12. Yasuda H, Shima N, Nakagawa N, et al. Osteoclast differentiation factor is a ligand for osteoprotegerin/osteoclastogenesis-inhibitory factor and is identical to TRANCE/RANKL. *Proc Natl Acad Sci USA* 1998; 95: 3597-3602

13. Luger NM, Honore R, Sabino MAC, et al. Osteoprotegerin diminishes advanced bone cancer pain. *Cancer Research* 2001; 61: 4038-4047

14. Honore P, Luger NM, Sabino MAC, et al. Osteoprotegerin blocks bone cancer—induced skeletal destruction, skeletal pain and pain related neurochemical reorganization of the spinal cord. *Nature Medicine* 2000; 6: 521-528

15. Schwel MJ, Honore P, Rogers SD, et al. Neurochemical and cellular reorganization of the spinal cord in a murine model of bone cancer pain. *J Neuroscience* 1999; 19: 10886-10897

16. Gravallese EM, Goldring SR. Cellular mechanisms and the role of cytokines in bone erosions in rheumatoid arthritis. *Arthritis Rheumatism* 2000; 43: 2143-2137

17. Viereck V, Emons G, Lauck V, et al. Bisphosphonates pamidronate and zoledronic acid stimulate osteoprotegerin production by primary human osteoblasts. *Biochem Biophys Res Commun* 2002; 291: 680-686

18. Walker K, Medhurst SJ, Kidd BL, et al. Disease modifying and antinociceptive effects of the bisphosphonate, zoledronic acid in a model of bone cancer pain. *Pain* 2002; 100: 219-229

19. Vierick V, Grundker C, Blaschke S, et al. Phytoestogen genistein stimulated the production of osteoprotegerin by human trabecular osteblasts. *J Cell Biochem* 2002; 84: 725-735

20. Gruber R, Karerth F, Fischer MB, et al. Platelet-released supernatants stimulate formation of osteoclast—like cells through a prostaglandin/RANKL—dependent mechanism. *Bone* 2002; 30: 726-732

21. Fleishmann R, Sheldon E, Maldonado-Cocco J, et al. Lumiracoxib is effective in the treatment of osteoarthritis of the knee: a prospective randomized 13-week study versus placebo and celecoxib. *Clin Rheumatol* 2006; 25: 42-53

22. Wittenberg RH, Schell E, Krehan G, et al. First-dose analgesic effect of the cyclo-oxygenase-2 selective inhibitor lumiracoxib in osteoarthritis of the knee: a randomized, double-blind, placebo-controlled comparison with celecoxib. *Arthritis Res Ther* 2006; 8: R35

23. Fox A, Medhurst S, Courade JP, et al. Anti-hyperalgesic activity of the COX-2 inhibitor-lumiracoxib in a model of bone cancer pain in the rat. *Pain* 2004; 107(1-2): 33-40

24. Ghilardi JR, Rohrich H, Lindsay TH, et al. Selective blockade of the capsaicin receptor TRPV1 attenuates bone cancer pain. *J Neurosci* 2005; 25: 3126-3131

25. Sevcik MA, Ghilardi JR, Halvorson KG, et al. Analgesic efficacy of bradykinin B1 antagonists in a murine bone cancer pain model. *J Pain* 2005; 6: 771-775

26. Peters CM, Lindsay TH, Pomonis JD, et al. Endothelin and tumorigenic component of bone cancer pain. *Neuroscience* 2004; 126: 1043-1052

27. Sevcik MA, Ghilardi JR, Peters CM, et al. Anti-NGF therapy profoundly reduces bone cancer pain and the accompanying increase in markers of peripheral and central sensitization. *Pain* 2005; 115: 128-141

Chapter 23

Pain Arising from Tendons and Tendon Sheaths

Gary McCleane

Pain arising from tendons and tendon sheaths can be severe, incapacitating, and chronic. Its onset may be spontaneous, associated with overuse or with other contributory factors such as degenerative disease. While background pain may be a feature, the worst excesses of pain are associated with movement and the ability to treat such movement-related, sudden-onset pain is not particularly good. While general methods such as the use of acetaminophen and mild opioids can be helpful, their generalized affect contrasts with the localized nature of the condition.

In this chapter a variety of tried and tested pharmacological options will be considered along with some other options that have been found useful but which, as yet, lack the firm evidence base. At the end, this discussion on options will be synthesized into a suggested treatment approach for this range of conditions. It is accepted that surgical intervention may be of benefit; the focus of this chapter is on nonsurgical options.

When options are considered, they can be divided into those with a localized effect or those with a more generalized mode of action. Alternatively, options can be considered according to their mode of administration. Consequently, options can be divided into those applied topically, orally, or peritendinously. The possession of a list of alternatives is important, as management of tendon-related pain can

Clinical Management of Bone and Joint Pain
© 2007 by The Haworth Press, Inc. All rights reserved.
doi:10.1300/5771_25

be difficult and no one option comes with a guarantee of success. Therefore, it may be necessary to work through a list of options before an effective remedy is obtained.

TOPICAL OPTIONS

Nonsteroidal Anti-Inflammatory Drugs

Despite widespread medical scepticism, it does seem that the topical application of nonsteroidal anti-inflammatory drugs (NSAIDs) is associated with pain relief. Mason and colleagues (2004) have published the results of their meta-analysis of the results of published studies on the use of topical NSAIDs in chronic musculoskeletal pain. They conclude, "Topical NSAIDs were effective and safe in treating chronic musculoskeletal conditions for two weeks. Larger and longer trials are necessary to fully elucidate the place of topical NSAIDs in clinical practice."

While the studies under analysis were not specifically carried out in patients with tendon-related pain, there is no reason to suppose that the results obtained in patients with other chronic musculoskeletal conditions do not extend to tendon-related pain.

Glyceryl Trinitrate

We have seen in Chapter 5 that the topical application of nitrates in the form of glyceryl trinitrate (GTN) can have both an analgesic and anti-inflammatory effect and that this effect is achieved by a mechanism distinct and different to that of the NSAIDs. Therefore, as well as being potentially efficacious, it lacks the peptic and other side effects of conventional NSAIDs.

An example of the potential efficacy of GTN in the treatment of the pain of tendinopathy comes from the study of Hunte and Lloyd-Smith (2005). They studied 65 patients whose average duration of pain from their Achilles' tendon condition was 16 months, with a range of 4 to 147 months, emphasizing the potentially chronic nature of this condition. They used a topical patch formulation of GTN, which was divided into segments for application over the painful area. When pain and a variety of measures of ankle mobility were considered, those treated with GTN had a greater chance of achieving symptom alleviation than the placebo group. Interestingly, headache, an expected side effect of nitrate use, was reported in 53 percent of the GTN group and by 45 percent of the placebo group.

Paoloni and colleagues (2004) also studied patients with Achilles' tendinopathy. They found that, after 6 months of treatment, 78 percent in the GTN group were asymptomatic as compared with 49 percent in the placebo group. The fact that after 6 months use patients continued to gain relief suggests that the tachyphylaxis described when nitrates are used to treat angina pectoris may not be encountered when they are used in pain treatment.

GTN is not effective only in the treatment of Achilles' tendon pain. Berrazueta and colleagues (1996) studied 20 patients with supraspinatus tendonitis. The subjects were randomized to receive either a GTN patch (5 mg per 24 hours) or a placebo patch. Within 48 hours of commencement of treatment, those patients receiving GTN patch treatment recorded a fall of just over 2.5 points on a 10 cm visual analog score of pain. Those in the placebo group recorded no change in pain. Only two patients in the GTN group reported headache. This study confirms that the pain-relieving effect of topically applied GTN can be rapid, and when taken in conjunction with the results of the previously described studies, which confirm a long-term effect, it suggests that topical GTN can be both a treatment for the acute and chronic pain associated with tendon pathology.

Lidoderm Patch

Lidocaine-containing patches have a verified effect in certain pain conditions and, in particular, in postherpetic neuralgia. While no trial evidence confirms a pain-relieving effect in tendon-related pain, anecdotal evidence, and indeed logic, suggests that it can have such an effect. Only a small amount of the lidocaine contained within the patch is actually released, and therefore its effect is local, not systemic. Consequently, side effects are relatively uncommon and innocuous. Skin rash and irritation at the application site are perhaps the most frequent complications of use.

Capsaicin

Again, capsaicin has a verified effect in a broad range of conditions from neuropathic pains to osteoarthritis, but not specifically tendon-related pain. That said, there is no reason to suggest that it is ineffective in those with tendon-related pain, and practical experience confirms this. Capsaicin achieves its effect by reversibly depleting the neurotransmitter substance P and also decreasing the density of epidermal nerve fibers, again in a reversible fashion. Repeated application is required for effect to be achieved, and so a trial of application for up to 1 month is required to gauge success. Burning discomfort at the application site usually decreases with sustained use and can also be reduced by the coadministration of glyceryl trinitrate.

Tricyclic Antidepressants

Oral tricyclic antidepressants (TCAs) are frequently used in the treatment of chronic pain conditions. However, their use is frequently associated with a variety of side effects including dry mouth, sedation, and weight gain. Recent evidence suggests that TCAs can have a peripheral, as well as central, effect and that this effect is achieved by interaction with peripheral adenosine receptors and sodium channels. Therefore, topical application of a TCA can be used as a method of pain relief, although this pain-relieving effect can take several weeks to become apparent. Side effects with topically applied TCAs are infrequent and nonserious. If overapplied, however, systemic side effects, as seen with oral TCAs, can occur. Currently the TCA doxepin is available in a 5 percent topically applied formulation.

INJECTIONS

Steroids

Local injection of corticosteroids is a widespread and apparently effective method of treatment for a broad range of painful tendon conditions. Usually this corticosteroid is coadministered with a local anesthetic such as lidocaine or bupivicaine. If a local anesthetic is used, then a fairly rapid reduction in pain confirms that the injection has been placed sufficiently close to the painful area for the corticosteroid to have a chance of alleviating the condition. However, this reduction in pain is often temporary as the effect of the local anesthetic wears off before the corticosteroid has a chance to begin its effect.

While corticosteroid injection is a well-tried method of treatment, a number of side effects can accrue from its use:

- Local lipoatrophy producing a depression in the skin at the site of injection
- Tendon weakening (especially relevant in weight-bearing tendons such as the Achilles' tendon)
- Local telangectasia at the injection site
- Systemic effects if corticosteroid injection is repeatedly carried out

In terms of the evidence of effect of this form of treatment, an example is given in the meta-analysis of the use of corticosteroid injections for painful shoulders carried out by Arroll and Goodyear-Smith (2005). They found that the "numbers needed to treat" (NNT), that is the number of patients needed to receive the treatment for one to gain a 50 percent reduction in symptoms, was 3.3 when this injection was used for rotator cuff tendonitis. The relative risk for improvement, when corticosteroid injection was compared with an oral NSAID, was 1.43, suggesting that corticosteroid injection (subachromial or intra-articular) was, on balance, more effective than an oral NSAID.

So evidence and clinical experience suggest that corticosteroid injection is a potentially effective treatment for tendon-related pain. However, there are many unanswered questions:

- Does the addition of a local anesthetic make any difference to the long term results of corticosteroid injection?
- Which corticosteroid produces maximum effect (triamcinolone, prednisolone, methylprednisolone, hydrocortisone, depomedrone, or betamethasone)?
- What dose of corticosteroid produces maximum benefit and minimal risk?
- What is a safe dosing interval for corticosteroid injection?

Hyaluronidase

Hyaluronidase is currently most frequently used in conjunction with local anesthetics in peribulbar eye blocks, where it helps the spread of the local anesthetic. It acts by breaking down soft tissue adhesions and as such can help breakdown the adhesions that occur with inflammatory conditions of tendons and their sheaths. Injection of hyaluronidase into a tendon sheath can achieve results comparable with those of corticosteroid injection, but without the potential adverse effects of corticosteroid use. That said, evidence for such an effect is currently lacking.

Tropisetron

Tropisetron belongs to the $5HT_3$ antagonist group of drugs. This group has been marketed for their antiemetic effect, which is most well established in the fields of postoperative nausea and vomiting and in chemotherapy-induced nausea. More recently it has been shown that $5HT_3$ antagonists, when given systemically, can also have an analgesic effect on the pain associated with fibromyalgia and irritable bowel syndrome and even in patients with neuropathic pain. This effect is produced by their specific action on the NK1-expressing neurones in the superficial laminae of the dorsal horn. These NK1-expressing neurones contain receptors for substance P.

However, Stratz and colleagues (2002) have shown that local, as opposed to systemic, administration of tropisetron can reduce the pain associated with tendinopathies. They compared local injection of tropisetron with an injection of a combination of dexamathasone (10 mg) and lidocaine, and assessed pain daily for 7 days and then after 3 months. They found that injection of tropisetron produced the same relief as dexamathasone at all measurement times and that this effect was on rest and movement pain. They speculated that the effect of tropisetron was due to its blocking of $5HT_3$ receptors and an inhibition of substance P release.

The potential advantage of such use of tropisetron would be that steroid-related side effects can be avoided. There are, however, a number of unanswered questions. Is this effect shared by all $5HT_3$ antagonists? How does the effect of tropisetron compare with other steroids such as triamcinolone or depomedrone? Is there a bell-shaped dose–response curve when tropisetron is used in this fashion as there is when it is used systemically in the treatment of fibromyalgia? And is the effect of tropisetron when used to treat the pain associated with a tendinopathy a purely local effect, or is there a central effect as well?

Tenoxicam

One would expect that the NSAID tenoxicam, when given systemically, would have the same chance of giving pain relief as any other NSAID. Itzkowitch and colleagues (1996) report that weekly periarticular injections of tenoxicam (20 mg) gave significant pain relief to patients with painful shoulders, including those with rotator cuff tendonitis, when compared with placebo injections. This interesting result leaves a number of questions unanswered. First, is this a local effect or an effect consequent on systemic absorption of tenoxicam? Second, is this effect individual to tenoxicam, or is it shared by other NSAIDs? Still, the fact that weekly injections of this NSAID gave significant relief when the half-life of the drug can be measured in hours, not days, is intriguing.

ORAL OPTIONS

Nonsteroidal Anti-Inflammatory Agents

Perhaps the first option in many patients is the NSAID. Which particular NSAID is chosen is largely a matter of personal preference. If this group were universally efficacious, then there would be no need for other options. Therefore, when contraindications do not exist, a short trial on a NSAID is warranted. Failure to respond is an indication for its withdrawal and substitution by another option. It is arguable whether failure to respond to one NSAID should be reacted to by a substitution by another NSAID. Perhaps it is better to select an entirely different option.

Cimetidine

It is known that the H_2 antagonist cimetidine decreases calcium levels and can be used with advantage in patients with hyperparathyroidism. When calcium is deposited in the shoulder joint region, impairment of function and pain commonly result. Yokoyama and colleagues (2003) describe 16 patients with chronic calcific tendinitis treated with cimetidine for 3 months. They found that pain scores (100 mm visual analog scale) fell from 63 to 14 mm and that 63 percent of the patients became pain free. In 56 percent of their patients, calcium deposits disappeared, while in only 25 percent did they remain unchanged. While this was not a randomized placebo-controlled trial, the results certainly merit consideration if only because no other pharmacological therapy offers the hope of decalcification of previously calcified tendon.

OTHERS

Nerve Blocks

When a noxious event occurs, and particularly when that irritation is prolonged, a number of changes occur, which include a "sensitization" of the nerve that travels to that area. Therefore, in the case of tendon pain, while the inflammation is around the tendon and its enveloping structures, the nerve to that region becomes sensitized, excitable, and ultimately contributes to the pain experienced. Therefore, interventions of that nerve can reduce the overall experience of pain. This is best exemplified by suprascapular nerve blocks. Shanahan and colleagues (2003) describe the results of their study on 83 people with shoulder pain who were randomized to receive either a suprascapular nerve block with bupivicaine and methylprednisolone or subcutaneous saline injection. They found that, after 1, 4, and 12 weeks, the group that received the suprascapular nerve block showed significant improvement in all pain and disability pain scores measured.

Dahan and colleagues (2000) randomized patients to receive either 3-weekly suprascapular nerve blocks with bupivicaine alone or saline as a placebo. Two weeks after the last injection there was a 64 percent reduction in pain scores in the active treatment group as compared with 13 percent in the placebo group. What the long-term results were is not clear, and therefore the issue of the benefit, or lack of benefit of the addition of corticosteroid to the local anesthetic, is not addressed.

Extracorporeal Shock Wave Therapy

A number of studies and case reports have suggested that extracorporeal shock wave therapy can be useful in the treatment of calcific rotator cuff tendonitis but not in the noncalcific variety. In addition to providing symptom alleviation, a reduction or complete removal of the calcific deposit may occur. For example, Wang and colleagues (2003) found that, after treatment with extracorporeal shock wave therapy in patients with calcific rotator cuff tendonitis, complete dissolution of calcium deposits occurred in 57 percent, with a further 15 percent of the subjects having a partial dissolution. In contrast, in the control group, 83 percent of the subjects had no change in their calcium deposits.

Harniman and colleagues (2004) have undertaken a systematic review of the use of extracorporeal shock wave therapy in patients with calcific and noncalcific tendonitis of the rotator cuff. As is common with such reviews, they found that many studies were weakened by small sample size, randomization issues, blinding and treatment provider bias, and inadequate outcome measures. They concluded that there is moderate evidence that high-energy extracorporeal shock wave therapy is effective in treating chronic calcific rotator cuff tendonitis when the shock waves are focused at the calcific deposit. They also concluded that there is moderate evidence that low-energy extracorporeal shock wave therapy is not effective for treating chronic noncalcific rotator cuff tendonitis, although that conclusion was based on only one high-quality study that was underpowered.

One word of caution is offered by Durst and colleagues (2002), who report a single patient who appeared to develop osteonecrosis of the humeral head after extracorporeal shock wave therapy.

Hyperbaric Oxygen

A single animal study suggests that hyperbaric oxygen may have a beneficial effect on tendinopathy. Hsu and colleagues (2004) induced tendinopathy in rabbits' patellar tendons and treated the animals with either hyperbaric oxygen, delivered at 2.5 atm for 120 min on 30 daily sessions, or with normobaric room air. After treatment for 6 weeks, the animals were sacrificed and examined histologically. Those treated with hyperbaric oxygen showed cellular changes that indicated healing with greater frequency than animals treated with normobaric room air. They suggested that hyperbaric oxygen may have increased collagen synthesis and collagen cross-link formation during the early healing process.

Perhaps the greatest problem with this form of treatment, if the results can be validated in humans, is the repetitive nature of the treatment with multiple sessions of hyperbaric oxygen being necessary for improvement to occur.

SUGGESTED TREATMENT
FOR TENDON-RELATED PAIN

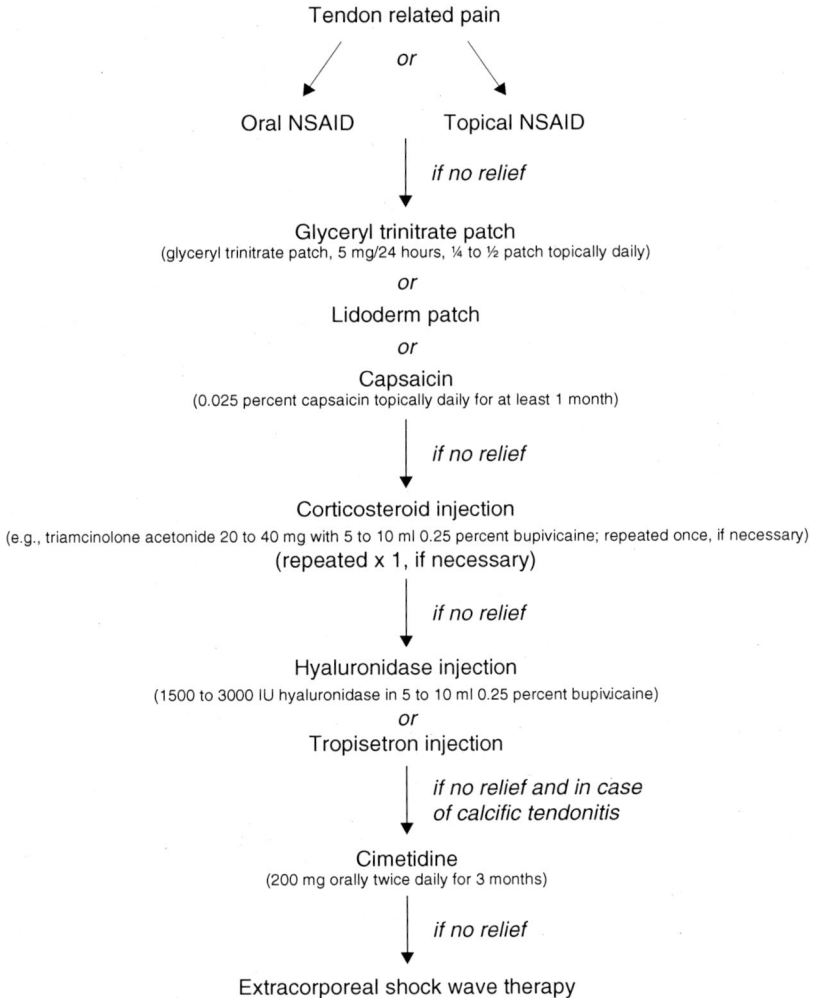

Tendon related pain

or

Oral NSAID   Topical NSAID

if no relief

Glyceryl trinitrate patch
(glyceryl trinitrate patch, 5 mg/24 hours, ¼ to ½ patch topically daily)

or

Lidoderm patch

or

Capsaicin
(0.025 percent capsaicin topically daily for at least 1 month)

if no relief

Corticosteroid injection
(e.g., triamcinolone acetonide 20 to 40 mg with 5 to 10 ml 0.25 percent bupivicaine; repeated once, if necessary)
(repeated x 1, if necessary)

if no relief

Hyaluronidase injection
(1500 to 3000 IU hyaluronidase in 5 to 10 ml 0.25 percent bupivicaine)

or

Tropisetron injection

*if no relief and in case
of calcific tendonitis*

Cimetidine
(200 mg orally twice daily for 3 months)

if no relief

Extracorporeal shock wave therapy

SELECTED REFERENCES

Topical NSAIDs

Mason L, Moore RA, Edwards JE, Derry S, McQuay HJ. Topical NSAIDs for chronic musculoskeletal pain: Systematic review and meta-analysis. *BMC Musculokelet Disord* 2004; 5: 28.

Glyceryl Trinitrate

Berrazueta JR, Losada A, Poveda J, Ochoteco A, Riestra A, Salas E, Amado JA. Successful treatment of shoulder pain syndrome due to supraspinatus tendonitis with transdermal nitroglycerin. A double blind study. *Pain* 1996; 66: 63-67.
Hunte G, Lloyd-Smith R. Topical glyceryl trinitrate for chronic Achilles tendinopathy. *Clin J Sport Med* 2005; 15: 116-117.
Paoloni JA, Appleyard RC, Nelson RC, Murrell GA. Topical nitric oxide application in the treatment of chronic extensor tendinosis at the elbow: A randomized, double-blinded, placebo-controlled clinical trial. *Am J Sports Med* 2003; 31: 915-920.
Paoloni JA, Appleyard RC, Nelson J, Murrell GA. Topical glyceryl trinitrate treatment of chronic noninsertional Achilles tendinopathy. A randomised, double-blind, placebo-controlled trial. *J Bone Joint Surg Am* 2004; 86: 916-922.

Corticosteroids

Arroll B, Goodyear-Smith F. Corticosteroid injections for painful shoulder: A meta-analysis. *Br J Gen Pract* 2005; 55: 224-228.

Tropisetron

Stratz T, Farber L, Muller W. Local treatment of tendinopathies: A comparison between tropisetron and depot corticosteroids combined with local anesthetics. *Scand J Rheumatol* 2002; 31: 366-370.
Stratz T, Varga B, Muller W. Treatment of tendopathies with tropisetron. *Rheumatol Int* 2002; 22: 219-221.

Tenoxicam

Itzkowitch D, Ginsberg F, Leon M, Bernard V, Appelboom T. Peri-articular injection of tenoxicam for painful shoulders: A double-blind, placebo controlled trial. *Clin Rheumatol* 1996; 15: 604-609.

Cimetidine

Yokoyama M, Aona H, Takeda A, Morita K. Cimetidine for chronic calcifying tendinitis of the shoulder. *Reg Anesth Pain Med* 2003; 28: 248-252.

Nerve Blocks

Dahan TH, Fortin L, Pelletier M, Petit M, Vadeboncoeur R, Suissa S. Double blind randomized clinical trial examining the efficacy of bupivicaine suprascapular nerve blocks in frozen shoulder. *J Rheumatol* 2000; 27: 1464-1469.

Shanahan EM, Ahern M, Smith M, Wetherall M, Bresnihan B, FitzGerald O. Suprascapular nerve block (using bupivicaine and methylprednisolone acetate) in chronic shoulder pain. *Ann Rheum Dis* 2003; 62: 400-406.

Extracorporeal Shock Wave Therapy

Cosentino R, De Stefano R, Selvi E, et al. Extracorporeal shock wave therapy for chronic calcific tendinitis of the shoulder: Single blind study. *Ann Rheum Dis* 2003; 62: 248-250.

Durst HB, Blatter G, Kuster MS. Osteonecrosis of the humeral head after extracorporeal shock-wave lithotripsy. *J Bone Joint Surg Br* 2002; 84: 744-746.

Gerdesmeyer L, Wagenpfeil S, Haake M, et al. Extracorporeal shock wave therapy for the treatment of chronic calcifying tendonitis of the rotator cuff: A randomized controlled trial. *JAMA* 2003; 290: 2573-2580.

Harniman E, Carette S, Kennedy C, Beaton D. Extracorporeal shock wave therapy for calcific and noncalcific tendonitis of the rotator cuff: A systematic review. *J Hand Ther* 2004; 17: 132-151.

Perlick L, Luring C, Bathis H, Perlick C, Kraft C, Diedrich O. Efficacy of extracorporeal shock-wave treatment for calcific tendinitis of the shoulder: Experimental and clinical results. *J Orthop Sci* 2003; 8: 777-783.

Peters J, Luboldt W, Schwarz W, Jacobi V, Herzog C, Vogl TJ. Extracorporeal shock wave therapy in calcific tendinitis of the shoulder. *Skeletal Radiol* 2004; 33: 712-718.

Speed CA, Richards C, Nichols D, et al. Extracorporeal shock-wave therapy for tendonitis of the rotator cuff. A double-blind, randomised, controlled trial. *J Bone Joint Surg Br* 2002; 84: 509-512.

Wang CJ, Yang KD, Wang FS, Chen HH, Wang JW. Shock wave therapy for calcific tendonitis of the shoulder: A prospective clinical study with two-year follow-up. *Am J Sports Med* 2003; 31: 425-430.

Hyperbaric Oxygen

Hsu RW, Hsu WH, Tai CL, Lee KF. Effect of hyperbaric oxygen therapy on patellar tendinopathy in a rat model. *J Trauma* 2004; 57: 1060-1064.

Chapter 24

When Is Pain Felt Over a Bone or Joint, Not Bone or Joint Pain?

Gary McCleane

While the primary focus of this book is the clinical management of bone and joint pain, in reality clinicians will often encounter patients whose primary complaint is pain felt over a bone or joint but their the underlying problem is not bone or joint disease. A realization of the nature of this pain may allow a more accurate diagnosis with a corresponding improvement in the chances of providing adequate pain relief.

Three examples of conditions, or groups of conditions, that give rise to limb pain, but are not primarily conditions caused by abnormalities of bone or joint in the limb, are considered.

RADIATED PAIN/NEUROPATHIC PAIN

A characteristic feature of neural injury is that symptoms are experienced distally, and at times proximally, to the site of the injury. For example, when an intervertebral disc prolapses and impinges of a nerve, neuropathic pain may be experienced in the distribution of that nerve. Such pain may comprise any of the constituent features of neuropathic pain, which include lancinating or shooting pain, numbness, paraesthesia, burning pain, and allodynia (pain created by a normally nonpainful stimulus). When this neuropathic pain is experienced

Clinical Management of Bone and Joint Pain
© 2007 by The Haworth Press, Inc. All rights reserved.
doi:10.1300/5771_26

in a limb, it is quite easy for it to be confused with bone or joint pain. However, the features of neuropathic pain have distinct differences with those encountered with bone or joint pain. Paraesthesiae are common with neuropathic pain, but not present with bone or joint pain, similarly with numbness. The situation with allodynia is a little more confusing. Where joint pathology exists and gives rise to pain, localized joint tenderness can be elicited and pressure on that joint gives rise to pain. When neuropathic pain is felt over a joint, allodynia may exist. This can seem to be joint tenderness, but more detailed assessment will show that this allodynia is more extensive than just the joint margin. Allodynia can be elicited by light touch or stroking the skin whereas joint tenderness requires more firm pressure to become apparent.

The presence of other signs arising over the joint or bone would further mitigate a referred pain. Therefore, the presence of swelling or edema, increase in temperature, joint crepitus, or localized erythema would collectively suggest a local joint problem.

Differentiation between a localized joint or bone problem and a radiated pain is essential for appropriate treatment. A radiated, neuropathic pain is more likely to be responsive to specific treatment modalities, which would unlikely be helpful if the pain was primarily arising from bone or joint. Neuropathic pain is typically treated with the following:

- Tricyclic antidepressants (e.g., amitriptyline, imipramine, and clomipramine)
- Antiepileptic drugs (e.g., carbamazepine, oxcarbazepine, lamotrigine, gabapentin, and pregabalin)
- Opioids
- Membrane stabilizing drugs (e.g., topical, oral, parenteral, and perineural)

Suggested Treatment of Neuropathic Pain

Many treatment options exist, and there are differing perspectives on treatment. This is one perspective: If symptoms remain despite an adequate trial of the medication in question, it should be discontinued.

Drug	Dose	Time to effect	Common side effects
Pregabalin	75 mg bid orally	Days	Somnolence Nausea
Lamotrigine	Dose increasing to 300 mg/day orally	When 300 mg/day is achieved	Skin rash Insomnia
Oxcarbazepine	150 mg qid	Days	Sedation Weight gain
Tramadol	50 mg qid	Days	Sedation Nausea
Lidoderm patch	One topically	Days	Local skin irritation
Capsaicin cream 0.075 percent	Topically qid	1 Month	Burning at site of application
Doxepin cream 5 percent	Topically qid	1 Month	Sedation Dry mouth if over applied

REFERRED PAIN

Referred pain can be defined as pain perceived as occurring in a region of the body topographically distinct from the region in which the actual source of the pain is located. The shoulder tip pain experienced with diaphragmatic irritation or the left arm and jaw pain with angina pectoris are well-known referred pains. But often, referred pain is felt in the arm or leg with sources in the back or neck, and can be confused with local processes in the arm or leg. Alternatively, such arm or leg pain can be confused with radiated neuropathic pain.

When referred pain is present, it is often possible to identify the source from which it emanates. On the one hand, the presence of source of irritation can give rise to a predictable distribution of referred pain, while on the other hand description of a referred pain is often predictive of its origin.

The differentiation between a referred and radiated pain is based on the descriptive quality of the pain. Referred pain is described in terms of an aching, constant, deep pain that is not altered by movement of the affected part. No matter what posture that affected part assumes, the referred pain remains unaltered. In contrast, radiated neuropathic pain is described in terms of shooting or lancinating pain, burning pain, paraesthesia, skin sensitivity, and numbness. Furthermore, referred pain is not associated with neurological aberrations such as diminution of sensation or alteration in muscle strength and reflexes, again in contrast to radiated pain.

When a source of irritation arises in the midline, bilateral referred pain results. When the irritation is on one side, unilateral referred pain results. For example, when an interspinous ligament is inflamed, the referred pain is found over the dermatome associated with that interspinous ligament, and since it is midline, the pain may be bilateral. In the case of facet joint inflammation, since it is found to one side of the midline, the referred pain produced is unilateral.

Undoubtedly the situation may be confusing. Hip joint inflammation can cause referred pain in the knee. Since knee osteoarthritis is a relatively common accompaniment of hip osteoarthritis, radiological investigation may not help understanding of the origin of the pain. However, referred pain does not give rise to joint tenderness, and so the presence of hip joint tenderness in the absence of knee joint tenderness can help in diagnosis.

Despite the commonness of referred pain, few studies have been carried out that give definitive information on effective treatments. That said, common sense would suggest that the most effective way to treat any referred pain is to provide effective treatment for the causal condition that gives rise to the referred pain. Where this source of irritation is longstanding, there may be a lag time between effective treatment being instituted for the source irritation and the referred pain diminishing. On occasions it may be weeks and even months before the referred pain disappears. In addition, it is not uncommon for patients to rate their referred pain as being more unpleasant and disabling that their source pain.

Anecdotal evidence suggests that the antiepileptic drugs are the most efficacious group of compounds for the management of referred pain.

Treatment for Referred Pain

Pain	Treatment
Source	Conventional treatment (e.g., NSAID, opioid, etc.)
Referred pain	Lamotrigine in dose increasing to 300 mg daily, *Or*
	Gabapentin in dose increasing to 2400 mg daily, *Or*
	Pregabalin 75 mg bid, *Or*
	Oxcarbazepine 150 mg qid

COMPLEX REGIONAL PAIN SYNDROME

The understanding of any condition is not aided if it is also known by a variety of other names and when the terminology continues to change with the passage of time and when there is no clear understanding of the cause of that condition. A prime example of this is complex regional pain syndrome (CRPS). This has been known in the past by a variety of other names, for example:

- Sudeks osteodystrophy
- Reflex sympathetic dystrophy
- Shoulder-hand syndrome
- Posttraumatic algodystrophy

Perhaps the best-known name for this condition was reflex sympathetic dystrophy, a term now discouraged because of its implication that the symptoms and signs associated with the condition are produced by a disorder of the sympathetic nervous system and that sympathetic blocks will be of value. It is certainly true that interventions that have a sympatholytic effect can be of real value in some, but a proportion of patients who exhibit features of the condition do not gain symptom alleviation (sympathetic independent pain).

Distinction must be made between CRPS type 1 (previously, reflex sympathetic dystrophy) and CRPS type II (causalgia).

The International Association for the Study of Pain have defined CRPS type I in the following terms:

> CRPS type I is a syndrome that usually develops after an initiating noxious event, is not limited to the distribution of a single peripheral nerve, and is apparently disproportionate to the inciting event. It is associated at some point with evidence of edema, changes in skin blood flow, abnormal sudomotor activity in the region of the pain, or allodynia or hyperalgesia.

In contrast, they define CRPS type II as: Burning pain, allodynia and hyperpathia usually in the hand or foot after partial injury or a nerve or one of its major branches.

A diagnosis of CRPS type I may be considered in the presence of at least three of the cardinal five features of the condition, which are these:

1. Allodynia (pain created by a normally nonpainful stimulus)
2. Burning pain
3. Local hyperhidrosis
4. Swelling or edema (which may be intermittent)
5. Discoloration (blue/dark, which again may be intermittent)

Allodynia associated with this condition may be static (that is precipitated by touch) or dynamic (by stroking), or mechanical or thermal (that is brought on by changes in temperature). Allodynia and burning pain are nondermatomal, in contrast to CRPS type II, in which there is a definite dermatomal distribution of pain. In further contrast to CRPS type II, nerve conduction studies are normal in type I.

The presence of other symptoms does not exclude the diagnosis. For example, paraesthesia or numbness may encountered where the CRPS type I is precipitated or found alongside neural injury. Localized osteoporosis is also frequent accompaniment, is used by some to support the diagnosis, and may be the result of either the condition itself or the underuse of the limb precipitated by the severity of the pain experienced.

Muscle contractures that cause clawing of fingers or toes often accompany the other features of this condition. When seen at their worst, the pressure of deformed fingers pressing on the palm of the hand, for example, can cause skin necrosis. Use of splints can prevent this, as can a constant attention to efforts to maintain movement of the limb. On occasion, the discoloration of an affected part can be so intense as to raise the possibility that the contractures are due to muscle ischemia, and therefore efforts to augment circulation should be instituted.

While most would associate CRPS type I with the upper limbs, this condition can affect almost any area of the body. Lower limb CRPS type I is not that uncommon, and case reports describe it as affecting other regions including the breast, face, and even the testicle.

Undoubtedly, CRPS type I is a difficult condition to treat. Mobilization of the affected part is fundamental to success. That said, such attempted mobilization against a backdrop of unremitting pain with a strong allodynic component is difficult. Therefore, any pharmacological intervention that lessens pain may be a significant aid to mobilization. To many, the treatment of CRPS type I is associated with sympathetic blocks. These include intravenous regional sympathetic blocks (IVRSBs) with guanethidine, local anesthetic stellate ganglion blocks, and local anesthetic or lytic lumbar sympathetic blocks. These are all in the realms of specialist practice. There are, however, a number of simple interventions that any practitioner can institute which may alleviate the symptoms of this condition. It is accepted that the evidence for many of the options outlined is anecdotal, but since most are low risk strategies, their use is commended.

Suggested Treatment for CRPS Type I

Drug	Dose	Specific indication
Glyceryl trinitrate	One patch topically	Blue/black limb discoloration
Lidoderm patch	One patch topically	Allodynia
Doxepin 5 percent	Topically qid	Pain, allodynia, burning pain
Capsaicin 0.075 percent	Topically qid	Pain
Pregabalin	75 mg bid	Pain
Lamotrigine	Dose increased to 300 mg daily	Pain, edema
Gabapentin	Dose increased to 2400 mg daily	Pain
Ondansetron	4 mg tid	Pain

Other Treatments for CRPS Type I

Calcitonin

Intravenous phentolamine

Intravenous regional sympathetic block with

- Guanethidine
- Atropine
- Magnesium
- Bretylium

Ketansarin

Corticosteroids

Epidural clonidine

Phenoxybenzamine

Local anesthetic stellate ganglion and lumbar sympathetic blocks

Lytic lumbar sympathectomy

Lumbar epidural injection and infusion of local anesthetic

Spinal cord stimulation

AID TO DIAGNOSIS

Symptom or Sign	Bone or joint disorder	CRPS	Neuropathic pain	Referred pain
Localized tenderness	+	−	−	−
Swelling/edema	+	+	−	−
Skin redness	+	−	−	−
Skin blueness	−	+	−	−
Pain on movement	+	+	−	−
Paraesthesia	−	−	+	−
Burning pain	+	+	+	−
Allodynia	−	+	+	−
Numbness	−	−	+	−
Aching pain in dermatomal distribution	−	−	+	+
Identifiable source of pain at proximal site	−	−	+	+

Index